REHABILITATION: MOBILITY, EXERCISE AND SPORTS

Assistive Technology Research Series

The Assistive Technology Research Series (ATR) aims to disseminate and archive assistive technology research summaries widely through publishing proceedings, monographs, and edited collective works. The series aspires to become the primary world-wide source of information in assistive technology research, through publishing state-of-the-science material across all continents. ATR defines assistive technology (AT) as any tool, equipment, system, or service designed to help develop, maintain or improve a person with a disability to function in all aspects of his or her life. Assistive technology helps people of all ages who may have a broad range of disabilities or limitations. The ATR series will accept manuscripts and proposals for a wide range of relevant topics.

Volume 26

Recently published in this series

ISSN 1383-813X

Rehabilitation: Mobility, Exercise and Sports

4th International State-of-the-Art Congress

Edited by

L.H.V. van der Woude

*Centre for Human Movement Sciences, University Medical Centre Groningen,
University of Groningen, The Netherlands
Centre for Rehabilitation, University Medical Centre Groningen,
University of Groningen, The Netherlands*

F. Hoekstra

Faculty of Human Movement Sciences, VU University Amsterdam, The Netherlands

S. de Groot

*Centre for Human Movement Sciences, University Medical Centre Groningen,
University of Groningen, The Netherlands
Rehabilitation Centre Amsterdam, The Netherlands*

K.E. Bijker

*Research Institute MOVE, Institute for Fundamental and Clinical Human Movement Sciences,
Faculty of Human Movement Sciences, VU University Amsterdam, The Netherlands*

R. Dekker

*Centre for Rehabilitation, University Medical Centre Groningen,
University of Groningen, The Netherlands*

P.C.T. van Aanholt

Department of Rehabilitation, Scheperziekenhuis, Emmen, The Netherlands

F.J. Hettinga

*Centre for Human Movement Sciences, University Medical Centre Groningen,
University of Groningen, The Netherlands*

T.W.J. Janssen

*Research Institute MOVE, Institute for Fundamental and Clinical Human Movement Sciences,
Faculty of Human Movement Sciences, VU University Amsterdam, The Netherlands
Rehabilitation Centre Amsterdam, The Netherlands*

and

J.H.P. Houdijk

*Research Institute MOVE, Institute for Fundamental and Clinical Human Movement Sciences,
Faculty of Human Movement Sciences, VU University Amsterdam, The Netherlands
Rehabilitation Centre Heliomare, Wijk aan Zee, The Netherlands*

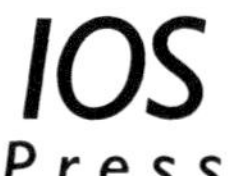

IOS
Press

Amsterdam • Berlin • Tokyo • Washington, DC

ISBN 978-1-60750-080-3
Library of Congress Control Number: 2009941383

Publisher
IOS Press BV
Nieuwe Hemweg 6B
1013 BG Amsterdam
Netherlands
fax: +31 20 687 0019
e-mail: order@iospress.nl

Distributor in the USA and Canada
IOS Press, Inc.
4502 Rachael Manor Drive
Fairfax, VA 22032
USA
fax: +1 703 323 3668
e-mail: iosbooks@iospress.com

LEGAL NOTICE

The publisher is not responsible for the use which might be made of the following information.

PRINTED IN THE NETHERLANDS

Sponsors

Hosted by:

Research Institute MOVE
Faculty of Human Movement Sciences (FBW)
Institute for Fundamental and Clinical Human Movement Sciences (IFKB)
VU University, Amsterdam, The Netherlands

Co-sponsored by:

Body@Work
Heliomare
KNAW
RCA
UMCG-RUG
VRA
ZonMw

Commercial sponsors:

Berkelbike
Biometrics Europe BV
Cardinal Health
Delsys
Double Performance
ForceLink
Human Kinetics
Informa Healthcare
IOS Press
JRRD
Max Mobility
McRoberts
OIM Orthopedie
Össur Europe
Otto Bock
Procare
RS Scan
Trike - Diamond Semi Conductor
Xsens
3W-Infomed

Rehabilitation: Mobility, Exercise and Sports
L.H.V. van der Woude et al. (Eds.)
IOS Press, 2010

Introduction to the 4th International State-of-the-art-Congress 'Rehabilitation: Mobility, Exercise & Sports'

L.H.V. VAN DER WOUDE[a,e], S. DE GROOT[a,c], K.E. BIJKER[b], R. DEKKER[e],
P.C.T. VAN AANHOLT[f], F. HOEKSTRA[b], F.J. HETTINGA[a], T.W.J. JANSSEN[b,c]
and J.H.P. HOUDIJK[b,d]

[a] *Centre for Human Movement Sciences, University Medical Centre Groningen,
University of Groningen,*
[b] *Research Institute MOVE, Institute for Fundamental and Clinical Human Movement
Sciences, Faculty of Human Movement Sciences, VU University Amsterdam,*
[c] *Rehabilitation Centre Amsterdam,*
[d] *Rehabilitation Centre Heliomare, Wijk aan Zee,*
[e] *Centre for Rehabilitation, University Medical Centre Groningen,
University of Groningen,*
[f] *Department of Rehabilitation, Scheperziekenhuis, Emmen, the Netherlands*

1. Introduction

Rehabilitation medicine in the Netherlands was officially founded as a separate medical profession in 1955. Being a young multidisciplinary area of clinical practice and health care, rehabilitation medicine evolved from an initially clinically-founded discipline towards a more academic-based discipline at the start of this millennium. In 2008 clinical rehabilitation care was offered in 24 specialized rehabilitation centers, in university hospitals and in many of the larger general hospitals in the Netherlands.[1] Rehabilitation medicine and care is based upon the conceptual framework of the International Classification of Functioning, Disability and Health (ICF [2]), and on an integral, structured and multidisciplinary team approach. The rehabilitation medical doctor is trained (in a 4 yr specialization program) largely towards the concepts and aims stated in the 'Whitebook on Physical and Rehabilitation Medicine in Europe' [3], published by the governing bodies of European specialists in physical and rehabilitation medicine. The rehabilitation medical specialist is a clinical specialist, yet part of the training program is directed towards research methodological content and skills.

Human Movement Sciences has been intimately linked to rehabilitation from its inception as an academic discipline in Amsterdam in the early seventies. As distinct from other Western countries, in the Netherlands the professional training of paramedical and nursing staff is outside the university teaching program and part of a separate system of higher education that primarily offers professional bachelor and

---

[1] www.revalidatie.nl/english

master programs. This is where physio-, occupational, vocational therapists, physical education and sports teachers are trained, also for rehabilitation practice. Human movement scientists follow a research-oriented university-based training program, focussed on the study of human movement, both with a fundamental and an applied connotation. 'Human movement sciences' (HMS) is an interdisciplinary study, encompassing a wide range of disciplines such as (exercise) physiology, psychology, anatomy, biomechanics, motor control & learning etc. It is offered as an independent scientific bachelor-master program at two universities (Amsterdam[2] and Groningen[3]) and as a Master specialization in two other universities (Nijmegen and Maastricht) in the Netherlands today. Among the most important applied contexts are the fields of sports, health care, and labor. Within the context of health, rehabilitation has from the beginning of HMS been of great interest to staff and students and has led to active collaborations between rehabilitation professionals and human movement scientists from the outset. It has generated two professors in human movement sciences and rehabilitation, in Amsterdam and Groningen. As such HMS has – together with the technical and social sciences – almost by nature contributed to the continued metamorphosis of rehabilitation from a clinical field of (para)medical care and practice, towards a much more evidence-based academic and clinical-research (multi-) disciplinary environment. Today in the Netherlands human movement scientists are in many cases the link between the programs of their schools and those of research institutes on the one hand and the rehabilitation centers/ departments on the other. Human movement scientists are often the knowledge managers and/or brokers [4] in multidisciplinary research networks and are trained to be the research-focussed liaison between clinical practice and academia.

2.   The Dutch rehabilitation–research situation

The academic or research performance of the rehabilitation discipline in the Netherlands and Europe has been described briefly by Stam [5]. The survey involved the input in 4 key-rehabilitation sciences journals (Archives of Physical Medicine and Rehabilitation, Clinical Rehabilitation, Journal of Rehabilitation Medicine and Disability and Rehabilitation) throughout the year 2004. All publications were ranked to country of origin of the research and authors. The Netherlands ranked 3rd, among a group of 12 countries, and was responsible for 8% of the total number of publications. At (31%) the USA headed the list. However, the list would be quite different if the population size of each country were taken into account, as is indicated by Coppen and Bailey for a similar ranking on clinical medicine [6], where the USA ranked 9 and the Netherlands 6 on the number of citations per 1000 population. The impact of the contribution of the Netherlands to the field of rehabilitation research in an international context is considerable and in part explains the active organization of the current congress.

With the 4th International congress we also in part celebrate the 2nd lustrum and the success of the Rehabilitation program of the Netherlands Organization for Health Research and Development (ZonMw)[4] which started some ten years ago. This very

---

[2] www.fbw.vu.nl

[3] www.umcg.nl

[4] www.ZonMw.nl/english

successful research stimulation program initiated 8 rehabilitation research networks. In particular, the national rehabilitation research network 'Restoration of mobility in SCI rehabilitation' has benefitted greatly from the research stimulation program, which has also been highly productive in terms of the number and diversity of research projects initiated, as well as in terms of successful PhD projects and publications.[5] A continued effort for the implementation of research findings in practice is sought through the joint effort of rehabilitation physicians, paramedical professionals and researchers. An important example of this collaboration is the patient monitoring project, where individual patients are monitored both clinically and through regular tests to further structure their individual status, rehabilitation strategy and program, and their prognosis [7].

Many rehabilitation centers and university departments, and thus the rehabilitation field and the patients, benefit to this day from the success of the ZonMw funding program. It has boosted the scientific infrastructure of rehabilitation centers, both in personel as well as in technical facilities. It has – above all – stimulated the academic observation and thinking processes in rehabilitation practice and boosted the number of rehabilitation professionals with a research background. This is clearly of crucial importance for the quality of rehabilitation treatment and outcome. The importance of such a rehabilitation research and sciences agenda was very clearly stipulated recently by Frontera and colleagues with their analysis of the North American rehabilitation situation [8,9]; the bottom line of their statement being that: "…survival of the (…rehabilitation…) specialty, may depend, among other things on the quality of the knowledge base. Very few things could be more important for our patients."

3. 4th International State-of-the-art-Congress 'Rehabilitation: mobility, exercise & sports'

It is indeed in the context of this brief history that the 4th International Congress 'Rehabilitation: Mobility, Exercise & Sports' is taking place, as a multidisciplinary event and team effort, and as a natural outcome of the continued collaboration between (local and international) rehabilitation professionals, human movement, social and engineering sciences. The current congress program follows the preceding congresses in 1991 [10], 1998 [11] and 2004 [12–14] and the academic evolvement of the organizing team in a very natural way.

The theme 'Rehabilitation: Mobility, Exercise & Sports' of the 4th International Congress has also evolved from the continued research work in recent years in the (inter)national context. The program follows the intricate collaboration between human movement sciences and rehabilitation professionals and practice, which among others have evolved in the working group 'Rehabilitation' of the Netherlands Society of Human Movement Sciences (VvBN)[6] and 'Human Movement & Sports' of the Dutch Association of Physical Medicine and Rehabilitation (VRA).[7] The latter stresses the recognition of exercise, active lifestyle and sports, not only as an important part of clinical rehabilitation, but much more also as a lifetime commitment, assumed to increase health and quality of life [15–20].

---

[5] www.scionn.nl

[6] www.bewegingswetenschappen.org/english/english.html

[7] vra.artsennet.nl

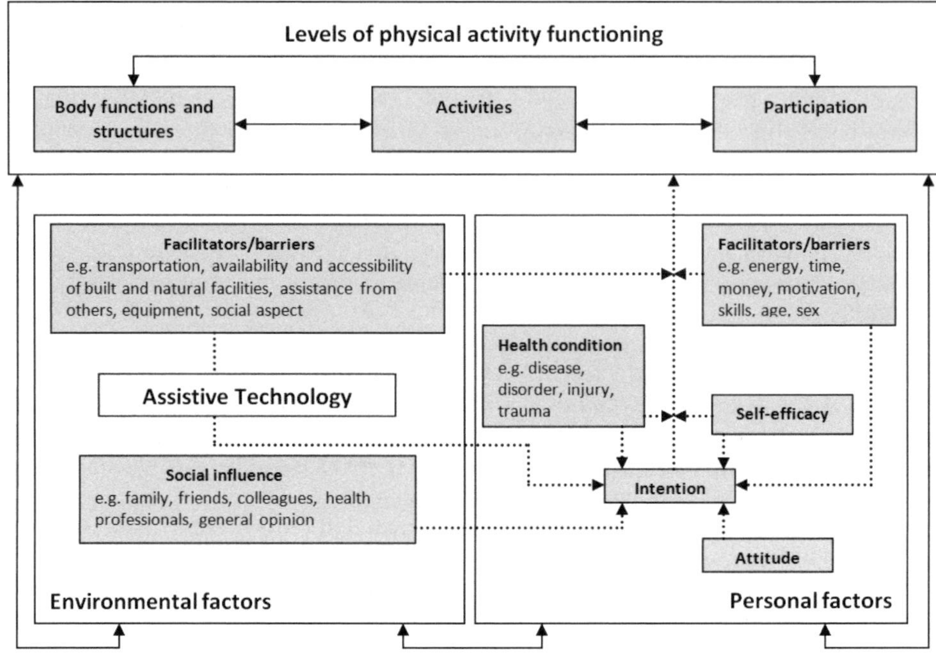

(Adapted from Van der Ploeg et al., 2004) [1]

Figure 1. The Physical Activity for People with a Disability.

4. Mobility, Exercise & Sports

The theme of the congress, mobility exercise and sports in the context of rehabilitation practice, is of extremely great interest to human movement scientists, and rehabilitation professionals. It is indicated to be of key importance in the process of recovery in persons with chronic disease and in the context of long-term health [1,16,18–21].

Mobility is defined in the ICF as '...the ability moving by changing body position or location or by transferring from one place to another, by carrying, moving or manipulating objects, by walking, running or climbing, and by using various forms of transportation.'[2]. Being a mobile individual is crucial for function, participation and quality of life. The extent of mobility will be dependent on the structures and functions and the capacities of the individual, availability and quality of assistive technology and environmental optimization, as well as the interfacing between these and the individual. Above all, personal qualities will impact the final outcome (Figure 1) [1,2,15].

Important questions revolve not only around the functions and structures of individuals with different diagnoses but also around how these impact activities, participation and quality of life. Beyond that the role of assistive technology, environmental barriers and questions of their fine-tuning to individuals in the light of daily functioning (and sports) are issues for technologists and ergonomists, as well as for rehabilitation professionals and human movement scientists.

Rehabilitation practice, and the individual, can and will try to affect mobility through exercise, training and learning of motor skills and overall functional and physical capacities. Sports introduce a natural environment of physical exercise and skill learning as well as a social context of participation and enjoyment. Yet, diagnosis-specific guidelines for exercise and training as well as motor learning are often still limited in their scientific evidence-base [16,17]. Optimal strategies for rehabilitation have to be established in the context of long-term preservation of function, health and quality of life. Moreover, exercise and sports are supposed to have benefits, but the combination of impairment, assistive technology and intensity of daily activities, exercise and sports must also be viewed in the context of risks of overuse and secondary impairment, as has been described for manual wheelchair use [14,22–24]. Fine-tuning between assistive technology and individual functions and structures as well as the regular supervision and feedback of exercise and training in rehabilitation, activities of daily living and sports require a thorough understanding of underlying mechanisms and processes in a wide range of individuals, with different diagnoses, and at different levels of expertise and performance, from daily practice to elite sports at the Paralympics.[8] The research agenda for that is wide, detailed and long, as was described for the Paralympic movement by Vanlandewijck [25]. The current congress intends to contribute to this important debate and to knowledge provision and development.

5. What we seek for…

The current and future congresses seek for the evidence-base of mobility, exercise and sports in the context of rehabilitation diagnosis, treatment and strategy and also of long-term functioning, participation, health and quality of life. The ICF [2] is the leading contextual framework in the development of research activities, the organization of knowledge, understanding and clinical practice. The importance of the congress lies in the exchange of the state-of-the-art knowledge, lively debates and the exchange of experiences among a diversity of clinical professionals and researchers from different disciplines, backgrounds and countries, leading to a continued cross-cultural debate and exchange, as has been recently advocated as a necessity to further the international field of physical medicine and rehabilitation [26].

The keynote speakers, the oral program and the poster sessions assure such a formal and informal debate, during exhibition time, breaks, the social program and in leisure time. The congress model of a 'one-track event for all' has proved to be effective in that perspective and will lead to international exchange and collaboration.

As previously [10,11], and apart from the 3 day program, the congress will provide a congress book with 3-page summaries of all oral and poster contributions, which you see here in front of you. A set of 10–12 highlights of the congress will also be published in the well-established journal 'Disability and Rehabilitation' as a special issue. This will support the outcome of the congress as a tool in the international communication of rehabilitation and human movement sciences.

References

[1]   Van der Ploeg, H.P., et al., *Physical activity for people with a disability: a conceptual model.* Sports Med, 2004. **34**(10): p. 639–49.
[2]   WHO, *International Classification of Functioning, Health and Disability.* 2001, Geneva: WHO.
[3]   Gutenbrunner, G., A.B. Ward, and M.A. Chamberlain, *White book on Physical and Rehabilitation Medicine in Europe.* J Rehabil Med, 2006. **39**: p. 1–48.

---

[8] www.paralympic.org

[4]   Fletcher, R.W. and S.W. Fletcher, *Knowledge Management*, in *Clinical Epidemiology, the essentials*. 2005, Lippincott Williams & Wilkins: Philadelphia. p. 221–231.

[5]   Stam, H.J., *Research in physical and rehabilitation medicine in Europe: how are we doing?* J Rehabil Med, 2006. **38**(1): p. 1–2.

[6]   Coppen, A. and J. Bailey, *20 most-cited countries in clinical medicine ranked by population size*. Lancet, 2004. **363**(9404): p. 250.

[7]   de Groot, S., et al., *Patient monitoring during inpatient spinal cord injury rehabilitation: implementation experiences of periodical testing*. Disability & Rehabilitation. **submitted**.

[8]   Frontera, W.R., *Research and the survival of physical medicine and rehabilitation*. Am J Phys Med Rehabil, 2006. **85**(12): p. 939–44.

[9]   Frontera, W.R., et al., *Rehabilitation medicine summit: building research capacity. Executive summary*. Arch Phys Med Rehabil, 2006. **87**(1): p. 148–52.

[10] Van der Woude, L., et al., eds. *Ergonomics of Manual Wheelchair Propulsion, State of the Art*. 1993, IOS press: Amsterdam. 366.

[11] Van der Woude, L.H.V., M.T.E. Hopman, and C.H. Van Kemenade, eds. *Biomedical Aspects of Manual Wheelchair Propulsion: State of the Art II*. 1999, IOS press: Amsterdam. 392.

[12] JRRD, S.I., *3rd International Congress Restiration on (wheeled) mobility in sci rehabilitation*. J Reh Res & Dev, 2004. **41**(2, supplement 2): p. 1–85.

[13] JRRD, S.i., *Background on the 3rd International Congress*. J Reh Res Dev, 2005. **42**(3, supplement 1): p. 1–110.

[14] T&D, *3rd international Congress 'Restoration of (wheeled) mobility in SCI rehabilitation, State of the art II'I: its background*. Technology and Disability, 1005. **17**: p. 55–123.

[15] Rimmer, J.H., *Use of the ICF in identifying factors that impact participation in physical activity/rehabilitation among people with disabilities*. Disabil Rehabil, 2006. **28**(17): p. 1087–95.

[16] Frontera, W.R., D.M. Slovnik, and D.M. Dawson, eds. *Exercise in rehabilitation medicine*. 2nd ed. 2006, Human Kinetics Publishers. 454.

[17] Durstine, J.L. and G.E. Moore, *ACSM's Exercise management for persons with chronic diseases and disabilities*. 2003, Chapaign: Human Kintecs, ACSM.

[18] Durstine, J.L., et al., *Physical activity for the chronically ill and disabled*. Sports Med, 2000. **30**(3): p. 207–19.

[19] Cooper, R.A., et al., *Research on physical activity and health among people with disabilities: a consensus statement*. J Rehabil Res Dev, 1999. **36**(2): p. 142–54.

[20] Nash, M., *Exercise as a health-promoting activity following spinal cord injury*. J Neurological Physical Therapy, 2005. **29**(2): p. 87–93.

[21] Rimmer, J.H. and D. Braddock, *Health promotion for people with physical, cognitive and sensory disabilities: an emerging national priority*. Am J Health Promot, 2002. **16**(4): p. 220–4, ii.

[22] Nichols, P.J., P.A. Norman, and J.R. Ennis, *Wheelchair user's shoulder? Shoulder pain in patients with spinal cord lesions*. Scand J Rehabil Med, 1979. **11**(1): p. 29–32.

[23] van Drongelen, S., et al., *Upper extremity musculoskeletal pain during and after rehabilitation in wheelchair-using persons with a spinal cord injury*. Spinal Cord, 2006. **44**(3): p. 152–9.

[24] van Drongelen, S., et al., *Glenohumeral joint loading in tetraplegia during weight relief lifting: a simulation study*. Clin Biomech (Bristol, Avon), 2006. **21**(2): p. 128–37.

[25] Vanlandewijck, Y., *Sports Science in the Paralympic movement*. J Rehab Res & Devel, 2006. **43**(7): p. XVII–XXIV.

[26] Negrini, S. and W.R. Frontera, *The Euro-American rehabilitation focus: a cultural bridge across the ocean*. Am J Phys Med Rehabil, 2008. **87**(7): p. 590–1.

Contents

Chapter 2. Handcycling

2.1 Oral Presentations

Chapter 5. Exercise Capacity

5.1 Keynote

5.2 Oral Presentations

Chapter 7. Training Strategies

7.1 Keynote

7.2 Oral Presentations

7.3 Poster Presentations

Chapter 8. FES

8.1 Oral Presentations

11.3 Poster Presentations

Chapter 1

Wheeled Mobility

1.1

Keynote

Rehabilitation: Mobility, Exercise and Sports
L.H.V. van der Woude et al. (Eds.)
IOS Press, 2010

doi:10.3233/978-1-60750-080-3-3

Wheeled mobility: current and future developments

R.A. COOPER

Department of Rehabilitation Science & Technology, University of Pittsburgh,
Pittsburgh, USA and Human Engineering Research Laboratories, Department of
Veterans Affairs Rehabilitation Research and Development Service, Pittsburgh, USA

World-wide this is an interesting time to participate in wheeled mobility research. The population of people who could benefit from wheeled mobility is growing at a rate of 5% percent per year by some estimates and at a rate of 22% per decade by more conservative numbers. Currently, about 100 million people around the planet use or would use a wheelchair if one were available. To this end, the World Health Organization commissioned a report to clarify best practices for wheelchair design, service delivery, and outcome measurement for low-income countries. In many respects this report is a model for all countries. Globally, there are pressures to reduce the costs associated with providing wheeled mobility, which is stifling innovation in some respects, but fueling the drive for greater scientific evidence. This is coupled with greater participation of people with disabilities as designers, engineers, scientists, and clinicians as the impact of accessibility and human-rights egislation begins to take effect. The future likely will require a much higher degree of scientific and medical evidence in order for quality wheeled mobility to be reimbursed by insurance companies. Fortunately, forward thinking clinicians and scientists have already started incorporating greater instrumentation and outcomes data collection. Consumers are becoming more involved in designing and selecting wheeled mobility through web-based tools that allow for wide-spread democratization of information. More educated and engaged clinicians and wheelchairs users who are or who work closely with scientists will eventually lead to greater mobility, community participation, and higher quality designs.

1.2

Oral Presentations

Rehabilitation: Mobility, Exercise and Sports
L.H.V. van der Woude et al. (Eds.)
IOS Press, 2010
© *2010 The authors and IOS Press. All rights reserved.*
doi:10.3233/978-1-60750-080-3-7

Outcomes after wheelchair configuration changes for postural support in persons with truncal paralysis; a pilot study

J.D. HASTINGS[a,1], K.G. SCHEPP[b], B. GOLDSTEIN[b], R. LOGSDON[b],
D. DEMONBREUN[c]
[a] *University of Puget Sound, Tacoma WA USA*
[b] *University of Washington, Seattle WA USA*
[c] *Department of Veterans Affairs, Tucson AZ USA*

Abstract. Purpose: To determine whether pain, posture and satisfaction with life change in persons with spinal cord injury after improvement in sagittal plane alignment via customized orthotic wheelchair configuration. Methods: Prospective repeated measure study. Participants: Eleven men with T1-T10 motor complete spinal cord injury. Main Outcome Measures: Seated Height (SH), Wheelchair User's Shoulder Pain Index (WUSPI), Posture Scale for Wheelchair Users (PSWU), pain intensity, and Satisfaction with Life Scale (SWLS). Results: Increase in SH was significant (p=. 03), mean change of 2.57 centimeters (1.01 inches); 95% C.I.: 0.33 to 4.82. At two weeks, participants reported significantly less pain (-9.6) on the WUSPI (p=. 03); C.I.: -18.34 to -0.87, and significantly lower 'worst pain' intensity (-1.18) (p=. 04); C.I.: -2.3 to -0.4. Remaining outcomes did not show significant change. Conclusion: The results of this study support the use of wheelchair configuration to provide orthotic stabilization in the sagittal plane to the paralyzed trunk. Improved postural alignment was shown to decrease shoulder pain and intensity of pain measured two weeks post intervention. Early orthotic postural support via wheelchair configuration may prevent the negative sequelae of postural deviations and promote improved health outcomes.

Keywords. posture, wheelchair, spinal cord injury, seating, pain.

1. Introduction

This study tests the theory that musculoskeletal pain and discomfort reported in wheelchair users with truncal paralysis is related to inadequate postural support. Conceptually the wheelchair is a truncal orthosis (an external device providing support through specifically located points of control)[1]. If the wheelchair is configured to provide support to spinal alignment, then there is less aberrant muscular work required for postural stability. If this aberrant muscular work is a source of musculoskeletal pain, then there will be less pain and this may lead to improved quality of life. Because

---

[1] Corresponding Author. Jennifer D. Hastings PT, PhD, University of Puget Sound,1500 N. Warner CMB 1070, Tacoma, WA 98416 (p) 253 879 3526, (f) 253 879 2933, (e) jhastings@ups.edu

the mechanics of the upper limb are predisposed by the alignment of the spine there is an expectation that upper limb musculoskeletal pain should also be lessened by improved spinal postural alignment[2, 3].

2. Methods

A convenience sample of full time manual wheelchair using veterans with truncal paralysis caused by SCI was recruited. Participants were interviewed and then photographed while seated in their personal wheelchairs. Physical examination included lower extremity passive range of motion and trunk flexibility and specific measurements of the personal wheelchair. Participants then completed the outcome measure questionnaires. A seating specialist (JH) synthesized the physical examination data with the observed seated postural alignment and prescribed changes to optimize postural support. The goal was to establish a sagittal plane pelvic stabilizing orthotic system[1] Changes generally moved the backrest out of recline (more vertical), lowered the backrest and increased the seat slope (front above horizontal). The participants were photographed again in the new configuration. After two weeks and 3 months participants returned additional sets of questionnaires. Baseline and post intervention photographs were measured for Seated Height (SH) which was the outcome measure for actual physical postural change (measured from seat rail to top of head).

3. Results

Participants aged 40 to 84 (median 54); years since injury 5 to 33 (median 18.6). The mean change in composite inside seat-to-back angle was a decrease of 3.4 degrees,(p=.001 95% confidence interval [C.I.] 1.85 to 4.87). The resulting configuration had an acute inside seat-to-back angle averaging 86 degrees.

SH showed a significant increase with a mean change of 2.57 centimeters (p=. 03; C.I.: 0.33 to 4.82). At two weeks after changes, participants reported a mean decrease of 9.6 on the WUSPI (p=. 03; C.I.: -18.34 to -0.87), and lower (-1.18) 'worst pain' intensity (p=. 04; C.I.: -2.3 to -0.4). One selected item from the PSWU; "my chair is not supportive enough" showed significant improvement (p=.01; C.I.: 0.10 to 0.81).

Participants indicated any current pain on a schematic. At baseline, all participants reported pain, many reported multiple sites. 83% of the pain sites were located in the axial trunk with indication at the neck, upper thoracic, lower thoracic and lumbar regions. Two weeks after wheelchair adjustment there were 20% fewer indications of pain reported in the axial trunk with no pain sites indicated in the neck.

3-month follow up: Pain reported continued to decline in axial trunk, with no pain reported in the neck and now two participants with no current pain. The PSWU item change continued significant all other changes were no longer significant at three month follow up. Two participants lost to follow up.

4. Discussion

Limitations include a small sample size, however the tested intervention is intended for individuals with truncal paralysis and the sample was clinically specific to this aim. Participants were not specifically recruited to have pain. However, SCI literature consistently reports that upper extremity pain is prevalent in the population[4-10] therefore it is appropriate to look for change in prevalence post any intervention which is theorized to relate to causal mechanisms of pain. The age of the participants does not reflect the general population of SCI. Yet this should be considered strength; the fact that this sample with an average of nearly 20 years of living with paralysis and a median age over 50 showed positive changes is impressive. The benefit from the postural intervention may be better appreciated in these quotes from participants:

"....my new position has changed the way I sit and push with my arms and I can push farther without my shoulders aching."

"I never knew that comfortable and being in a wheelchair were compatible. I just assumed they weren't. It is like being reborn."   *this subject injured for 29yrs

5. Conclusion

The results of this study support the use of wheelchair configuration to provide orthotic stabilization in the sagittal plane to the paralyzed trunk. Improved orthotic support was shown to increase erect sitting and improved postural alignment was shown to decrease the amount of pain reported in the axial trunk and neck, decrease shoulder pain and decrease reported intensity of musculoskeletal pain measured two weeks post intervention. Early orthotic postural support via wheelchair configuration may prevent the negative sequelae of postural deviations, reduce musculoskeletal pain above the level of spinal cord injury and promote improved health outcomes.

References

[1]   J.D. Hastings, E.R. Fanucchi, S.P. Burns: Wheelchair configuration and Postural Alignment in Persons with Spinal Cord Injury. *Archives of Physical Medicine Rehabilitation* **84** (April) (2003), 528-534.

[2]   B. Goldstein, J. Young, E.M. Escobedo, Rotator Cuff Repairs in Individuals with Paraplegia. *Am J Phys Med Rehabil* **76**(July/August no.4) (1997), 316-322.

[3]   M. Boninger, R.L. Waters, T. Chase, et al. Preservation of Upper Limb Function Following Spinal Cord Injury: A Clinical Practice Guideline for Health-Care Professionals. Washington DC: Paralyzed Veterans of America Consortium for Spinal Cord Medicine, 2005.

[4]   J. Silfverskiold, R.L. Waters, Shoulder pain and functional disability in spinal cord injury patients, *Clin Ortho Rel Res* **272** (1991), 141-145.

[5]   I.H. Sie, R.L Waters, R.H. Adkins, H. Gellman, Upper extremity pain in the postrehabilitation spinal cord injured patient. *Arch Phys Med Rehabil* **73(1)** (1992), 44-48.

[6]   M. Dalyan, D.D. Cardenas, B. Gerard, Upper extremity pain after spinal cord injury. *Spinal Cord* **37**(3) 1999, 191-5.

[7]   D.A. Ballinger, D.H. Rintala, K.A. Hart, The relation of shoulder pain and range-of-motion problems to functional limitations, disability, and perceived health of men with spinal cord injury: a multifaceted longitudinal study. *Arch Phys Med Rehabil* **81**(12) (2000), 1575-81.

[8]   J.A. Turner, D.D. Cardenas, C.A. Warms, C.B. McClellan, Chronic pain associated with spinal cord injuries: a community survey. *Arch Phys Med Rehabil* **82**(4) (2001), 501-9.

[9]   T.A. Dyson-Hudson, S.C. Kirshblum, Shoulder pain in chronic spinal cord injury, Part I: Epidemiology, etiology, and pathomechanics. *J Spinal Cord Med* **27**(1) (2004), 4-17.

[10] M. Alm, H. Saraste, C. Norrbrink, Shoulder pain in persons with thoracic spinal cord injury: prevalence and characteristics. *J Rehabil Med* **40**(4) (2008), 277-83.

Rehabilitation: Mobility, Exercise and Sports
L.H.V. van der Woude et al. (Eds.)
IOS Press, 2010
© 2010 *The authors and IOS Press. All rights reserved.*
doi:10.3233/978-1-60750-080-3-10

Mechanical efficiency of asynchronous hand-rim wheelchair propulsion after 4-weeks of practice

J.P. LENTON[a,b], N.E. FOWLER[a], L.H.V. VAN DER WOUDE[c], V.L. GOOSEY-TOLFREY[a,b]

[a] *Department of Exercise & Sport Science, Manchester Metropolitan University, UK*
[b] *Peter Harrison Centre for Disability Sport, School of Sport and Exercise Sciences, Loughborough University, UK*
[c] *Centre for Human Movement Sciences, University Medical Centre Groningen, University of Groningen, The Netherlands*

Abstract. The purpose of this study was to investigate adaptations in gross mechanical efficiency during asynchronous hand-rim wheelchair propulsion of novice able-bodied participants following 4 weeks of practice. Twenty seven male participants performed a series of five, 4-minute sub-maximal exercise bouts at 1.7 $m \cdot s^{-1}$. Arm frequencies consisted of the freely-chosen frequency (FCF), followed by 4 counter-balanced paced trials pushing at 60, 80, 120, and 140% of the FCF. Gross efficiency (GE) was determined. Participants were divided into two experimental groups (FCF, N = 9; 80% FCF, N = 8) and a control group (N = 8). The experimental groups received a 4-week propulsion practice period (3$\cdot wk^{-1}$, 12 practice trials) at 1.7 $m \cdot s^{-1}$. Post practice period all groups repeated the five 4-minute sub-maximal exercise bouts. Over the practice period the mean GE for the FCF condition increased in both experimental groups (+1.0 & 0.9%) compared to the control group (+0.1%) (P = 0.001). Arm frequency decreased at FCF in both experimental groups (P = 0.001), however, larger changes were observed in the FCF experimental group. Four weeks practice had a beneficial effect on metabolic cost and GE in male novice participants. This improved GE associated to the resulting changes in the self-selected arm frequency in both experimental groups, as an overall indicator of propulsion technique.

Keywords. wheelchair ergometry, able-bodied, gross efficiency, skill.

1. Introduction

The skills required for hand-rim propulsion are more than often learned during rehabilitation as a completely novel task. Therefore, training and learning of manual hand-rim wheelchair propulsion would be deemed an essential part of the rehabilitation process. In a cross-sectional study, Lenton et al. (2) demonstrated that wheelchair experience significantly improves the efficiency of hand-rim propulsion as result of continued practice / training.

Previous research, de Groot et al. (1) reported that a low-intensity three week practice program resulted in a significant improvement in gross efficiency. The practice had favourable effects on timing parameters of the propulsion technique and mechanical efficiency, consequently highlighting the positive effect practice can have even when only conducted over a short period of time. The purpose of this study is to investigate adaptations in gross mechanical efficiency during asynchronous hand-rim propulsion.

2. Methods

Participants

Twenty five healthy, male, able-bodied participants (22 ± 4 years) volunteered for this study. Prerequisite for participation was no prior experience in wheelchair propulsion or training in upper body sports activities.

Procedure

Participants performed a series of five, 4-minute sub-maximal exercise bouts at a speed of 1.7 m·s^{-1}. Arm frequencies consisted of the freely chosen frequency (FCF), followed by 4 counter-balanced paced trials pushing at 60, 80, 120 and 140% of the FCF. Participants were divided into two experimental groups (FCF, N = 9; 80% FCF, N = 8) and a control group (N = 8). Experimental groups received a 4-week propulsion practice period (3 · wk^{-1}, 12 practice trials [4 · 4 min practice blocks]) on the wheelchair ergometer. One week post practice participants repeated sub-maximal exercise bouts at 1.7 m·s^{-1}.

Data Collection

Gross efficiency (GE) of propulsion was determined according to the ratio: GE = (External Work Accomplished / Total Energy Expended) · 100 (%).

Statistics

A 2 x 3 (time by group) mixed measures ANOVA with time as the within factor was applied to all physiological data. Significance for all tests was assumed at p ≤ 0.05. A Bonferroni *post hoc* test was applied to further analyse significant main effects.

3. Results

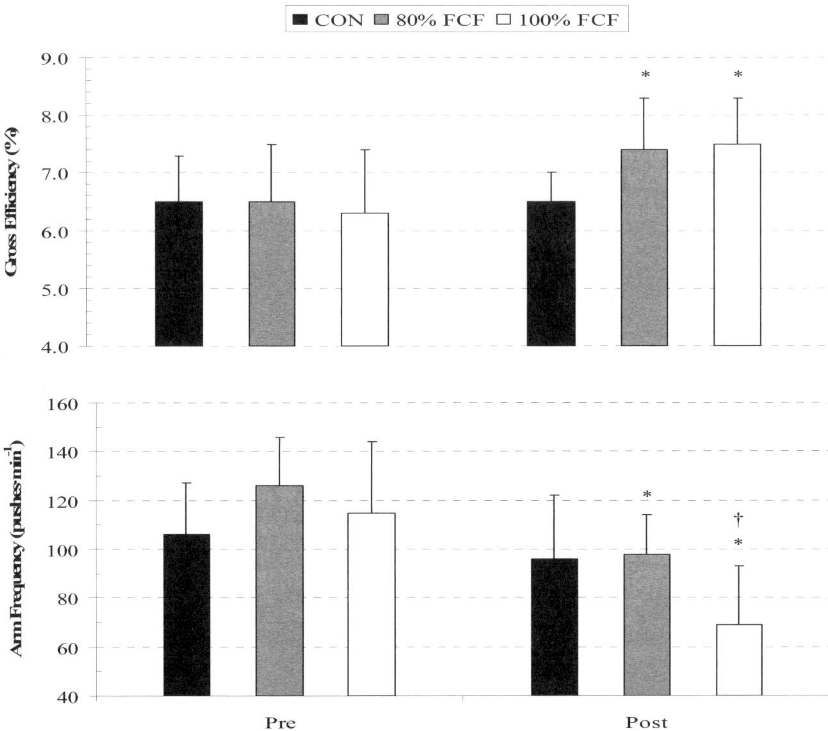

Figure 1. Gross efficiency and Arm Frequency results pre and post practice period of the FCF condition for three groups (mean and SD). * Significant difference between pre and post tests p < 0.01. † Significant difference between practice groups post practice p < 0.01.

4. Conclusion

Four-weeks of asynchronous hand-rim wheelchair propulsion practice had a beneficial effect on metabolic cost and GE in the experimental groups. An improved GE appeared to be associated to the changes in the self-selected arm frequency in both experimental groups of novices. Further analysis of kinematic and EMG data will help to understand the improvements of propulsion technique in more detail and in the light of the changes in GE.

References

[1]   S. de Groot, D.H.E.V. Veeger, A.P. Hollander, L.H.V. van der Woude. Wheelchair propulsion technique and mechanical efficiency after 3 wk of practice. Medicine and Science in Sports and Exercise. 34(5) (2002), 756-766.

[2]   J.P. Lenton, N.E. Fowler, L.H.V. van der Woude, V.L. Goosey-Tolfrey. Wheelchair propulsion: Effects of experience and push strategy on efficiency and perceived exertion. Applied Physiology, Nutrition and Metabolism. 33 (2008), 870-879.

Rehabilitation: Mobility, Exercise and Sports
L.H.V. van der Woude et al. (Eds.)
IOS Press, 2010

doi:10.3233/978-1-60750-080-3-13

Positioning the wheelchair close to the target surface reduces shoulder muscular demand for sitting pivot transfers

A.M. KOONTZ[a,b,1], D. GAGNON[c,d], E. BRINDLE[a,b], R.A. COOPER[a,b]

[a] *Human Engineering Research Laboratories, VA Pittsburgh HealthCare System, Pittsburgh, PA, USA*
[b] *Departments of Rehabilitation Science and Technology and Bioengineering, University of Pittsburgh, Pittsburgh, PA, USA*
[c] *School of Rehabilitation, University of Montreal, Montreal, Canada,* [d] *Center for Interdisciplinary Research in Rehabilitation of the Greater Montreal, Montreal, Quebec, Canada*

Abstract. For many wheelchair users, performing transfers is essential for achieving independence with daily activities. However, transfers are particularly straining on the upper limbs and may contribute to the development of pain and overuse injuries at the shoulder. The purpose of this study was to determine the muscular demands of seven bilateral muscles acting at the shoulder and elbow during level and non-level transfers with and without a gap separating the wheelchair and target surface. Fourteen men with spinal cord injury transferred from their own wheelchair to a 1) level bench, 2) level bench with a 10 cm gap, 3) higher bench (+10 cm), 4) higher bench with a 10 cm gap, 5) lower bench (-10 cm), and 6) lower bench with a 10 cm gap in a random order. The maximum surface EMG reached during transfers was normalized to the subject's maximum EMG value reached during maximum static contractions for each muscle. Gaps required greater recruitment of the biceps and anterior deltoid muscles ($p < 0.05$). The increased muscle activation observed with gaps is likely due in part to increased combined shoulder flexion and abduction and glenohumeral joint strain on the anterior wall. As a result, individuals with SCI should be advised to position their wheelchair as close as possible to the surface they intend to transfer.

Keywords. transfers, activities of daily living, spinal cord injury, electromyography.

1. Introduction

Achieving the highest level of societal participation after spinal cord injury (SCI) hinges on the ability to independently move the body from one surface to another. Performing routine transfers; however, are believed to contribute to the high prevalence of pain and injury reported among individuals with spinal cord injury (SCI) as the upper extremity was not designed for weight bearing [1]. Any loss of upper limb function significantly affects ability to transfer and function independently [2]. The purpose of this study was to investigate the muscular demands at the shoulder and

---

[1] Corresponding Author.

elbow during level and non-level transfers with and without a gap separating the wheelchair and target surface.

2. Methods

Participants

Informed consent was obtained from fourteen male manual wheelchair users with a SCI ranging from S1 to C6 (age: 46 ± 9 years, SCI duration: 12 ± 8 years, height 1.8 ± 0.8 m, and mass: 75.3 ± 11.3 kg.

Experimental Protocol

After attaching surface electrodes to seven muscles around the shoulder and elbow bilaterally, standardized manual muscle testing was performed to verify electrode position and generate the maximum voluntary contraction. Electromyographic signals were recorded while subjects performed a sitting pivot transfer (e.g., majority of body weight supported by their arms) from their wheelchair to a bench. Hand, feet, buttocks and wheelchair position were marked and used to establish a reference for setting up the following transfers which were performed in a random order: level with a 10 cm gap, higher bench (+10 cm) no gap, higher bench with a 10 cm gap, lower bench (-10 cm) no gap, and lower bench with a 10 cm gap. The maximum surface EMG reached during transfers was normalized to the subject's maximum EMG value reached during maximum static contractions for each muscle (peak %MVC).

Statistics

Wilcoxon signed rank tests were used to detect significant differences between the no gap and gap conditions for the low, level, and high transfer (adjusted $p = 0.0167$). As the sample was small and the muscle activity was highly variable among participants, we also denoted differences for $p < 0.05$. Results are presented for each arm separately as they serve different roles during the transfer.

3. Results

Leading arm

Muscular demand of the pectoralis major sternal (PMS), pectoralis major clavicular (PMC), anterior deltoid (AD) and biceps (BI) muscle groups was greater when a gap was introduced at all three transfer heights. The AD and BI peak %MVC reached statistical significance for the level and low transfers, respectively (Figure 1). The leading arm triceps (TRI) peak %MVC was higher for the level transfer with gap (72%) versus without gap (67%), similar for the low transfer (58% gap versus 58% no gap), and lower for the high transfer (68% gap versus 72% no gap).

Trailing arm

Higher or similar peak %MVC was found with gaps versus no gaps for the PMC and PMS for all three transfer heights. Muscle demand was significantly higher for the AD and BI muscles for the level transfer with gap versus no gap (Figure 1). Less muscle demand was found for the AD and BI muscle for high gap versus no gap transfers. The TRI muscle demand was higher for the gap transfers: level transfer (76% gap versus 71% no gap), low transfer (61% gap versus 59% no gap) and high transfer (99% gap versus 97% no gap).

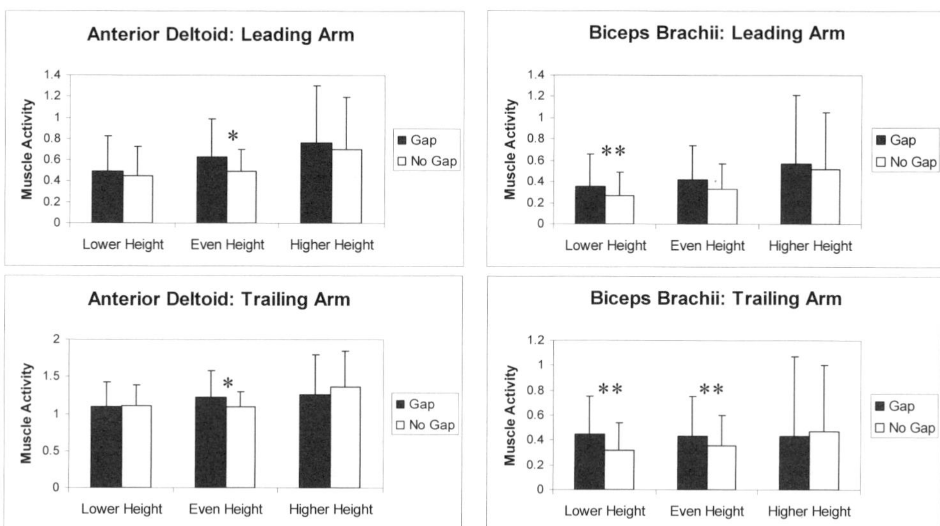

Figure 1. Average normalized peak EMG activity for the anterior deltoid and biceps brachii for the leading and trailing arm for all transfers. Key: $*= p < 0.05$; $** = p < 0.0167$

4. Conclusion

This study confirmed that a greater horizontal distance separating the wheelchair and the target surface increases muscular demand in both arms during sitting pivot transfers. Increased AD and BI muscle activation observed with gaps is likely due in part to increased combined shoulder flexion and abduction and glenohumeral joint strain on the anterior wall. As a result, individuals with SCI should be advised to position their wheelchair as close as possible to the surface they intend to transfer.

References

[1] Nichols, PJ et al. Wheelchair user's shoulder? Shoulder pain in patients with spinal cord lesions. Scand J Rehabil Med 1979;**11**:29-32.
[2] Curtis KA et al. Shoulder pain in wheelchair users with tetraplegia and paraplegia. Arch Phys Med Rehabil 1999;**80**:453-7.

1.3

Poster Presentations

Rehabilitation: Mobility, Exercise and Sports
L.H.V. van der Woude et al. (Eds.)
IOS Press, 2010
© 2010 The authors and IOS Press. All rights reserved.
doi:10.3233/978-1-60750-080-3-19

19

Automatic filtering and phase detection of propulsive and recovery phase during wheelchair propulsion

R. AISSAOUI[a,b,1]
*[a] Laboratoire de Recherche en Imagerie et Orthopédie,
École de technologie supérieure, Montreal, Canada
[b] Centre de Recherche Interdisciplinaire en Réadaptation de Montréal*

Abstract. The determination of propulsive and recovery phases of manual wheelchair propulsion are important in estimating the efficacy of manual propulsion. With the actual potential of collection of database by different research team, manual determination of propulsive and recovery phases of each wheelchair cycle represents a tremendous amount of time. Automatic detection with only a single threshold and low-pass filtering is insufficient to detect initial and terminal phases during propulsion. The purpose of this work is to present a new adaptive method based on short-time spectral analysis (STSA) of forces and moment acting at the handrim level. Eight able-bodied subjects were asked to propel on ergometer with 3 slopes, while forces and moments were recorded with an instrumented rear wheels. The STSA was applied to raw signal and automatic detection was based on priori and a posterior probability of absence and presence of propulsive signal. Better results are obtained with the new adaptive method when compared to the classical method with one single threshold and one cut-off frequency per signal. This method will prove useful when monitoring manual propulsion for a long term, and with different types of propulsion and classification of pattern of daily activities.

Keywords. wheelchair propulsion, short-time spectral analysis, decision-directed method.

1. Introduction

Dynamic rolling platforms are now widely used in the measurement of handrim forces and moments during manual wheelchair propulsion [1]. The determination of propulsive and recovery phases of manual wheelchair propulsion are important when estimating potential risk injury, the effect of positioning as well as shoulder kinetics [2-3]. When dynamic platform are in movement: i.e. without any forces exerted at the handrim level, the channels that are acting out of the plane of the wheel exhibit generally a constant offset, whereas those acting on the plane of the wheel exhibit a sine-wave offset with varying frequency. The variation in frequency is due to the wheel's angular velocity in time-domain (Fig.1). This apparent sine-wave is due essentially to the mechanical misalignment of the longitudinal axis of each beam and the axle centre of the wheel speed, as well as the linear bearing length. In their

---

¹ Corresponding Author. Aissaoui Rachid, Dépt. Génie de la production automatisée, École de Technologie Supérieure, 1100, Rue Notre-Dame Ouest, Montréal, Canada, H3C 1K3. Email: rachid.aissaoui@etsmtl.ca.

pioneered work, Cooper et al. [4] attempted to analyze the frequency content of pushrim forces and moments during manual wheelchair propulsion and proposed a manual clustering method to differentiate between the frequency content of the noise acting at the pushrim during recovery phase and the signal acting during the propulsive phase. The method proposed in [4] for the estimation of the optimal cut-off frequency depends mainly on the bias introduced by the distorted sine-wave of the noise and is a speed dependent in time-domain. This bias will affect the frequency content of the propulsive and recovery phase since the distorted sine-wave is at low frequency and the separation between noise and signal spectrum will be difficult. In this paper we propose new method to automatically remove the baseline first from the loaded signal and then use a decision-directed estimation approach to enhance a signal to noise ratio in the propulsive phase and to reduce signal variation during the recovery phase.

2.   Methods

Kinetic data from SmartWheel (240 Hz) were provided from study which investigated the physical strength needed for a manual wheelchair user to climb a access ramps: one with a slope of 1 in 10, that is, a ramp that rises one unit every 10 units in length, one with a coefficient of 12 and 20 [6]. The data from 8 able-bodied subjects were used in this study. The subjects sat on the same manual wheelchair (Prima, Orthofab, Canada), and were asked to propel at the natural speed for a distance of 10 m in the custom-made ergometer [3]. First, the sine-wave signal was removed from the raw data using a least-square approach in the geometric domain, and then the decision-directed (DD) estimation approach was applied to the signal [5]. The second (COO) approach was to apply a Butterworth filter designed with cut-off frequencies as defined in [4]. For each stroke we defined the duration of the recovery and propulsion using a threshold of 5% for [4] and 0.01% in our method. We also estimated the noise level in dB in the recovery phase

3.   Results

Figure 1 shows the behavior of the DD method with respect to the COO one in the recovery phase. The DD method is able to recognize the silent part of the propulsion by reducing the noise whereas it enhances the signal during the first dip at the beginning of the propulsion phase. Table 1 shows the time duration of the propulsion phase for 8 subjects when propelling in 3 different ramps 10, 12 and 20. There was a statistical significant ramps effect on the duration of the propulsion phase. In general, the COO method underestimates the propulsion duration-time by a maximum of 37 frames. Even though, this tendency was not statistically significant due to the large variability of the subjects. Normalization should be done in the future to alleviate this problem. However there was a statistical significant method effect on the SNR parameters. The latter indicates clearly the effectiveness of the method to extract the propulsion phase from the noisy signal even if the threshold used by the DD method (0.01%) is five hundred times lower than the one used (5%) for the COO method.

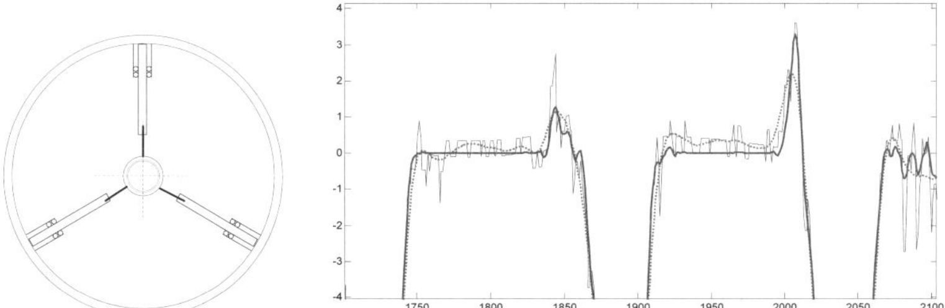

Figure 1. Left, representation of the SmartWheel. Right, typical sagittal moment during a recovery phase of one subject, DD (thick), Butterworth (dotted), raw (thin)

Table 1. Results of the experiment analysis for 8 subjects and for each ramp. The ramp columns correspond to the frame duration of the propulsion phase whereas the SNR correspond to the level of the noise in the recovery phase of movement.

| ramp | DD | | | | | | COO | | | | | |
subject	10 frame	SNR dB	12 frame	SNR dB	20 frame	SNR dB	10 frame	SNR dB	12 frame	SNR dB	20 frame	SNR dB
1	93.73	-3.20	54.62	-10.48	40.68	-11.21	79.13	-2.98	46.62	-1.50	35.87	-3.81
2	126.56	-11.68	85.58	-7.05	46.19	-3.10	113.71	-7.34	77.97	-6.18	41.69	-1.64
3	147.06	-7.18	98.71	-27.31	59.50	-12.18	110.21	-7.47	101.71	-2.87	52.75	-8.99
4	74.73	-8.42	69.10	-4.17	52.51	-8.05	72.69	-0.64	58.67	-2.64	44.80	-6.89
5	132.09	-10.32	140.70	-16.40	64.39	-15.68	114.63	-8.18	129.22	-10.31	57.05	-10.44
6	117.25	-12.57	106.85	-11.79	77.32	-13.77	104.16	-2.80	94.94	-7.41	71.06	-5.98
7	84.09	-4.56	77.91	-5.07	49.58	-8.15	75.79	-3.83	69.76	-4.36	37.15	-6.80
8	83.27	-14.13	73.51	-7.46	47.44	-14.52	80.63	-2.38	70.53	-5.45	41.18	-5.56

4. Conclusion

The new developed decision-directed method proves useful in reducing the level of the noise in the recovery phase whereas it keeps all information close to the real measured data. This is due essentially to the adaptive nature of the Wiener filtering and time frequency approach. This method can be helpful in the clear determination of the nature of the dip at the beginning of the propulsion phase. This is important since this portion of the propulsion phase controls the transmission of the energy to the handrim.

References

[1]   K.S. Asato, R.A. Cooper, R.N. Robertson, J.F. Ster, SMARTWheels development and testing of a system for measuring manual wheelchair propulsion dynamics. *IEEE Trans. BME..* **40**, (1993), 1320-1324.

[2]   R.A. Cooper, Boninger M.L, Shimada S.D, Lawrence B.M, Glenohumeral joint kinematics and kinetics for three coordinate system representations during wheelchair propulsion, *Am. J. Phys. Med. Rehabil.* **78**, (1999), 435-446.

[3]   R. Aissaoui, G. Desroches, Stroke pattern classification during manual wheelchair propulsion in the elderly using fuzzy clustering, *J. Biomech.* **41**, (2008), 2438-2445.

[4]   R.A. Cooper, C.P. Digiovine, M.L Boninger, S.D. Shimada, R.N. Robertson, Frequency analysis of 3-dimensional pushrim forces and moments for manual wheelchair propulsion, *Automedica* **16**, (1998), 355-365.

[5]   Y. Ephraim, D. Malah, Speech enhancement using a minimum mean-square error short-time spectral amplitude estimator, *IEEE Trans. ASSP,* **32**, (1984), 1109-1121.

[6]   J. Rousseau, R. Aissaoui, D. Bourbonnais, *Measuring the effort needed to climb access ramps in manual wheelchair users.* Canadian Mortgage and Housing Corporation, dec (2003), 60 p.

Rehabilitation: Mobility, Exercise and Sports
L.H.V. van der Woude et al. (Eds.)
IOS Press, 2010

doi:10.3233/978-1-60750-080-3-22

Effect of seat height on the propulsion effectiveness and the glenohumeral joint load in handrim wheelchair propulsion

U. ARNET[a], S. VAN DRONGELEN[a,1], H.E.J. VEEGER[b], L.H.V. VAN DER WOUDE[c]

[a] *Swiss Paraplegic Research, Nottwil, Switzerland*
[b] *Research Institute MOVE, IFKB, VU University, Amsterdam, The Netherlands*
[c] *Center for Human Movement Sciences, University Medical Center Groningen, Groningen, The Netherlands*

Abstract. The purpose of this study was to evaluate the effectiveness of force application and the load on the glenohumeral joint during handrim wheelchair propulsion at two different seat heights. In a research laboratory able-bodied male subjects propelled a wheelchair fitted with a SmartWheel on a treadmill at 3 different speeds, while power output was kept constant at 25 W by a pulley system. There was no effect of seat height on the propulsion effectiveness and the glenohumeral joint load under the current experimental conditions.

Keywords. wheelchair, seat height, effectiveness, shoulder load, able-bodied.

1. Introduction

Physical activity and an active lifestyle are important to prevent long term health problems for those people who are wheelchair dependent. Handrim wheelchair propulsion is the most commonly used mode of transportation in this population, however it has been shown to be an energetically and mechanically straining form of transportation. To prevent overuse problems as well as to maintain a physically active lifestyle, an optimal wheelchair-user configuration has to be found.

Regarding mechanical efficiency and oxygen cost, it is known that seat height is optimal if the elbow angle is between 100° and 120° [1]. Additional to these two variables, mechanical load on the upper extremities and effectiveness of force application are important outcomes to be evaluated for an optimal wheelchair-user configuration. Veeger et al. introduced the fraction of effective force (FEF) to describe how effective forces are applied to the handrim in wheelchair propulsion [2]. At low power outputs, a decrease in FEF has been found with an increase in seat heights in persons with a spinal cord injury [1].

The mechanical load on the upper extremity is expressed as the glenohumeral contact force (GH contact force) which expresses the sum of the external and the

---

[1] Corresponding Author: Ursina Arnet, Swiss Paraplegic Research, Guido A. Zächstrasse 4, CH-6207, Nottwil, Switzerland. E-mail: ursina.arnet@paranet.ch

muscle forces around the joint. This is assumed to be an important factor in the risk for overuse injuries.

The purpose of this study was to evaluate whether an absolute change in seat height influenced the effectiveness of force application and the load on the glenohumeral joint during submaximal handrim wheelchair propulsion.

2. Methods

Subjects and protocol

Ten able-bodied male subjects participated in this study after having given written informed consent. Subjects' characteristics (mean ± SD): age 29 ± 4 years, height 1.80 ± 0.08 m and body mass 81 ± 16 kg. All subjects were non-experienced wheelchair users. The study protocol was approved by the local medical ethics committee.

The subjects were asked to propel a wheelchair fitted with a SmartWheel on a treadmill at a velocity of 0.83, 1.11 and 1.38 ms^{-1} for one minute. Each condition was performed with a standard seat height (0.5 m from the floor) and an elevated seat height (0.6 m). Power output was kept constant at 25 W over the 3 speeds by a pulley system.

Data acquisition

The kinetic and kinematic data were measured during the last 30 seconds of each exercise bout. Propulsion forces were obtained by a SmartWheel (Three Rivers Holdings LLC). Kinematics were recorded with 6 infra-red-cameras (Oqus, Qualisys AB). Five unique clusters of reflective markers (4 markers each) were attached to the subject's hand, forearm, upper arm, acromion and thorax. These clusters were related to the anatomical landmarks and local coordinate systems of the upper limbs [4].

Data analysis and statistical analysis

Kinetic variables were calculated as the mean over all completed pushes. FEF was calculated as the ratio between the tangential force and the total force during the push phase. The Delft Shoulder and Elbow model (DSEM) was used to study the glenohumeral joint loading (n = 4). Input data to the model were the 3D forces, moments and kinematics of five regular consecutive push cycles of each condition.

A two-factor (seat height & speed) repeated measures ANOVA was performed to evaluate the effect of seat height on FEF and GH contact force. Level of significance was set at $p < 0.05$.

3. Results

Average elbow angle (internal angle between upper and lower arm) in a standardized sitting posture was 100° ± 7 for the standard and 132° ± 11 for the elevated seat height.

Mean calculated power output was 28.8 ± 1.7 W. Mean values of GH contact force and FEF are listed in Table 1. Over all speed conditions, seat height had no effect on GH contact force and FEF.

Table 1. Mean values and standard deviation of the outcome parameters during the push phase: FEF (fraction of effective force) from 10 subjects, GH force (glenohumeral contact force) during 5 pushes from 4 subjects.

Seat height	standard			elevated		
	0.83 ms^{-1}	1.11 ms^{-1}	1.38 ms^{-1}	0.83 ms^{-1}	1.11 ms^{-1}	1.38 ms^{-1}
mean GH force [N]	663 ± 200	616 ± 132	540 ± 140	596 ± 170	479 ± 128	559 ± 157
max GH force [N]	1313 ± 382	1352 ± 336	1155 ± 418	1346 ± 633	980 ± 258	1058 ± 283
FEF [%]	78.5 ± 9.5	77.1 ± 9.5	74.3 ± 10.2	71.1 ± 8.4	72.1 ± 8.1	71.5 ± 7.8

4. Discussion and conclusion

The means of the GH forces were between 479 and 663 N, which is below 100 % body weight. These results were lower than values from Veeger et al. who found mean GH forces of 850 N for wheelchair propulsion at 20 W with 1.38 ms^{-1} [6]. For the four measured subjects, there is no seat height-related difference for mean and peak GH force. This would indicate that seat height has no direct contribution to the risk of overuse symptoms.

Over all speed conditions, there were no significant seat height-related differences for the FEF. This is in accordance with the results from Kotajarvi et al. [5], who also measured FEF with different standardized seat heights above ground. If the seat height is individually adjusted (standardized to elbow angle) instead of a standardized height above ground, an influence of seat height on FEF was found; van der Woude et al. reported lower FEF at higher seat heights [1, 3]. In the current study, the anthropometry of different subjects was not taken into account with the fixed absolute seat height. Therefore the effects of muscle length between subjects ruled out the effects of muscle length within subjects (seat heights). This might be an explanation why there is no effect of seat height on FEF in this study. Since there is an effect of seat height with standardized elbow angles but not with standardized seat height, the results indicate that individual adjustment of the wheelchair is important.

References

[1] L.H.V. van der Woude, et al., Seat height in handrim wheelchair propulsion, *J Rehabil Res Dev* **26** (1989), 31-50.

[2] H.E.J. Veeger, et. al.,Load on the upper extremity in manual wheelchair propulsion, *J Electromyogr Kinesiol* **1** (1991), 270-280.

[3] L.H. van der Woude, et al., Seat height: effects on submaximal hand rim wheelchair performance during spinal cord injury rehabilitation, *J Rehabil Med* **41** (2009), 143-149.

[4] G. Wu, et al., ISB recommendation on definitions of joint coordinate systems of various joints for the reporting of human joint motion--Part II: shoulder, elbow, wrist and hand, *J Biomech* **38** (2005), 981-992.

[5] B.R. Kotajarvi, et al., The effect of seat position on wheelchair propulsion biomechanics, *J Rehabil Res Dev* **41** (2004), 403-414.

[6] H.E. Veeger, et al., Load on the shoulder in low intensity wheelchair propulsion, *Clin Biomech (Bristol Avon)* **17** (2002), 211-218.

Rehabilitation: Mobility, Exercise and Sports
L.H.V. van der Woude et al. (Eds.)
IOS Press, 2010
© 2010 The authors and IOS Press. All rights reserved.
doi:10.3233/978-1-60750-080-3-25

Rolling resistance analysis during wheelchair movement

J.C. CABELGUEN[a], F. LAVASTE[a,1]

[a] *Laboratoire de BioMécanique, UMR 8005 CNRS, Ecole Nationale Supérieure d'Arts et Métiers, 151 Bd de l'Hôpital 75013 Paris, France*

Abstract. The purpose of this study is to present an analysis of wheelchair's rolling resistance which can be explain by the two wheel's rolling resistance factor $\lambda 1/r1$ and $\lambda 2/r2$, of the back wheel and of the front wheel respectively. Deceleration tests of manual wheelchair allowed calculating $\lambda 1/r1$ and $\lambda 2/r2$ from accelerometer measurements. For a rigid ground, $\lambda 2/r2$ is almost 8,5 times higher to $\lambda 1/r1$; so, the value of the wheel's rolling resistance factor is higher on front wheels. In this case, for a velocity of 1m/s and a total weight of 1000N, the power rolling resistance could be 11watt. This information shows the importance of the wheel's rolling resistance factor and of the centre of gravity position to study wheelchair locomotion.

Keywords. manual wheelchair locomotion, wheel's rolling resistance, power rolling resistance.

1. Purpose

Wheelchair's locomotion leads to various specific pathologies, which are mainly neurological and osteoarticular. The purpose of this study is to present an analysis of wheelchair's rolling resistance phenomenon. During movement, wheel and ground are deformed. The ground reaction forces resultant is not applied on the theoretical contact point between the wheel and the ground, but at the distance λ of this point. λ is the rolling resistance parameter.

2. Methods

The analysis of the wheel chair propulsion show that the power rolling resistance (PRR) is defined by:

$$PRR = \left(\frac{\lambda_1}{r_1} \frac{P_1}{P} + \frac{\lambda_2}{r_2} \frac{P_2}{P} \right) PV_f \tag{1}$$

where $\lambda 1$ respectively $\lambda 2$ are the rolling resistance parameter of the back wheel and of the front wheel, r1 respectively r2 are the radius of the back wheel and of the front

---

[1] Corresponding Author: francois.lavaste@paris.ensam.fr

wheel, P1 respectively P2 are the load applied on the back wheel and on the front wheel with P=P1+P2, and Vf the wheel chair's speed (Figure 1).

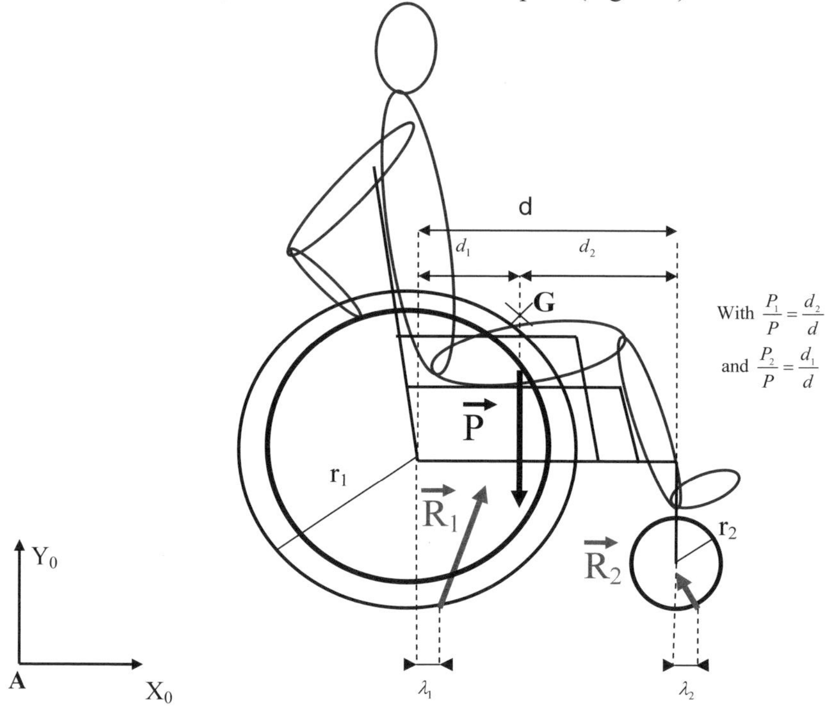

Figure 1. Mechanical parameters of rolling resistance for a manual wheelchair.

The factors λ/r are called wheel's rolling resistance factor (WRRF). To determinate λ1 and λ2, we express it in the deceleration's equation of wheelchair in movement during drag test:

$$\gamma_f = -\left[\frac{\lambda_1}{r_1}\frac{P_1}{P} + \frac{\lambda_2}{r_2}\frac{P_2}{P}\right]g \tag{2}$$

Deceleration values are obtained by an instrumented wheelchair called FRET1 (Figure 2) during drag test experimentations [1, 2].

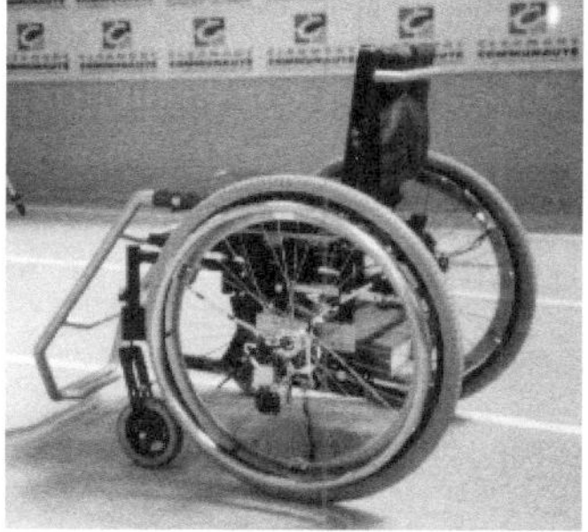

Figure 2. FRET1 used for deceleration tests.

3.   Results

For a rigid ground, λ for back wheels and front wheels are respectively 1mm and 2mm. So with r2=70mm and r1= 300mm, $\lambda2/r2$ is almost 8,5 times higher to $\lambda1/r1$ With this data and Vf=1m/s and P= 1000N, and P2/P= 30% the PRR=11watt and is a linear function of P2/P (Figure 3).

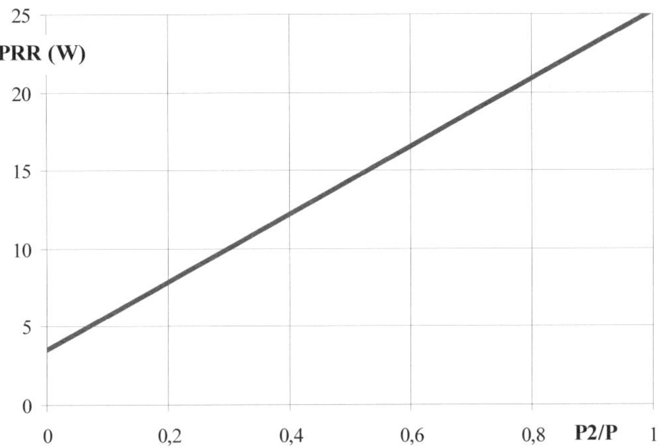

Figure 3. Linear relationship between P2/P and PRR.

4.   Conclusion

When we know $\lambda1$ and $\lambda2$ we can calculate the PRR for a wheel chair. We show that the PRR depends of the load repartition between the back wheel and the front wheel and so of the WRRF. The value of the WRRF is higher on front wheels. This information shows the importance of the WRRF and of the centre of gravity position for the rolling resistance.

References

[1]   M. Dabonneville, Ph. Vaslin, Ph. Kauffmann, N. de Saint Rémy, Y. Couétard & M. Cid. A self-contained wireless wheelchair ergometer designed for biomechanical measures in real life conditions. *Technology and Disability* **17**, 2 (2005), 63–76.
[2]   L.H.V. van der Woude, C. Geurst, H. Winkelman & H. Veeger. Measurement of wheelchair rolling resistance with a handle bar push technique. *Journal of Medical Engineering and Technology* **27**, 6 (2003), 249-258.

Rehabilitation: Mobility, Exercise and Sports
L.H.V. van der Woude et al. (Eds.)
IOS Press, 2010

doi:10.3233/978-1-60750-080-3-28

Estimating the caster wheels' orientation of a manual wheelchair during level ground propulsion

F. CHÉNIER[1], P. BIGRAS, R. AISSAOUI
*Imaging and Orthopedics Research Laboratory, École de Technologie Supérieure
de Montréal, Québec, Canada*

Abstract. Purpose: In order to build a realistic manual wheelchair simulator, an accurate dynamic model of the wheelchair-user system is needed. Besides, the characterization of this model necessitates the continuous knowledge of each caster wheel's orientation (CWO). The aim of this work is to propose a method that predicts these orientations based on the rear wheels' kinematics. Methods: A standard wheelchair equipped with two instrumented wheels was moved following straight and curvilinear patterns. A first-order model expressing the variation rate of the CWOs with respect to the rear wheels' kinematics was developed. The numerical integration of the model leads to an estimate of the CWOs. Simultaneously, the orientation of a caster wheel was measured using a three-dimensional optoelectronic system. Results: The estimated and the observed orientation values were compared. The estimation error was very low (<5 deg) when the orientation does not abruptly change, and stayed below 10 degrees at all times. Conclusion: Based on our data, it is possible to predict the CWOs with a fairly good accuracy using only the geometrical parameters of the wheelchair and the data from the instrumented rear wheels. This method is promising since it will help characterizing the wheelchair-user dynamic model in the future.

1. Introduction

Most wheelchair ergometers use an inertia and a resistive force as the wheelchair user dynamic model. Although this is sufficient for most applications, it is inaccurate when the caster wheels have a significant impact on the dynamics of the wheelchair, for example when executing turning maneuvers. It is possible to include the caster wheels in the model [1], but the caracterization of the model remains difficult because of its high number of parameters. As a solution, parameter estimation techniques can be used, in the condition of acquiring simultaneous real-life recordings of (1) the applied torques on the rear wheels, (2) the rear wheels' kinematics, and (3) the caster wheels' orientation (CWOs). While (1) and (2) are commonly recorded using instrumented wheels [2], the CWOs are more difficult to obtain.

---

[1] Corresponding Author: felix.chenier.1@ens.etsmtl.ca

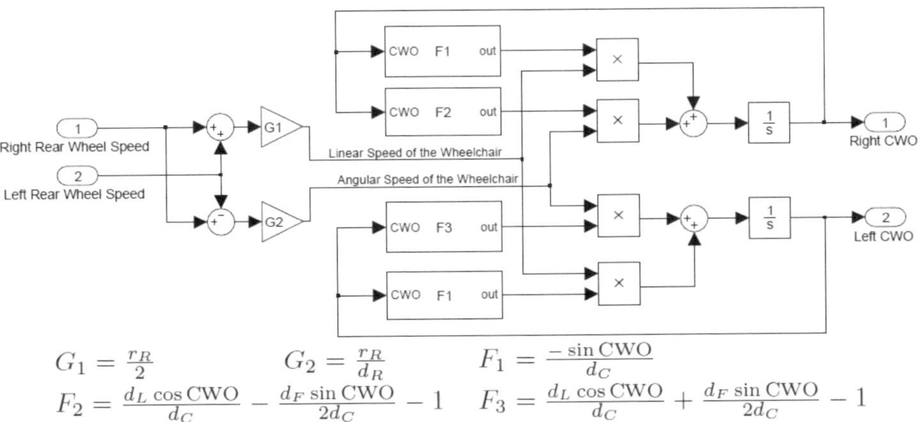

$$G_1 = \frac{r_R}{2} \qquad G_2 = \frac{r_R}{d_R} \qquad F_1 = \frac{-\sin \mathrm{CWO}}{d_C}$$

$$F_2 = \frac{d_L \cos \mathrm{CWO}}{d_C} - \frac{d_F \sin \mathrm{CWO}}{2d_C} - 1 \qquad F_3 = \frac{d_L \cos \mathrm{CWO}}{d_C} + \frac{d_F \sin \mathrm{CWO}}{2d_C} - 1$$

Figure 1. First order model used to estimate the CWO from the rear wheels' angular speeds.

Table 1. List of symbols

Symbol	Definition	Symbol	Definition
r_R	Radius of the rear wheels	d_L	Length of the wheelchair
d_R	Distance between the rear wheels	d_C	Caster trail length
d_F	Distance between the front wheels	CWO	Caster Wheel Orientation

2. Hypothesis

We made the hypothesis that if at every moment, none of the wheels are slipping laterally, it is possible to obtain a good estimate of the CWOs without any additional instrumentation. Using a kinematic model of the wheelchair, we obtained a first-order model linking the CWOs to the angular speed of the rear wheels (Fig.1).

3. Validation methods

Experimental design: A standard manual wheelchair equipped with two instrumented wheels (3rivers Inc., USA) were used for the experiment. In order to represent the mass distribution of a small person, a weight of 34 kg was placed on the seat whereas 11.3 kg were placed on the foot rest. Additionally, a Visualeyez II VZ4000 3D optoelectronic system was used to collect the 3D position of four markers fixed onto the wheelchair: two on the frame and two on the right caster fork. After starting the data acquisition from both wheels and the optoelectronic system, an external operator pushed the wheelchair following different patterns: straight line, regular oscillations and random oscillations. When the wheelchair was not in the field of view of the optoelectronic system anymore, it was brought back to its starting point and a new pattern was started.

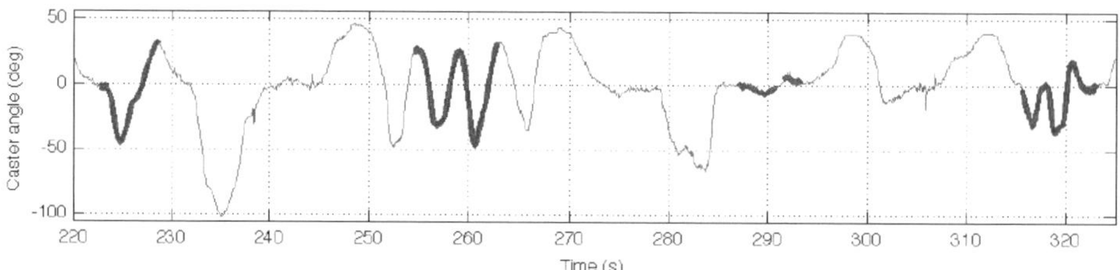

Figure 2. Concordance between the measured CWO (bold) and the estimated CWO (thin).

Data processing

Optoelectronic System: The three-dimensional position of the markers was sampled at 120Hz, then filtered at 6Hz by G(s), which is a 4th-order low-pass Butterworth filter. This cutoff frequency is known to be the maximal useful frequency for the wheelchair propulsion [3]. The reference CWO was then calculated from the filtered positions of the four markers.

Instrumented Wheels: The angular position of each rear wheel was sampled at 240Hz, then filtered by sG(s) in order to obtain the angular speeds. The system in Fig. 1 was processed using a ode45 Runge-Kutta integration technique in order to find the estimated CWO.

4. Results and discussion

A preliminary result is shown in Fig. 2. The error between the measured and the estimated CWO is inferior to 5 degrees when the caster orientation does not abruptly change, and stays below 10 degrees at all times. We made the hypothesis that the floor friction would be high enough to avoid wheel slipping. This was verified by performing the experiment on a clean, hard and freshly waxed floor with only 11.3 kg on the foot rest, which constitutes a low-friction setup.

However, future research must be done in order to generalize these results for any conventional hard floor.

Acknowledgments

This project receives support from the National Sciences and Engineering Research Council of Canada (NSERC). There is no conflict of interest in this project.

References

[1]   Johnson and Aylor, "Dynamic modeling of an electric wheelchair," IEEE Transactions on Industry Applications, vol. IA-21, no. 5, pp. 1284 – 1293, 1985.

[2]   Asato, Cooper et al., "Smart wheels: development and testing of a system formeasuring manual wheelchair propulsion dynamics," Biomedical Engineering, IEEE Transactions on, vol. 40, no. 12, pp. 1320–1324, 1993.

[3]   Cooper, DiGiovine et al., "Filter frequency selection for manual wheelchair biomechanics," Journal of Rehabilitation Research and Development, vol. 39, no. 3, pp. 323 – 336, 2002.

Rehabilitation: Mobility, Exercise and Sports
L.H.V. van der Woude et al. (Eds.)
IOS Press, 2010

doi:10.3233/978-1-60750-080-3-31

Quality measure in service delivery of mobility devices

S. KARDAM, R. COOPER, B.E. DICIANNO, R.A. COOPER, T. BOBISH
Human Engineering Research Laboratories,
Highland Drive VA Medical Center, Pittsburgh, PA 15260
Dept. Rehab. Science &Technology, University of Pittsburgh, Pittsburgh, PA 15261
Dept. PM&R, University of Pittsburgh Medical Center, PA 15261

Abstract. The goal of this project is to analyze data from the tracking sheets of therapists of the Center for Assistive Technology (CAT) at the University of Pittsburgh Medical Center to determine how much time is taken for delivery of manual or power wheelchairs and scooters. Executing the process in a timely manner is a necessary part of client satisfaction and quality of service. The average total days taken for delivering the mobility device were calculated as 110 .00 +/- 70.11 days, which conforms to the goal of 100 days set by CAT. A total of 257 out of 549 (46.8%) devices delivered in 2007 and 2008 were delivered in 51-100 days. The longest time period in the delivery process was the period between when the report was completed and final delivery of the device which consisted heavily of insurance review. Therapists seemed to be able to facilitate delivery time by shortening the time for report writing as well as shortening times of vendor responsibilities. Manual wheelchairs had the longest delivery time, likely due to the need for customization and fitting. More research is needed to determine how diagnosis, insurance type, and vendors may influence delivery time.

Keywords. wheelchair, power mobility, quality assurance, scooter, service delivery.

1. Introduction

In the client centered service delivery model, client satisfaction with the device is critical and time to delivery is a crucial part of client satisfaction. [1][2].While it is obvious that mobility devices should be delivered within a reasonable timeframe, there is very little literature that documents the average time from client assessment to delivery of equipment.

Service quality is a measure of how well the service level delivered matches the consumers' expectations [3][4],[5]. Delivering quality service means conforming to customer expectations on a consistent basis. The quality measure is a comparison between expectation and performance. Expectation from the client is how soon a client anticipates a delivery, and performance is the actual time it takes from the initial evaluation to the final delivery.

At the University of Pittsburgh, Center for Assistive Technology (CAT), the seating and mobility evaluation team includes physical therapists and/or occupational therapists, physiatrists, rehabilitation engineers, technicians and vendor representatives. The evaluation process centers on the development of standards of practice to monitor performance and should lead to improvements in: (i) service delivery practices; (ii) mobility device users' participation; and (iii) accountability and justification of service delivery [6]. The therapist and the physician compile the medical justification within a comprehensive report (letter of medical necessity) and work closely with the vendor to monitor the timelines of the process. To assure a timely delivery process, CAT has set a target of under 100 days from the initial visit to the final delivery of the mobility device which is considered to be a challenging but realistic time line. This descriptive study is to evaluate how close CAT meets the target timeline and to analyze the efficiency of a service delivery organization.

2. Methodology

This descriptive project measures an aspect of quality of service delivery of mobility devices at CAT; no institutional review board protocol was needed. Information was collected by reviewing client charts and the internal tracking databases. Outcome variables collected included total time in days from the initial visit to the final delivery of manual and power wheelchairs and scooters from Jan 2007 to May 2008. This period was divided into 3 sub-periods, labeled as vendor's time, therapist's time, and insurance's time.

The tracking sheet captures the start date of the evaluation process (the day of the client's initial evaluation), the end date of the evaluation process (the day the therapist receives the specifications of the mobility device), and the date that the report is completed, and the delivery date of the mobility device. **Vendor's time** (sub-period 1) is defined as the initial evaluation date to the end date of the evaluation process. During this time the vendor has to complete a home evaluation and forward final specifications for the mobility device to the therapist. The CAT policy requests the vendor to complete this within 30 days. **Therapist's time** (sub-period 2) is from receipt of the final specifications i.e. end date of the evaluation to completion of the letter of medical necessity. The CAT policy requests the therapist to complete this within 14 days. **Insurance's time** (sub-period 3) is from the date of the report to the delivery of the mobility device.

Alpha values were set at 0.05 a priori. Descriptive statistics were used to compute average time in days for each time period. A Kruskal-Wallis test was utilized to examine for differences among therapists and among wheelchair types with respect to length of sub-periods.

3. Results

We collected data from 549 cases. Figure 1 show the average time in days for each sub-period. The average total days taken for delivering the mobility device were calculated as 110 .00 +/- 70.11 day. Therapist's time was shortest, followed by vendor's time, then by insurance's time. A total of 52 (9.5%) mobility devices were delivered less than or equal to 50 days, 257 (46.8%) from 51-100 days, 153 (9.7%) from 101-150 days, 57 from 151 to 200 days, 19 (3.5%) from 201-300 days, 7 (1.3%) from 301-400 days and 5 (1.0%) from 401-876 days.

Length of vendor's time, therapist's time, and total time were significantly associated with the therapist (p<.0001, p=0.003 and p=0.02, respectively). Insurance's time was not significantly associated with the therapist. The therapists present at the CAT clinic 1 day a week had longer sub-periods than those present 2 days a week.

Manual wheelchairs had significantly longer delivery times followed by power wheelchairs and scooters (p<0.0001).

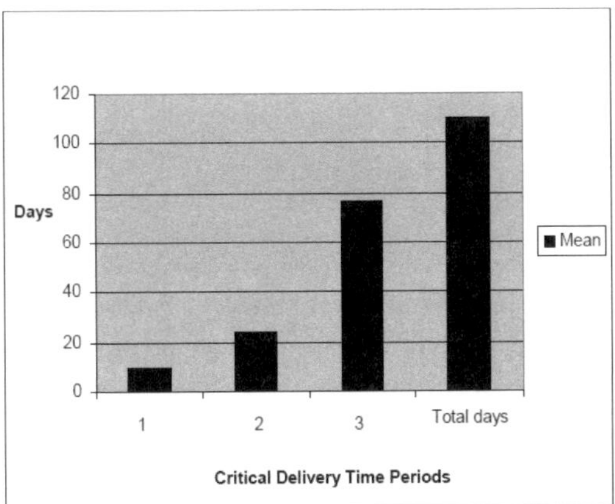

Figure 1. Time taken to deliver the mobility device

Figure 1 depicts the mean time and the standard deviation in days taken by the vendor's, therapists and insurance which is denoted by sub period 1, sub period 2 and sub period 3 respectively. By this table we get to know that the total average time taken is 110.00 +/- 70.11 days.

The individual time is 24.11 +/- 27.75 for sub period 1, 9.51 +/- 10.71 for sub period 2, and 76.54 +/- 64.52 for sub period 3.

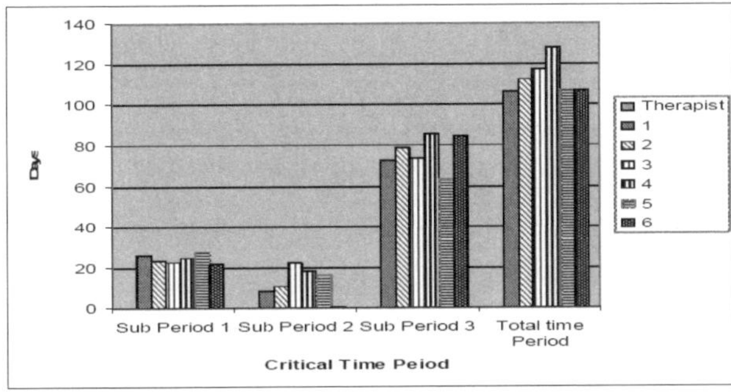

Figure 2. Sub-periods broken down by individual therapist

Figure 2 shows the time taken by therapists, vendors and insurance for the clients by each therapist. Therapist 1, 2 and 6 are for 2 days a week in the clinic and other 3 are only for a day per week. So the therapists present at the CAT clinic 1 day a week had longer sub-periods than those present 2 days a week

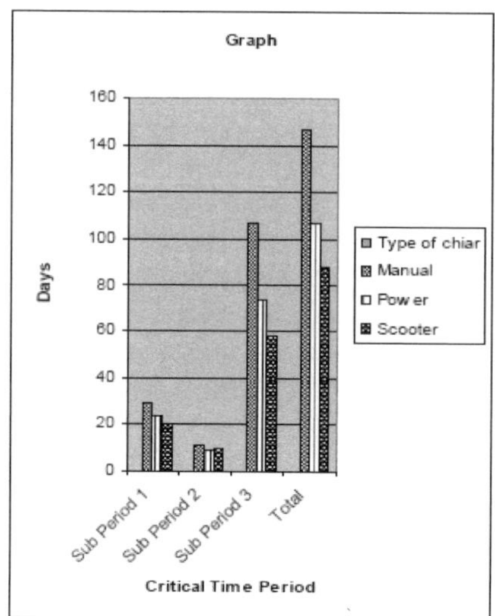

Figure 3. Sub-periods broken down by type of mobility device

In Figure 3 the sub period 1, 2, and 3 are mentioned for the type of mobility device i.e. manual wheelchair, power wheelchair and the scooters. By this table it can be inferred that the manual wheelchair take more time to be delivered as the total time for manual wheelchair is 147.19 +/-94.49 than others in all the 3 sub periods. It is 29.57 +/- 45.88 days for sub period 1 and 11.20 +/-11.22 and 84.32 +/- 106.60 for sub period 2 and 3 respectively

4. Discussion/Conclusion

The process of acquiring an appropriate mobility device in a timely manner is a collaborative team effort at CAT. Executing the process in a timely manner is a necessary part of client satisfaction. To assure a timely delivery process, CAT had set a target time of under 100 days from the initial visit to the final delivery of the mobility device. Average delivery time of 110 days comes close to that measure. Sub-periods 1 and 2, in which vendors and therapists are primarily responsible for service, had lower times than what our policy requests. However, it is important to keep in mind that sub-period 3 is tracked from report date to final delivery. This includes time that is dependent on insurance approval but also time that is not dependent upon the insurance company, such as the time from the vendors receiving the letter of medical necessity to sending it to the insurance company, as well as the time from when the vendor receives insurance approval to when the mobility device is ordered and then received by the client. The time it takes manufacturers to produce and deliver wheelchairs needs to be studied in the future.

The therapist assigned to a client seemed to influence the length of time of the sub-period in which the vendor primarily has responsibility; thus the therapist may have a significant influence on vendor time by fostering better communication and facilitating workflow. Some therapists were able to complete reports more quickly than others.

Therapists who attend clinic once a week generally have less time to finish their reports than the therapists who visit clinic 2 days a week, which likely explains the differences in sub-period lengths that were therapist dependant. Most of the manual wheelchairs prescribed at CAT are high end ultra-light chairs and require complex fitting and customization for users, which likely explains why their delivery times take significantly longer than other devices. Further work needs to be done to analyze the associations between length of time in acquiring a mobility device and diagnosis, insurance type, and vendor.

References

[1]　Harris F, Sprigle S., Outcome measurement of a wheelchair intervention. *Disabil Rehabil Assist Technol.* 2008 Feb 8;1-10. PMID: 18608441 [PubMed - as supplied by publisher]

[2]　Lemaire E, Necsulescu L, Greene G., Service Delivery Trends for a Physical Outreach program. *Disabil Rehabil.* 2006 Nov 15;28(21):1349-59.PMID: 17083183 [PubMed indexed for MEDLINE]

[3]　Parasuraman A, Zeithaml V and Leonard L. Berry, A Conceptual Model of Service Quality andIts Implications for Future Research. *Journal of Marketing*, Vol. 49, No. 4 (Autumn, 1985), pp. 41-50

[4]　Cook A, Hussey: Assistive Technologies: Principles and Practice, St Louis, 1995, Mosby.

[5]　 RESNA: Giuidelines for basic knowledge and skill for assistive technology service provision, Arlington, VA, April 1996, RESNA

[6]　Long,T, Huang L , Woodbridge, M, Woolverton, M, Minkel, J MA, PT, Integrating AssistiveTechnology Into an Outcome-Driven Model of Service Delivery *Infants and Young Children* Lippincott & Wilkins, Inc Vol. 16, No. 4, pp. 272–283c 2003

Rehabilitation: Mobility, Exercise and Sports
L.H.V. van der Woude et al. (Eds.)
IOS Press, 2010
© *2010 The authors and IOS Press. All rights reserved.*
doi:10.3233/978-1-60750-080-3-36

Mechanical and physiological assessment of pressure ulcer-preventing cushions in a population with spinal cord injury

B. CRESPO-RUIZ[1], A. DE LA PEÑA-GONZÁLEZ, S. PÉREZ-NOMBELA, A. GIL-AGUDO

Biomechanical and Technical Aids Department of National Hospital for Spinal Cord Injury, Toledo (SESCAM), Spain

Abstract. Purpose: To develop a multimodal procedure for evaluating pressure ulcer-preventing cushions and conduct a comparison of the biomechanics and tissue response induced by 4 pressure ulcer-preventing cushions most commonly prescribed to patients with spinal cord injury in our hospital. Methods: Firstly, the distribution of pressures at the user-cushion interface was analyzed (Xsensor), and secondly, tissue viability was assessed by transcutaneous oxygen pressure (TcPO2) (Radiometer TCM 400) in 22 people with thoracic complete spinal cord injury (T1-T2). The variables analyzed were related with the distribution of pressures and contact surface at the user-cushion interface (Pmax, Pm, Psd, Stot, S>60 and % S>60) and tissue response (TcPO2). Results: The dual-compartment air cushion produced the best Pmax, Pm, Psd and Stot results compared to the other cushions (P<0.05). TcPO2 values did not differ significantly between cushions. Conclusion: A method was developed for the multimodal evaluation of pressure ulcer-preventing cushions that enhances our understanding of how these cushions behave and can help to prevent pressure ulcers in both sports and rehabilitation.

Keywords. ulcer pressure, spinal cord injury, transcutaneous oxygen pressure.

1. Introduction

Pressure ulcers (PU) are zones of damage to the skin and underlying tissue due, among other factors, to sustained pressure on the skin and soft tissues. In population groups such as older adults and people with spinal cord injury, the risk of developing PUs is greater [1]. Among all the treatments proposed for the treatment of PUs, consensus exists that prevention is the best option [2]. Different studies have indicated that the use of pressure-relieving surfaces, which are designed to conserve tissue integrity, reduces the incidence of PUs induced by prolonged periods of sitting [3,4].

One of the physiologic parameters most closely related to tissue viability status seems to be TcPO2 [5]. In view of these facts, we decide to study the possible relations between the biomechanical behavior of different pressure-relieving seating surfaces and the viability of tissues subjected to pressure in the ischial areas of 4 cushions

---

[1] Beatriz Crespo Ruiz. Biomechanics and Technical Aids Department. Hospital Nacional de Parapléjicos. Finca la Peraleda s/n. 45071 Toledo. Spain, +34925247763 E-mail: bcresporuiz@fundacionhnp.org

frequently used in our populations with spinal cord injury: the single-compartment, low-profile, Kineris air cushion (cushion 1); single-compartment, high-profile Askle Santé model, WinncareGroup, air cushion (cushion 2); dual-compartment Roho Enhancer model, The Roho Group, air cushion (cushion 3); and the Jay-2 model, Medical Sunrise, gel and semi-firm foam cushion (cushion 4).

2. Methods

Subjects and protocol. Twenty-two male patients with complete thoracic spinal cord injury (T1-T12) ASIA A, mean age 35.4 ±9.1 years and BMI 22.4± 3.5, participated in the study. Before inclusion, all subjects signed the corresponding informed consent form. The ethical guidelines of the declaration of Helsinki were adhered to.

Measurement of mechanical parameters. In first place, the distribution of pressures in the user-cushion interface in static position was analyzed using a pressure sensor mesh (Xsensor) with four pressure ulcer-preventing cushions. The order in which the cushions were tested was properly randomized.

Measurement of physiologic response in the bilateral ischial. A Radiometer TCM 400 oximeter was used. The electrodes were placed on the areas of interest and the patient was transferred to the wheelchair with the test cushion. The TcPO2 value was recorded every minute during the first 5 minutes.

Variables analyzed. The variables analyzed were variables related with the pressure distribution and contact surface at the user-cushion interface, such as right ischial pressure (Prt.isch), left ischial pressure (Plf.isch), maximum pressure (Pmax), mean pressure (Pm) and its standard deviation (Psd), total contact surface (Stot), the surface with a pressure superior to 60 mmHg (S>60), the percentage of S>60 with respect to Stot (%S>60), and transcutaneous oxygen pressure (TcPO2).

3. Statistical Analysis

All statistical analyses were made with SPSS 12.0. The data distribution and descriptive statistics for each variable were obtained. Due to the sample size, nonparametric analyses followed by a Bonferroni correction were made. The Friedman test allowed us to evaluate the null hypothesis of similar behavior between cushions, followed by pairwise comparison using the Wilcoxon rank test (significance level $p<0.05$).

4. Results

Statistically significant differences were observed in many variables between the 4 types of cushions. For the variables related with the pressure distribution at the user-cushion interface, analyses a posteriori by multiple comparisons showed that the dual-compartment air cushion (cushion 3) offered the best results because it had lower central values for the variables Pmax ($p<0.001$ vs. cushion 1, $p< 0.001$ vs. cushion 2, and $p< 0.001$ vs. cushion 4), Pm ($p=0.005$ vs. cushion 1, $p=0.001$ vs. cushion 2, and $p=0.001$ vs. cushion 4), and Psd ($p=0.005$ vs. cushion 1, $p=0.001$ vs. cushion 2, and $p=0.001$ vs. cushion 4).

The dual-compartment air cushion also was the cushion with which the best results were obtained on analyzing the total user-cushion contact surface (Stot), with statistically significant results compared to the other 3 cushions (p<0.001 vs. cushion 1, p<0.001 vs. cushion 2, and p=0.005 vs. cushion 4) (Table 1).

In the comparative analysis of the 4 cushions for tissue response to the mechanical effect of sitting, 2 variables were analyzed. No significant differences were found between any of the cushions.

Table 1. Results of the variables related with pressure distribution and contact surface for each cushion.

	Cushion 1	Cushion 2	Cushion 3	Cushion 4
Pmax	141± 95	153.0± 73.8	96.0 ± 33.0	144.5 ± 105.8
Prt.isch	120.5 ± 57.8	144.0 ± 65.0	84.0 ± 36.1	103.5 ± 100.3
Plt.isch	118 ± 90.3	124.0 ± 53.8	92.0 ± 17.8	100.5 ± 51.5
Pm	38.7 ± 6.6	38.2 ± 6.9	33.9 ± 5.0	37.8 ± 8.7
Psd	19.4 ± 8.9	20.2 ± 9.1	15.1 ± 4.8	21.6 ± 7.0
Stot	1208,9 ±223.0	1271.8 ± 177.5	1599.2 ± 471.0	1416.9 ± 233.5
S>60	126.6 ±122.2	156.5 ± 110.1	83.9 ± 115.3	175.0± 212.5
%S>60	10.0 ±10.3	12.5 ± 8.8	5.8 ± 9.2	10.8 ± 15.3

* Data expressed as medians ±interquartile range.

5. Conclusion

Thanks to the experience accrued in the present study, we completed a procedure for evaluating different seating surfaces by simultaneous analysis of the distribution of pressures on the user-cushion interface and the status of tissue viability by means of TcPO2. On the other hand, the data obtained allow us to affirm that in the sample analyzed in the conditions described in this experiment, the dual-compartment air cushion had the best mechanical behavior compared to the other cushions analyzed.

References

[1]   C.A. Salzberg, D.W. Byrne, C.G. Cayten, Predicting and preventing pressure ulcers in adults with paralysis. *Adv Wound Care* **11** (1998), 237-46.
[2]   R.E. Sachse, S.A. Fink, B. Klitzman, Multimodality evaluation of pressure relief surfaces. *Plast Reconstr Surg* **102** (1998), 2381-7.
[3]   R. Lim, Sirett. Clinical trials of foam cushions in the prevention of decubitus ulcers in elderly patients. *J Rehabil Res Dev* **25** (1988), 19-26.
[4]   T.A. Conine, C. Hershler, D. Daechsel et al., Pressure ulcer prophylaxis in elderly patients using polyurethane foam or Jay wheelchair cushions. *Int J Rehabil Res* **17** (1994), 123-37.
[5]   J. Thorfinn, F. Sjöberg, D. Lidman. Sitting pressure and perfusion of buttock skin in paraplegic and tetraplegic patients, and in healthy subjects: a comparative study. Scand *J Plast Reconstr Surg Hand Surg* **36** (2002), 279-83.

Rehabilitation: Mobility, Exercise and Sports
L.H.V. van der Woude et al. (Eds.)
IOS Press, 2010

doi:10.3233/978-1-60750-080-3-39

39

Effect and process evaluation of implementing patient monitoring in spinal cord injury rehabilitation

S. DE GROOT[a,b,1], G. BEVERS[c], M.W.M. POST[d], F. WOLDRING[e],
G.A. MULDER[e], L.H.V. VAN DER WOUDE[b]

[a] *Rehabilitation Center Amsterdam*
[b] *Centre for Human Movement Sciences, University Medical Centre Groningen,
University of Groningen*
[c] *Research Institute MOVE, Faculty of Human Movement Sciences, VU University
Amsterdam*
[d] *Rehabilitation Center De Hoogstraat and Rudolf Magnus Institute for Neuroscience,
Utrecht*
[e] *Centre for Rehabilitation, Location Beatrixoord, University Medical Center,
Groningen*

Abstract. The purpose of this study was to evaluate the implementation of standardized physical and functional tests to individually monitor patients with a spinal cord injury (SCI) in 8 rehabilitation centers and to analyze enablers and barriers of the implementation process. A prospective effect- and process evaluation was performed. Team members responded to mailed questionnaires at the start (n=115) and end (n=82) of the one-year implementation period. Furthermore, a questionnaire was administered to managers (n=8), coordinators (n=8) and 32 persons with SCI in 4 centers. Outcome of the effect evaluation was the phase of implementation of standardized testing in each center. The process evaluation analyzed enablers and barriers of the implementation process. After a year of implementation, half of the centers shifted to higher implementation phases. None of the centers was classified in the highest phase. Enablers were the positive attitude of the team members regarding standardized testing and an encouraging local coordinator. Most important barrier was lack of time to implement standardized testing. It can be concluded that there is a large support for implementing standardized tests to monitor functioning of patients with SCI. During a year a positive shift was visible in the extent of implementation. Successful implementation of patient monitoring requires substantial amounts of time and effort of the rehabilitation centers involved.

Keywords. outcome and process assessment (Health Care), spinal cord injury, questionnaires, program evaluation.

1. Introduction

The use of objective standardized measurements to quantify results of rehabilitation and as part of evidence-based rehabilitation practice, is seen as an increasingly important

---

[1] Corresponding Author: Sonja de Groot; s.d.groot@rcamsterdam.nl

part of good clinical practice [1]. In the Netherlands, as part of the spinal cord injury (SCI) research program[2], 8 rehabilitation centers started to implement standardized physical and functional tests to individually monitor patients with a SCI. The aims of the present study are to investigate 1) the extent to which patient monitoring was implemented in SCI rehabilitation after 1 year; 2) the enabling factors and barriers of successful implementation of patient monitoring.

2. Methods

Participants

Process and effect evaluations were performed in all eight SCI-specialized rehabilitation centers in the Netherlands. Four questionnaires (for patients (n=32), coordinators (n=8), team members (n=115), managers (n=8)) were administered to measure the opinions of participants on the effect and process of implementing patient monitoring at baseline (T1) and at 1 year follow-up (T2).

Process and effect evaluation

For each rehabilitation center, the effect was described as phase of implementation (orientation, insight, acceptance, change or maintenance [2]) at T1 and T2, determined with the questionnaire filled out by the team members.

The process was described by 4 domains of enablers or barriers of the implementation: characteristic of the innovation itself, of the individual team member involved, of the group of team members and of the organization.

Statistics

A rehabilitation center has reached a particular phase of implementation (effect) if 75% of the team members have given a positive answer on questions belonging to that phase and also in the previous implementation phases.

To determine the relationship between the implementation phase and the enablers and barriers of the implementation process, the number of positive answers on the questions belonging to the 4 domains were analyzed. Thereafter, a Kruskal-Wallis non-parametric test was performed to analyze factors that were significantly different between the different implementation phases (p<0.05).

3. Results

Following the criteria of the effect evaluation, the number of centers in the different implementation phases were as follows: orientation (T1: 2 centers; T2: 1 center), insight (T1: 2 centers; T2: 1 center), acceptance (T1: 1 centers; T2: 1 center), change (T1: 3 centers; T2: 5 centers), maintenance (T1: 0 centers; T2: 0 centers). In summary, there was a shift towards higher implementation phases between T1 and T2.

The center in the orientation phase had a lower percentage positive answers on all 4 domains compared to the centers in the other implementation phases (Figure 1). Enablers were the positive attitude of the team members regarding standardized testing

---

[2] www.scionn.nl

and an encouraging local coordinator. Most important barrier was lack of time to implement standardized testing.

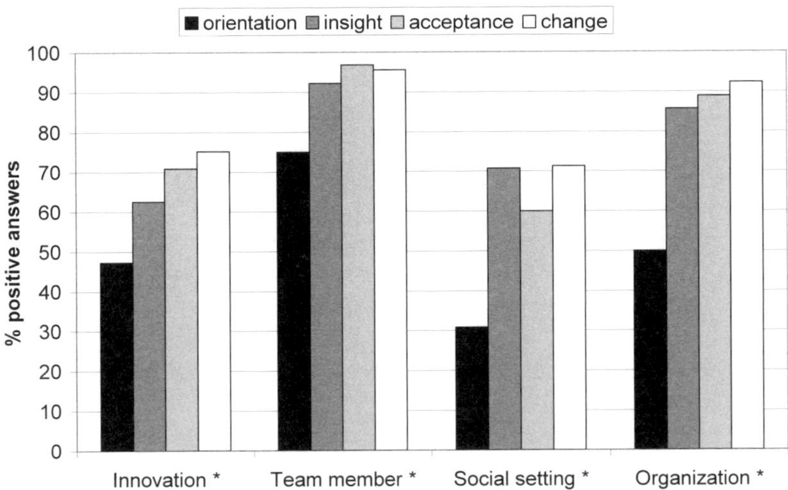

Figure 1. Results of the percentage positive answers of the team members on the 4 domains per implementation phase. * = Significant difference between implementation phases at p < 0.05.

4. Conclusion

There is a large support for implementing objective tests in SCI rehabilitation and after 1 year of implementation a positive shift was visible in the extent and level of implementation. Successful implementation of patient monitoring costs a lot of time and effort and needs financial and substantial support of the organization. SCI rehabilitation and patients are suggested to profit from more objective and structured monitoring.

References

[1]　R. Haigh et al., The use of outcome measures in physical medicine and rehabilitation within Europe. *J Rehabil Med* **33** (2001) 273-8.

[2]　R. Grol et al., *Improving patient care: the implementation of change in clinical practice*. Elsevier, Edinburgh, 2005.

Rehabilitation: Mobility, Exercise and Sports
L.H.V. van der Woude et al. (Eds.)
IOS Press, 2010

doi:10.3233/978-1-60750-080-3-42

Ergonomic indexes for upper limb musculoskeletal disorders risk quantification according to manual wheelchair kinematics

N. LOUIS [a], G. DESROCHES [b], R. DUMAS [b], P. VASLIN [c], L. CHEZE [b],
P. GORCE [a,1]

[a] *HANDIBIO-EA 4322, Laboratoire de Bio-modélisation et d'ingénierie des Handicaps,
Université du Sud Toulon-Var, La Garde, France*
[b] *LBMC UMR_T 9406, UCBL-INRETS, Université de Lyon, Villeurbanne, France*
[c] *LIMOS UMR 6158, CNRS Université Blaise Pascal Clermont 2, Aubière, France*

Abstract. Manual wheelchair propulsion is a well known factor of upper limb musculoskeletal disorders risk (ULMDR). Through a large bibliographic review, movement amplitude and repetition, proximity of joints limits, user overweight and vertical forces are commonly admitted as the main risk factors of upper limb injuries in wheelchair propulsion. Thus, we propose a clinically usable method to quantify ULMDR according to wheelchair kinematics. Through a synthesis of literature information, for the three upper limb joints, ergonomic indexes were grouped in a general equation to quantify ULMDR. A case study has been realized. A 3D analysis of upper limb motion during propulsion was made using a Vicon 460 system. Four different wheelchair configurations were tested: two seat heights and two anterior-posterior wheel positions. For both seat heights, computed ULMDR are less important for backward position. For both antero-posterior wheel positions, computed ULMDR are less important for the highest seat position. The results showed good promises at quantifying the impact of sitting changes on ULMDR. These ergonomic indexes could be helpful in clinical settings when prescribing a wheelchair. To validate this method, a longitudinal study will be performed. Forces applied on hand rims will be added in further development.

Keywords. musculoskeletal disorder, wheelchair, upper limb, kinematics.

1. Introduction

Manual wheelchair propulsion is a well known factor of upper limb musculoskeletal disorders risk (ULMDR) [1, 2]. Through a large bibliographic review, movement amplitude and repetition, proximity of joints limits, user overweight and vertical forces are commonly admitted as the main risk factors of upper limb injuries in wheelchair propulsion. Thus, we propose a clinically usable method to quantify ULMDR according to wheelchair kinematics.

---

[1] Corresponding Author : Philippe GORCE, HANDIBIO-EA 4322, Laboratoire de Bio-modélisation et d'ingénierie des Handicaps, Université du Sud Toulon-Var, La Garde, France; E-mail : philippe.gorce@univ-tln.fr

2. Ergonomic indexes for ULMDR

Through a synthesis of literature information [2-8], for the three upper limb joints, ergonomic indexes for ULMDR were grouped in a general equation Eq. (1). Equation parameters are depending on the articulation:

- Shoulder flexion-extension and then abduction are the main biomechanical risk factors of shoulder pain.
- Elbow ULMDR is link with the flexion-extension angle.
- Studies reporting on the wrist highlighted the importance of flexion-extension in carpal tunnel syndrome and tendinitis. Eq. (2) defined the wrist ergonomic index for ULMDR.

3. Case study: material and method

To illustrate ergonomic indexes for ULMDR, a case study have been realized on one able-bodied subject (age : 41 years old, weight : 71kg, height : 184cm, arm length : 35cm, forearm length : 28cm, hand : 21cm). Four different wheelchair configurations were tested: two seat heights (51cm and 54 cm) and two anterior-posterior wheels positions (1cm and 4cm). 3D analysis of upper extremity motion was made using a Vicon 460 system (Oxford Metrics, Oxford, UK). Fifty anatomical and technical markers were installed on the wheelchair and participant.

Upper body is considered as a rigid segment articulated system (trunk, arm, forearm and hand). For each segment, an anatomical frame is defined according to ISB recommendations [9]. Thus, Euler angles were chosen to describe upper body's relative movements. An inverse kinematic model permits to quantify the successive rotations corresponding to shoulder flexion-extension, shoulder adduction-abduction, shoulder internal-external rotation, elbow flexion-extension, wrist pronation-supination (WP), wrist flexion-extension (WFE) and wrist radio-ulnar deviation (WD). Respective rotation amplitudes have been computed (WPA, WFEA, WDA) for a propulsive cycle. Ergonomic indexes for ULMDR describe in Eq. (1), and for the wrist in particular in Eq. (2), were quantified.

4. Results

For both seat heights, computed ULMDR are less important for backward position. For both antero-posterior wheel positions, computed ULMDR are less important for the highest seat position. Figure 1 illustrates those results for the wrist.

5. Conclusion

The results showed good promises at quantifying the impact of sitting changes on ULMDR. These ergonomic indexes could be helpful in clinical settings when prescribing a wheelchair. To validate this method, a longitudinal study will be performed. Forces applied on hand rims will be added in further development.

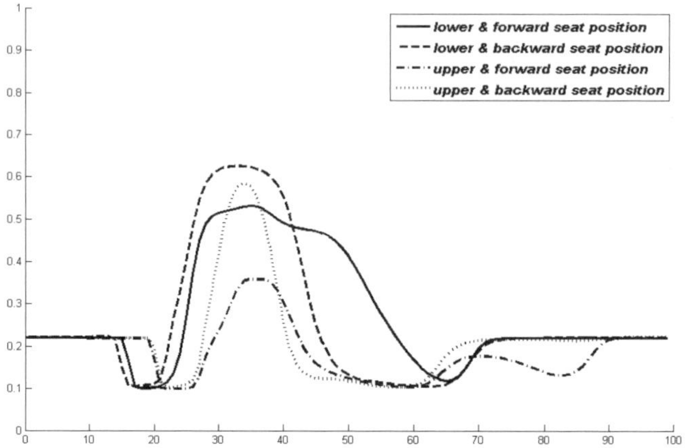

Figure 1. Wrist musculoskeletal disorder risk evolution according to propulsion cycle percentage.

$$ULMDR = \alpha(Movement\ Amplitude) + \beta(Articular\ Position) \tag{1}$$

$$Wrist\ ULMDR = 0.25[0.1(WFEA > 0.8*150) + 0.2(WDA > 0.8*65) +$$
$$0.7(WPA > 0.8*165)] + 0.75\left[0.1(WP > 0) + 0.2\left(\frac{\left(\tanh\left(\frac{|WD-2.5|}{2}-6\right)+1\right)}{2}\right) +\right.$$
$$0.7\left(\frac{\left(\tanh\left(\frac{|WFE|}{5}-5\right)+1\right)}{2}\right) \tag{2}$$

References

[1]   S.J. Mulroy, et al., Effects of spinal cord injury level on the activity of shoulder muscles during wheelchair propulsion : an electromyographic study. *Archives of physical medicine and rehabilitation* **85** (2004), 925-934.

[2]   H.E. Veeger, L.A. Rozendaal, and F.C. van der Helm, Load on the shoulder in low intensity wheelchair propulsion. *Clinical biomechanics* **17**(3) (2002), 211-8.

[3]   M.L. Boninger, et al., Shoulder and elbow motion during two speeds of wheelchair propulsion: a description using a local coordinate system. *Spinal Cord* **36**(6) (1998), 418-26.

[4]   M.L. Boninger, et al., Pushrim biomechanics and injury prevention in spinal cord injury: recommendations based on CULP-SCI investigations. *Journal of Rehabilitation Research & Development* **42**(3 Suppl 1) (2005), 9-19.

[5]   A.M. Koontz, et al., Shoulder kinematics and kinetics during two speeds of wheelchair propulsion. *Journal of Rehabilitation Research & Development* **39** (2002), 635-649.

[6]   P. Mukhopadhyay, L. O'Sullivan, and T.J. Gallwey, Estimating upper limb discomfort level due to intermittent isometric pronation torque with various combinations of elbow angles, forearm rotation angles, force and frequency with upper arm at 90° abduction. *International Journal of Industrial Ergonomics* **37** (2007), 313-325.

[7]   I.A. Murray and G.R. Johnson, A study of the external forces and moments at the shoulder and elbow while performing every day tasks. *Clinical biomechanics* **19**(6) (2004), 586-94.

[8]   S.D. Shimada, et al., Kinematic characterization of wheelchair propulsion. *Journal of Rehabilitation Research & Development* **35**(2) (1998), 210-8.

[9]   G. Wu, et al., ISB recommendation on definitions of joint coordinate systems of various joints for the reporting of human joint motion--Part II: shoulder, elbow, wrist and hand. *Journal of Biomechanics* **38**(5) (2005), 981-992.

Rehabilitation: Mobility, Exercise and Sports
L.H.V. van der Woude et al. (Eds.)
IOS Press, 2010

doi:10.3233/978-1-60750-080-3-45

The cutaneous reflex response during manual wheeling

M.K. MACGILLIVRAY [a,1], B. SAWATZKY[a], T. LAM[a], P. ZEHR[b]
[a] *University of British Columbia*
[b] *University of Victoria*

Abstract. Introduction: Approximately 155, 000 Canadians depend on manual wheelchairs for locomotion [1] and an estimated 31-73% of these people will experience shoulder pain as a result of manual wheeling [2]. Biomechanical research into the determinants of shoulder pain has been inconclusive. However, to date there has been very little research into the neural control of manual wheeling. One concept is that rhythmic upper limb movement (such as arm swing, swimming, and possibly manual wheeling) is regulated by a central pattern generator (CPG) and follows a similar pattern of sensory processing as described for walking. This study will explore this concept by investigating the modulation of cutaneous reflexes during manual wheeling. Purpose: The purposes of this study are to determine if the cutaneous reflex response to stimulation of the superficial radial nerve are phase-dependent during manual wheeling, to determine if there is evidence of task specificity between manual wheeling and upper arm cycling and to determine if manual wheeling experience changes the pattern of reflex modulation during wheeling. Methods: Subjects will include 15 manual wheelchair users (MWUs) with spinal cord injury and 15 non-MWUs. All subjects will complete two tasks in a randomized order including wheeling on a wheelchair treadmill at a self-selected speed and arm cycling using an arm ergometer. Electrical stimulation of the superficial radial nerve will be conducted pseudorandomly throughout the wheeling cycle eliciting cutaneous reflex responses. EMG responses will be measured in 6 muscles. The wheeling cycle will be broken up into phases using a custom made program utilizing SmartWheel and Optotrak data. Cutaneous reflex responses will be grouped and averaged depending on the phase of the wheeling cycle and be compared between MWUs and non-MWUs. Anticipated Results: It is anticipated that that the difference in cutaneous reflex amplitude between stimulated and un-stimulated EMG responses will vary dependending on the phase of the wheeling cycle. It is also anticipated that task-dependency will be evident by greater amounts of cutaneous reflex modulation of the wheeling task compared to the arm cycling task and that a greater amount of modulation will be observed in the MWU group compared to the non-MWU group.

Keywords. biomechanics, neuromechanics, manual wheelchair, shoulder injury, wheeling strategies, cutaneous reflex response, modulation, latency.

1. Introduction

Manual wheelchair use is one of the most common and more permanent forms of adapted mobility. There are an estimated 155,000 Canadians living in private

---

[1] Megan MacGillivray: MSc Candidate, School of Human Kinetics, University of British Columbia, Vancouver, British Columbia, Canada; E-mail: megank84@interchange.ubc.ca

households who require a wheelchair [1]. One of the largest populations using manual wheelchairs is people with spinal cord injuries. More than 41,000 Canadians are living with a spinal cord injury (SCI) with approximately 1100 new cases each year (Rick Hansen Foundation).

Although wheelchairs offer a means to improve mobility for people with lower limb disabilities, many manual wheelchair users will experience shoulder pain throughout their lives as a result of some element of wheelchair use. Manual wheeling as well as other wheelchair related tasks are thought to contribute to shoulder injury and pain. Any loss of upper arm function or associated problems places the independence of a manual wheelchair user at risk [3,4]. Previous studies have shown that anywhere from 31% to 73% of spinal cord injured MWUs will experience shoulder pain [5,2]. It has also been found that people who begin using manual wheelchairs as children report less shoulder pain than people who began using wheelchairs as adults during adulthood [6].

There is inconclusive evidence for possible biomechanical correlates to shoulder pain and it remains unclear whether there is a 'preferred' wheeling pattern for minimizing injury. To date, the majority of research has focused on the biomechanics of propulsion rather than understanding the neural strategies underlying manual wheeling. Studies to investigate the neural mechanisms underlying wheeling will help further our understanding of how the nervous systems adapts to long-term wheelchair use and provide a new perspective on rehabilitation training for manual wheelchair users.

Neural control, potentially consisting of a central pattern generator (CPG) or series of CPGs, of the upper limbs has been explored over the past decade. Rhythmic upper limb movements are of particular interest because they are thought to be vestigial movements maintained from an early evolutionary quadrupedal form of gait. Similar to what has been observed during walking, the processing of sensory input from cutaneous receptors in the upper limbs during rhythmic movement also exhibits phase dependent and task-dependent modulation.

2. Purpose

The purposes of this study are to (1) DETERMINE whether there is *phase-dependent* modulation of the cutaneous reflex response to electrical stimulation of the superficial radial nerve during manual wheeling (2) DETERMINE whether the cutaneous reflex response to electrical stimulation of the superficial radial nerve is *task-specific* between manual wheeling and upper limb cycling (3) INVESTIGATE the effects of manual wheeling experience on the pattern of reflex modulation in response to electrical stimulation of the superficial radial nerve.

3. Methods

Fifteen MWUs and 15 able-bodied subjects will be studied. All subjects will be a minimum of 19 years of age and capable of wheeling at a self-selected comfortable pace for 5 minutes without stopping. All subjects will be in good health. MWUs must have a history of spinal cord injury (due either to congenital or traumatic lesion) below T1. MWUs will also have spent a minimum of one year in a wheelchair.

A motion analysis system (Optotrak 3020) will be used to record sagittal-plane upper limb kinematics on the right side of the body during wheeling. The marker on the

3rd metacarpophalangeal joint will be used to define the wheeling strategy for each subject. EMG data will be collected on the right side of the body from the anterior, medial and posterior deltoids, triceps, biceps, and flexor carpi radialis.

The superficial radial nerve will be pseudorandomly electrically stimulated on the right side of the body not more than once per movement cycle. For each participant the radiating threshold will be identified. The stimulus amplitude for the experiment will be delivered at 2 times the radiating threshold.

The SmartWheel (Three Rivers Holdings, Inc., Mesa, AZ) will be attached to the right side of the wheelchair. The SmartWheel will be used to collect the 3-dimensional forces applied to the pushrim.

Custom-written software in MATLAB (Mathworks, Natwick, MA) will be used to separate the data into individual wheeling cycles. Data will then be separated into stimulated and non-stimulated trials. Both the stimulated and non-stimulated data will further be broken up into 8 bins (sections) for both arm cycling and wheeling trials. Subtracted EMG traces (non-stimulated response subtracted from the stimulated response) will be calculated for each bin and analyzed for phase dependency. A Modulation Index (subtracted EMGmax - Subtracted EMGmin)/EMGmax*100) will be calculated for early, middle and late cutaneous reflex response for each group (WMUs and able-bodied subjects) and each condition (manual wheeling and arm cycling).

4. Preliminary Data

Preliminary analysis has suggested that there is evidence of phase-dependent modulation. Further exploration will explore this concept more in-depth and determine if there is evidence of task specificity for manual wheeling.

References

[1] M. Shields, Use of wheelchairs and other mobility support devices, Health Reports/ Statics Canada **15** (3) (2004), 37-41.

[2] M.L. Boninger et al. Propulsion patterns and pushrim biomechanics in manual wheelchair propulsion, Arc Phys Med Rehabil **83** (5) (2002), 718-723.

[3] K.A. Curtis et al. Reliability and validity of the Wheelchair User's Shoulder Pain Index (WUSPI). Paraplegia **33** (10) (1995), 595-601.

[4] W.E. Pentlans and L.T. Twomey. Upper limb function in persons with long term paraplegia and implications for independence: Part II. Paraplegia **32** (4) (1994), 219-224.

[5] K.A. Curtis et al. Shoulder pain in wheelchair users with tetraplegia and paraplegia. Arch Phys Med Rehabil **80** (4) (1999), 453-457.

[6] B.J. Sawatzky et al. Prevalence of shoulder pain in adult- versus childhood-onset wheelchair users: a pilot study. J Rehabil Res Dev **42** (2005), 1-8.

Rehabilitation: Mobility, Exercise and Sports
L.H.V. van der Woude et al. (Eds.)
IOS Press, 2010
© 2010 The authors and IOS Press. All rights reserved.
doi:10.3233/978-1-60750-080-3-48

Pilot evaluation of a wheelchair accessible treadmill

A.T. CRAMER[a,b], A.P. KARPINSKI[a], R. RODRIGUEZ[a], L. GUO[a,b], N. WESTING[b], W.M. RICHTER[a,1]

[a] MAX mobility LLC
[b] Vanderbilt University

Abstract. This pilot study tested the hypothesis that exercising on a wheelchair accessible treadmill improves cardiovascular fitness for manual wheelchair users without adverse effects on propulsion biomechanics or shoulder pain. Three manual wheelchair users participated in 30 minute exercise sessions three times per week for six-weeks using self-selected programs on a wheelchair accessible treadmill. Exercise capacity and propulsion biomechanics were assessed before and after the six week program. On average, subjects displayed increases in maximum VO_2 (22.9%) and maximum heart rate (9.6%), while resting heart rate decreased (14.7%). Propulsion biomechanics and shoulder pain did not change. There were no adverse effects associated with extended use of the treadmill. The results suggest that persons with paraplegia can improve cardiovascular fitness through the regular aerobic exercise with a wheelchair accessible treadmill.

Keywords: biomechanics, cardiovascular fitness, exercise, paraplegia, propulsion, treadmill, wheelchair.

1. Introduction

The prevalence of obesity in manual wheelchair users (MWUs) exceeds that of the general population by more than 200% [1]. Obesity leads to secondary conditions such as cardiovascular disease, the leading cause of death for individuals with spinal cord injury[2,3].

Adapted treadmills have been shown to provide an effective means of improving the health of MWUs within the research environment[4]. A proof-of-concept wheelchair accessible treadmill prototype was developed by the investigators. This pilot study examines the effectiveness of the treadmill prototype in improving the health of three paraplegics.

2. Methods

Subjects signed and IRB-approved consent form prior to participation. Three subjects participated in the pilot and they were 33.7 ± 8.9 years old, 16.7 ± 9.7 years post injury, and ranged in neurologic level from T3 to T10.

During the initial and final visits, the subject's resting heart rate and blood pressure were taken. Propulsion biomechanics were recorded while the subject propelled

---

[1] Corresponding Author.

continuously on multiple grades for a period of 90 seconds. Maximal VO_2 and maximal heart rate were determined through a protocol of steadily increasing speed and grade, until maximum endurance, the point at which the subjects could not keep up with the treadmill. The maximum VO_2 and peak heart rate were determined as the maximum values during this protocol. The difference between peak heart rate and heart rate recorded 2 minutes after propulsion ceased was recorded as Heart Rate Recovery. Finally, subjects completed the Wheelchair Users Shoulder Pain Index (WUSPI) [5].

Subjects exercised three times per week for 30 minutes. They were free to choose their own exercise program(s) during the session, which included sprints, hills, random, fat burn, manual, and custom programs. The subjects were able to adjust the intensity level of the exercise programs to correspond to their own abilities.

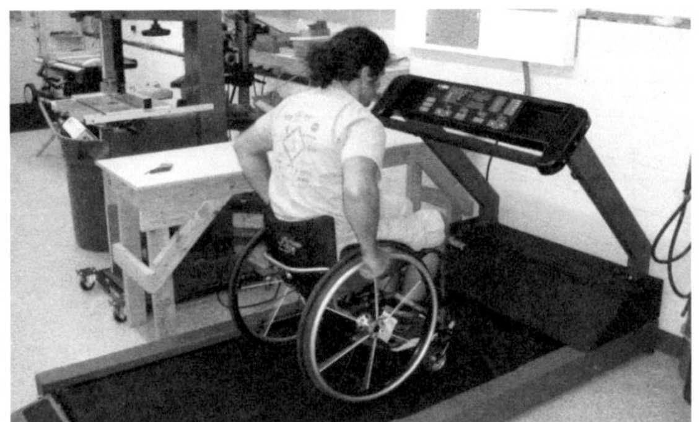

Figure 1: The treadmill has a large propulsion deck, a ramp for boarding, and a dynamic safety system.

3. Results

All subjects were able to independently board and operate the treadmill safely without encountering any adverse events. Metabolic and biomechanic measures were compared from the pre- and post-exercise assessment using a two-way ANOVA. With the small sample size, differences were determined to be significantly significant for P values less than 0.10.

Table 1: Metabolic Measures

Subject	*Maximum VO$_2$ (L/min)		*Maximum HR (bpm)		HR Recovery (bpm)		*Resting HR (bpm)	
	Pre	Post	Pre	Post	Pre	Post	Pre	Post
A	1.22	1.42	177	187	60	61	75	59
B	0.77	1.21	168	193	72	78	83	71
C	1.57	1.73	154	167	47	63	68	63
Mean	1.18	1.45	166	182	60	67	75	64
SD	0.40	0.26	12	14	13	9	8	6

indicates statistical significance at P < 0.1

Metabolic measures for the subjects are presented in Table 1. Maximum VO_2 increased following the 6 week exercise program. The VO_2 increase averaged 22.9% and was statistically significant (P=0.093). Maximum heart rate for each subject also increased by 9.6%, (P=0.073). In addition, resting heart rate of each subject decreased from pre- to post training an average of 14.7% (P=0.076). The resulting handrim propulsion biomechanics, shown in Table 2, showed no differences from the pre- to post testing. The pretest WUSPI evaluations presented an average score of 10.7 ± 17.6, ranging from 0 - 31. None of the subjects indicated that exercise on the treadmill induced, prolonged, or aggravated any form of shoulder pain that they possessed prior to participation.

Table 2: Propulsion Biomechanics

	Peak Force (N)		Push Angle (Deg)		Cadence (Push/min)	
Subject	Pre	Post	Pre	Post	Pre	Post
A	96	89	69	88	53	37
B	79	93	98	96	64	65
C	128	130	89	87	62	65
Mean	101	104	85	90	60	56
SD	25	23	15	5	6	16

4. Conclusion

MWUs face a higher risk for the developing cardiovascular disease as well as UE pain and injury. The results of this pilot study suggest that MWUs can improve cardiovascular fitness through regular aerobic exercise on a wheelchair accessible treadmill with no adverse side effects.

Acknowledgements

This study was funded by the National Institutes of Health grant #1R43 HD052311-01

References

[1] Weil E, Wachterman M, McCarthy EP, Davis RB, O'Day B, Iezzoni LI, Wee CC. Obesity Among Adults With Disabling Conditions. JAMA 2002; 288: 1265-1268.

[2] Myers J, Lee M, Kiratli J. Cardiovascular disease in spinal cord injury: an overview of prevalence, risk, evaluation, and management. Am J Phys Med Rehabil. 2007; 86: 142-153.

[3] Gass GC, Camp EM, Davis HA, Eager DD, Grout L. The effects of prolonged exercise on spinally injured subjects. Medicine and Science in Sports and Exercise. 1981;13(5):277-283.

[4] Whipp BJ, Wasserman K. Oxygen uptake kinetics for various intensities of constant-load work. Journal of Applied Physiology 1972; 33(3):351-356.

[5] Curtis KA, Roach KE, Applegate EB, Amar T, Benbow CS, Genecco TD, Gualano J. Development of the Wheelchair User's Shoulder Pain Index (WUSPI). Paraplegia. 1995;33(5):290-3.

Rehabilitation: Mobility, Exercise and Sports
L.H.V. van der Woude et al. (Eds.)
IOS Press, 2010
© 2010 The authors and IOS Press. All rights reserved.
doi:10.3233/978-1-60750-080-3-51

51

Comparison of wheelchair wheels in terms of vibration and spasticity in people with spinal cord injury

S.N.W. VORRINK[a,1], L.H.V. VAN DER WOUDE[a], A. MESSENBERG[b], P.A. CRIPTON[b,c], B. HUGHES[d], B.J. SAWATZKY[c]

[a]*Faculty of Human Movement Sciences, Vrije Universiteit, Amsterdam, the Netherlands; Departments of* [b]*MechanicalEngineering,* [c]*Orthopaedics, and* [d]*Rehabilitation Medicine, University of British Columbia, Vancouver, British Columbia, Canada*

Abstract. A wheelchair undergoes vibrations while traveling over obstacles and uneven surfaces, resulting in whole body vibration of the person sitting in the wheelchair. According to clinicians, people with spinal cord injury (SCI) report that vibration evokes spasticity. The relatively new Spinergy wheelchair wheels (Spinergy, Inc; San Diego, California) are claimed to absorb more road shock then conventional steelspoked wheelchair wheels. If this claim is true, this wheel might also reduce spasticity in people with SCI. We hypothesized that Spinergy wheels would absorb vibration, reduce perceived spasticity, and improve comfort in individuals with SCI more than standard steel-spoked wheels. To test this hypothesis, 22 nondisabled subjects performed a passive ramp test so that we could more closely examine the dampening characteristics of the Spinergy versus traditional wheels. Furthermore, 13 subjects with SCI performed an obstacle test with both wheel types. Vibrations were measured with accelerometers, and spasticity and comfort were assessed with subject-reported visual analog scales. The results of the study showed that, within the current experimental setup, the Spinergy wheels neither reduced vibration or perceived spasticity nor improved comfort in people with SCI more than the conventional steelspoked wheels.

Key words: obstacles, rehabilitation, spasticity, spinal cord injury, Spinergy, steel-spoked, vibration, visual analog scale, wheelchair wheels, whole-body vibration.

1. Introduction

The number of people using a wheelchair is estimated at 2.2 million in the United States, 750,000 in the United Kingdom, and 152,400 in the Netherlands [1]. These individuals spend a large part of their life in their wheelchair, so their quality of life depends highly on the quality and comfort of the wheelchair. A wheelchair vibrates while traveling over obstacles and uneven surfaces, resulting in whole-body vibration (WBV) of the person sitting in the wheelchair. People with spinal cord injury (SCI) have reported that rough surfaces and obstacles, such as bumps in sidewalks or rumble carpets, illicit spasms. However, in the literature, no research has been conducted to support these reports.

Spasticity and neuropathic pain can result after an SCI. Spasticity is defined as "a velocity dependent increase in the tonic stretch reflex (muscle tone) with exaggerated tendon reflexes, resulting from the hyper excitability of the stretch reflex, as one component of the upper motor neuron syndrome" [3]. The exact mechanisms underlying the development of spasticity are not fully understood [4–5]. Among individuals with SCI, 65 to 78 percent have symptoms of spasticity [4].

Spinergy wheelchair wheels (Spinergy, Inc; San Diego, California) are relatively new on the market. These wheels have specialized features, including a triple-cavity rim, an alloy hub with one-piece construction, and carbon-fiber spokes that originate from the hub (reverse spoking). Spinergy claims that as a result of these specialized features, the wheels absorb 25 percent more road shock than conventional steel-spoked wheels [6]. If true, this energy absorption would be highly advantageous in long-term wheelchair use and would suggest that these wheels could decrease the discomfort caused by WBV. More specifically, they might reduce spasticity caused by WBV in individuals with SCI.

The first purpose of this study was to verify Spinergy's claim that its wheelchair wheels absorb 25 percent more road vibration than other conventional wheelchair wheel designs. The second purpose was to assess whether Spinergy wheelchair wheels, as compared with standard steel-spoked wheelchair wheels, reduce spasticity triggered by wheeling over rough surfaces and obstacles and improve the comfort level of individuals with SCI.

2. Method

There were two parts in this study; part one addressed the first purpose and part two the second purpose of the study.

Subjects

Part 1: Twenty-two nondisabled subjects participated (12 men, 10 women). They had no previous experience with wheeling in a wheelchair.

Part 2: Thirteen subjects with SCI (10 men, 3 women).

Measurement of Vibration

Vibration was measured with two Mechworks MDS 203 two-dimensional accelerometers (Waterloo, Ontario, Canada). One accelerometer was mounted on the main axle and the other on the footplate.

Procedure

Part 1: the subjects sat passively in the wheelchair and rolled down a ramp with a slope of 8° after being released by the researcher. At the bottom of the ramp, the wheelchair and subject rolled over a small speed bump (0.025 m high × 0.080 m long) that caused vibration.

Part 2: the subjects were asked to wheel over each of the nine obstacles laid out in a gymnasium that represented obstacles people come across in daily life. They performed these nine trials with both the spinergy and steel-spoked wheel, using their own wheelchair.

3. Results

Part 1: No significant differences were found between the two wheel types for peak acceleration (Spinergy: 2.84 ± 1.16 *g*, steel-spoked: 2.81 ± 1.09 *g*), root mean square (Spinergy: 0.33 ± 0.10, steel-spoked: 0.33 ± 0.10), or peak power.

Part 2: The visual analogue scale (VAS) on spasticity and the VAS on comfort were not significantly different between the different wheel types for any of the obstacles (Figure 1).

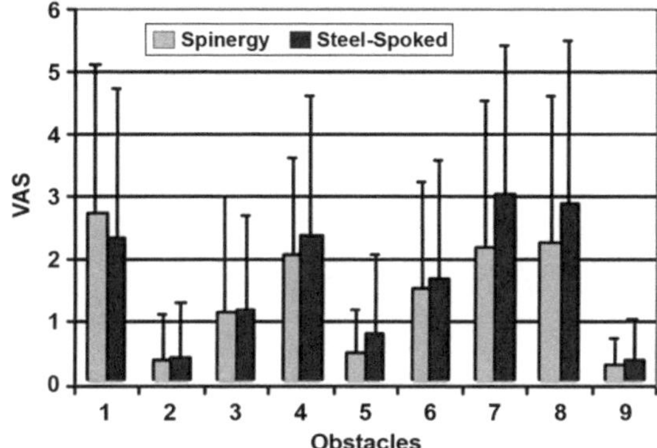

Figure 1. Subjective spasticity ratings (mean ± standard deviation) measured with 0–10 visual analog scale (VAS).

4. Conclusion

We can conclude that under the current standardized conditions, the Spinergy wheelchair wheels, as compared with the standard steel-spoked wheelchair wheels, neither absorb more vibration at the footplate or the axle nor reduce perceived spasticity or improve comfort in individuals with SCI wheeling over rough surfaces and obstacles.

References

[1] Van Drongelen AW, Van Roszek B, Hilbers-Modderman E, Kallewaard M, Wassenaar C. Wheelchair incidents. Bilthoven (the Netherlands): RIVM; 2002.
[2] Lance JW. Pathophysiology of spasticity and clinical experience with baclofen. In: Feldman RG, Young RR, Koella WP, editors. Spasticity: Disordered motor control. Chicago (IL): Year Book Medical Publishers; 1980. p. 185–220.
[3] Adams MM, Hicks AL. Spasticity after spinal cord injury. Spinal Cord. 2005;43(10):577–86.
[4] Burchiel KJ, Hsu FP. Pain and spasticity after spinal cord injury: Mechanisms and treatment. Spine. 2001;26(24 Suppl): S146–60.
[5] Spinergy [homepage on the Internet]. San Diego (CA): Spinergy; c2006 [updated 2006]. Frequently asked questions [about 3 screens]. Available from: http://www.spinergy.com/Wheelchair/faq.aspx
[6] S. N. W. Vorrink, L. H. V. Van der Woude, A. Messenberg, P. A. Cripton, B. Hughes, MD, B. J. Sawatzky. Comparison of wheelchair wheels in terms of vibration and spasticity in people with spinal cord injury. *Journal of rehabilitation research and development* **45 (9)**, (2008), 1269-1280

Rehabilitation: Mobility, Exercise and Sports
L.H.V. van der Woude et al. (Eds.)
IOS Press, 2010

doi:10.3233/978-1-60750-080-3-54

The leveraged freedom chair: a wheelchair designed for developing countries

A.G. WINTER[1], M. BOLLINI, D. DELATTE, G. JONES, H. O'HANLEY,
N. SCOLNIK
MIT Mobility Lab, Massachusetts Institute of Technology, Cambridge, MA, USA

Abstract. In this work we present the Leveraged Freedom Chair (LFC), a wheelchair-based mobility aid designed specifically for the developing world. People with disabilities in developing countries have needs that differ drastically from those of people in the developed world; they most often do not have access to public transportation and are forced to travel long distances on rough terrain. Existing mobility aids, such Western-styled wheelchairs, are inefficient to propel and difficult to use off-road. Hand-powered tricycles, although more efficient for long distance travel, are too large to use in the home. The LFC is designed to fully suit the needs of people with disabilities in developing countries by utilizing upper body power through a lever-drive system. The drivetrain, which is made from locally available bicycle components, enables the user to select different gear ratios by sliding his or her hand up and down the levelers. The levers are sized to optimally convert upper body power when traveling on the variety of terrains encountered in the developing world.

Keywords. lever-powered, lever wheelchair, lever drivetrain, multi-speed, variable speed, developing countries

1. Introduction

The Leveraged Freedom Chair (LFC) is a lever-propelled, wheelchair-based mobility aid that can be made anywhere in the world with off-the-shelf bicycle parts and cope with varied terrain ranging from steep hills to sandy roads to muddy walking paths. For indoor use, the LFC can operate as a regular push rim wheelchair by simply removing the levers. The motivation behind this project is to provide mobility to people with disabilities in developing countries no matter their location, travel requirements, or local environment. Currently available mobility products do not totally fulfill usage needs. Western-styled wheelchairs are inefficient to propel [2] and are exhausting to use for long distances on rough roads. Hand-powered tricycles are more efficient than wheelchairs [2-4] but are much too large to use within the home. Public transportation is rarely an option, as 70% of the disabled population live in rural areas [1].

---

[1] PhD Candidate in mechanical engineering and author of correspondence, Phone: +(617) 312-4207, Email: awinter@mit.edu

2. LFC drivetrain design

The LFC achieves a multi-speed, fixed gear ratio drivetrain with the lever system shown in Fig. 1. Unlike most gear trains, which operate in varied states to obtain multiple ratios, the LFC's drivetrain exists in only one state; it is the user who changes his hand position to change the mechanical advantage of the device. If more torque at the wheel is needed to climb a hill, the user simply slides his hands up the levers and away from the pivots, as shown in Fig. 1a. If more speed is required, the user moves his hands closer to the lever pivots, as shown in Fig. 1b, achieving a greater angular velocity of the drivetrain for a given hand speed.

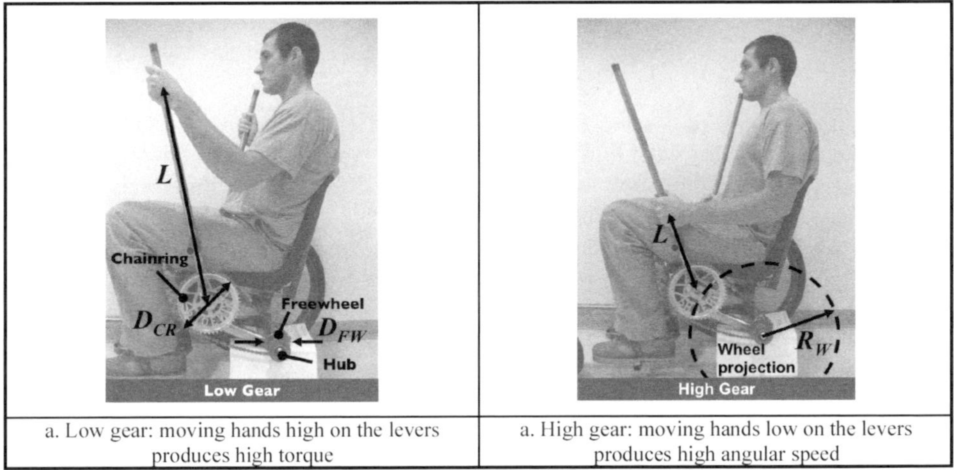

a. Low gear: moving hands high on the levers produces high torque	a. High gear: moving hands low on the levers produces high angular speed

Figure 1. LFC variable mechanical advantage drive train

3. LFC performance testing and comparison to existing mobility aids

The LFC was tested in various environments and operating conditions against an East African wheelchair and tricycle. Five test subjects, three male and two female, ranging from age 22-29, none of whom regular wheelchair users, rode each mobility aid. In a 0.87km (0.54 mile) endurance test on linoleum, the mean LFC velocity for the group was 1.89m/s, with the wheelchair 11.7% slower at 1.67 m/s and the tricycle 24.3% faster at 2.34m/s, shown in Fig. 2a. Percent increased heart rate from rest for the LFC, wheelchair, and tricycle were 44.5%, 40.5%, and 36.4%, respectively. This test demonstrates that the LFC can travel significantly faster than a wheelchair on smooth terrain for the same level of exertion. In a hill climb test on a stepped, concrete indoor ramp composed of 1:12 slope sections, with an overall run of 42.1m and rise of 2.9m, the LFC had the fastest group-averaged velocity up the ramp at 1.59m/s, with the wheelchair 22.7% slower at 1.23m/s and the tricycle 17.9% slower at 1.31m/s, shown in Fig. 2b. The exertion levels for each mobility aid were similar, with increased heart rate from rest for the LFC, wheelchair, and tricycle 55.3%, 50.8%, and 55.9%, respectively. These data demonstrate that, for a given level of exertion, more propulsion power can be produced with the LFC than with the wheelchair or tricycle.

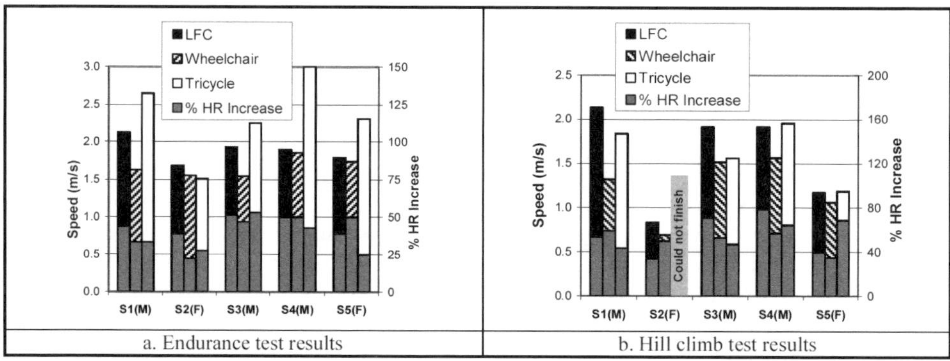

Figure 2. Performance test results of the LFC against a wheelchair and hand-powered tricycle

The final tests were conducted outdoors on ultra-high resistance surfaces in order to simulate the limits of what could be encountered in a developing country. The LFC was able to travel through snow, with a measured coefficient of rolling resistance that averaged from 0.21 to 0.34, with peaks as high as 0.48. It was also able to climb a 17.6° slope (1:3.1 rise) on wet, muddy grass. To put the formidability of this slope in perspective, the maximum allowable rise of a smooth wheelchair ramp is 1:12 according to ADA regulations [5]. Both the wheelchair and tricycle were not able to move through the snow. The wheelchair was able to make it up the steep slope, but with much more effort than was required with the LFC.

4. Conclusion

The LFC is capable of traveling virtually any road encountered in developing countries. The variable mechanical advantage attained from the lever drivetrain enables an LFC user to travel quickly and efficiently on smooth, flat roads and produce enough torque to conquer steep hills and soft ground. The single-speed, bicycle component drivetrain allows the LFC to be built and serviced anywhere in the world at prices similar to those of existing mobility aids. We are confident that the efficiency, compact size, and operational flexibility of the LFC will completely fulfill the mobility needs of people with disabilities in developing countries.

References

[1]   Groce, N.E., *Health beliefs and behaviour towards individuals with disability cross-culturally.* Introduction to Cross-Cultural Rehabilitation: An International perspective 1999.
[2]   van der Woude, L.H.V., et al., *Alternative Modes of Manual Wheelchair Ambulation: An Overview.* American Journal of Physical Medicine & Rehabilitation, 2001. **80**(10): p. 765-777.
[3]   Woude, L.H.V.v.d., et al., *Mechanical Advantage in Wheelchair Lever Propulsion: Effect on Physical Strain and Efficiency.* Journal of Rehabilitation Research and Development, 1997. **34**(3): p. 286-294.
[4]   Linden, W.L.v.d., et al., *The Effect of Wheelchair Handrim Tube Diameter on Propulsion Efficiency and Force Application (Tube Diameter and Efficiency in Wheelchairs).* IEEE Transactions on Rehabilitation Engineering, 1996. **4**(3).
[5]   ADA, *Accessibility Guidelines for Buildings and Facilities (ADAAG), 4.8 Ramps.* 2002, United States Access Board.

Rehabilitation: Mobility, Exercise and Sports
L.H.V. van der Woude et al. (Eds.)
IOS Press, 2010
© 2010 The authors and IOS Press. All rights reserved.
doi:10.3233/978-1-60750-080-3-57

Reliability and validity of the extended wheelchair circuit in persons with spinal cord injury

M.D.J. WOLVERS[a], M. ZWINKELS[a], S. DE GROOT[b,c], L.H.V. VAN DER WOUDE[c]

[a] *Research Institute MOVE Faculty of Human Movement Sciences, VU University, Amsterdam*
[b] *Rehabilitation Centre Amsterdam*
[c] *Centre for Human Movement Sciences, University Medical Centre Groningen, University of Groningen, The Netherlands*

Abstract. To evaluate the reliability and validity of the extended Wheelchair Circuit fifteen dependent subjects with Spinal Cord Injuries performed the extended Wheelchair Circuit two times with 9.3 ± 11.3 days between the trials. Test-retest reliability and validity were calculated for the three outcome measures: ability score, the performance time score and the physical strain score. Validity was assessed by analyzing the scores of the Wheelchair Circuit on age, lesion level and completeness of the lesion. The intraclass correlation coefficients of the Wheelchair Circuit were 0.94 for ability score, 0.99 for performance time score and 0.82 for physical strain score at confidence level $p<0.05$. Validity was good using lesion level on both ability and performance time scores: a significant difference between scores of persons with para- and tetraplegia was found ($p<.05$). Age did not correlate with any of the scores and also completeness of the lesion was no factor for wheelchair skill performance. Comparing the original Wheelchair Circuit with the ability score of the extended Wheelchair Circuit showed that the variability and discrimination between subjects and groups improved, but floor and ceiling effect remained. The Extended Wheelchair Circuit is a reliable research tool. The ability and performance time score are valid scores. Further research should focus on validity (especially of the physical strain score) and floor and ceiling-effect reducing tasks using a larger and more varied study population.

Keywords: extended wheelchair circuit, spinal cord injury (SCI), wheelchair skills.

1. Introduction

In the Netherlands approximately 60% of all persons with spinal cord injury (SCI) is completely wheelchair dependent and therefore might be restricted in independent living. Because quality of life is closely associated with independent living, mastering wheelchair skills is very important in daily life [1,2]. The actual training of these skills is therefore a vital part of the rehabilitation process. Wheelchair skill evaluation is equally important.

The original Wheelchair Circuit consisted of eight standardized tests [1,2] and has been proven to be both reliable and valid. The purpose of the current study was to reduce the ceiling and floor effects by adding 6 new tasks and check the Extended Wheelchair Circuit on reliability and validity.

2. Methods

The Wheelchair Circuit had three outcome measures: ability score, performance time score and physical strain score. In the original Wheelchair Circuit these scores were composed of eight tasks: figure-of-eight shape, crossing a doorstep, mounting a platform (10 cm), 15 meter sprint, 3% slope, 6% slope, 3 minutes wheelchair propulsion and making a transfer. The extended part consisted of 6 tests, namely another size doorstep (1.2 cm) and passing a door to reduce the floor effect, wheelchair propulsion on rough surface, cross slope, a wheelie and a driven wheelie (ceiling effect reducing tasks). All 14 tasks were related to activities in daily life. Fifteen wheelchair-dependent participants with SCI performed the Wheelchair Circuit twice at different occasions.

Data analysis: Heart-rate was registered and all tasks were judged by completeness and required time or reached distance. The ability score was a summation of the ability scores per task: each task was rated with zero (not able), half (partly able) or one (able). Performance time score was calculated as the time needed for three and six tasks, to compare both scores. The Delta Heart Rate (DHR) was used to calculate the physical strain score and calculated as the difference between resting heart rate and peak heart rate during each task.

Statistical analysis: For the three outcome measures test-retest reliability was calculated using the Intraclass Correlation Coefficients (ICC). Validity was assessed by analyzing the scores of the Wheelchair Circuit on age, lesion level and completeness of the lesion. A Pearson correlation was used to check the validity using age. Both lesion level and completeness of the lesion were analyzed using an independent t-test ($p < 0.05$).

3. Results

Table 1 gives a good impression of the Extended Wheelchair Circuit outcome measures.

Table 1. Descriptive Statistics.

	N	Minimum	Maximum	Mean	SEM	Standard Deviation
Ability 1 (14 tasks)	15	9.5	14.0	12.9	0.4	1.5
Ability 2 (14 tasks)	15	10.5	14.0	13.1	0.3	1.1
Ability 1 (8 tasks)	15	5.5	8.0	7.5	0.2	0.7
Ability 2 (8 tasks)	15	6.5	8.0	7.5	0.2	0.6
Performance time 1 (3 tasks)	15	15.1	47.6	25.9	2.3	8.9
Performance time 2 (3 tasks)	15	15.7	48.3	26.2	2.3	9.0
Performance time 1 (6 tasks)	15	24.5	80.0	42.8	4.0	15.5
Performance time 2 (6 tasks)	15	25.7	80.5	42.6	4.0	15.5
Physical strain 1	9	19	37	29.0	1.8	5.5
Physical strain 2	8	20	43	29.8	2.6	7.3
Age	15	20	70	44.9	4.1	15.9

The ability score according to Kilkens et al [1,2] as well as both performance time scores (3 and 6 tasks) are included.

Reliability: All three scores had high and significant test-retest reliability. The ICCs of the Wheelchair Circuit were 0.94 for ability score, 0.99 for performance time score and 0.82 for physical strain score.

Comparing Wheelchair Circuit versions: Both the original and the extended ability score are displayed in figure 1. This figure shows that the range of scores was larger in the extended version and therefore discrimination improved. Nevertheless, the ceiling and floor effect is still the same.

Validity: Age and completeness of the lesion did not show any difference and therefore could not prove validity of the extended Wheelchair Circuit. A t-test showed that people with paraplegia scored better than people with tetraplegia in the ability and performance time scores, but not in physical strain scores.

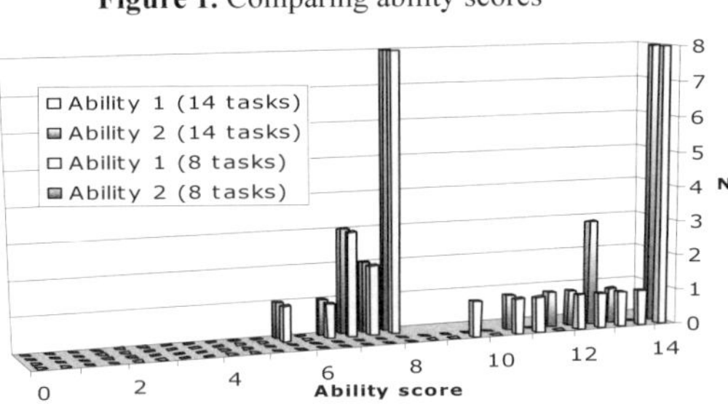

Figure 1. Comparing ability scores

4. Discussion

The desired reduction of the floor effect could not be analyzed. Also the ceiling effect has not been reduced. This is probably due to an insufficient number or too experienced (i.e. outpatient) participants that might have caused a too little varied population considering wheelchair skills. Essentially it is a multivariate problem.

5. Conclusion

The test is a practical tool to work with, is useful in all sorts of settings and environments and the materials are cheap and obtainable. The Wheelchair Circuit is a reliable research tool. The ability and performance time score are valid scores.

Further research must focus on validity (especially of the physical strain score) and on floor and ceiling-effect reducing tasks using a larger and more varied study population.

References

[1]   Kilkens, O.J., A.J. Dallmeijer, L.P. de Witte, L.H. van der Woude, M.W. Post. The Wheelchair Circuit: Construct Validity and Responsiveness of a Test to Assess Manual Wheelchair Mob:ility in Persons With Spinal Cord Injury. Archive of Physical Medical Rehabilitation 2004; 85:424-31.

[2]   Kilkens, O.J., M.W. Post, L.H. van der Woude, A.J. Dallmeijer, W.J. van den Heuvel. The Wheelchair Circuit: Reliability of a Test to Assess Mobility in Persons With Spinal Cord Injuries. Archive of Physical and Medical Rehabilitation 2002; 83:1783-8.

Rehabilitation: Mobility, Exercise and Sports
L.H.V. van der Woude et al. (Eds.)
IOS Press, 2010
© *2010 The authors and IOS Press. All rights reserved.*
doi:10.3233/978-1-60750-080-3-60

The segway personal transport as an alternative mobility device for people with disabilities: physiologic benefits?

G.BOUTILIER[1,a] B.J. SAWATZKY[b]
[a] *UBC Dept of Experimental Medicine*
[b] *UBC Dept of Orthopaedics*

Abstract. Introduction: The Segway Personal Transporter® is a self-balancing, electric-powered transportation device. While the Segway has not been marketed to individuals with mobility impairments, we wish to investigate the potential this technology offers to enhance quality of life in this population. Objectives: To determine the functional abilities that are necessary for successful use of the SegwayPT® as a personal mobility device and to asses how it compares to clients' current method of mobility. Methods: Participants (n=22) underwent three training sessions with the Segway to correlate their functional ability with their skill level on the device based on a Segway Task Assessment tool. Secondly, of the 22 subjects, 10 subjects navigated a 25m obstacle course with their current mobility devices and then the Segway. Outcome measures were the Wheelchair Outcomes Measure (WhOM) score and the difference in the time required to complete the obstacle course. Results: All participants successfully completed the Segway Task Assessment, regardless of scores on functional assessments. There was a significant increase in WhOM score between subjects' current mobility method and using the Segway for client specific goals. Interestingly, some subjects felt remarkable improvements with their spasticity after using the Segway. Conclusion: The Segway may be a useful device for a broad range of populations with functional disabilities to meet their mobility goals. We are now exploring possible therapeutic benefits of using the Segway with respect to spasticity and fatigue in SCI.

Keywords. Mobility Impairment, Segway, Spinal Cord Injury, Alternative Mobility

1. Introduction

The Segway Personal Transporter, introduced in 2001, is described as "the first self balancing, electric powered transportation device."[1] A rider stands on a small platform supported 20cm off the ground by 2 parallel wheels, and holds onto handlebars. A twist grip on the left bar is used to steer the device. When the rider leans forward, the Segway moves forward and when the rider leans back, it moves back, or stops. Balancing the Segway is possible because gyroscopes and other sensors constantly sense a person's center of gravity and make minute adjustments to ensure a balanced and upright posture. [1] The Segway is marketed as a revolutionary device that requires

---

[1] G. Boutilier. Email: boutilier@icord.org

no special skills and that "virtually anyone can use." [11] The Segway has been marketed to people as an alternative transportation device that can replace the automobile on short trips and commutes of less than 20km. [1,3]

Although there are no peer-reviewed articles regarding the Segway as a mobility aid for disabled populations, there are many personal accounts posted on the Internet by people with disabilities who use it for mobility purposes. These people include those with Parkinson's disease, multiple sclerosis, amputations, arthritis, cerebral palsy, postpolio syndrome (PPS), chronic fatigue syndrome, spinal cord injury (SCI), fibromyalgia, and hip replacement. [4] Segway users report that socially, there are fewer stigmas associated with using it for transportation than there are when using a wheelchair or scooter. [5, 6] The Segway is not regarded as a medical device and therefore users believe that it does not attract attention to their disability. [6] For some people, the Segway restores "a great sense of hope and meaning" in their life. [5] One person explained that when he uses his Segway, he is no longer "at fire hydrant height, [but] at human being height." [6] Powerful statements such as these demonstrate the need for more research into the appropriateness of the Segway as a safe alternative to other mobility aids.

Phase 1: Realizing Mobility

Currently, there are no standard assessments with which to determine a person's suitability for power mobility. [7] By compiling this information, a therapist can help prescribe appropriate power mobility for a particular patient's needs. [8] Our purpose in this study was to determine the functional abilities that are necessary for successful use of the Segway as a mobility device by people with disabilities, and to determine the functional measure(s), if any, that correlate with skills level. The experiences of study participants' in using the Segway were also explored to look further into its realistic use as a mobility device.

Therefore, we performed a prospective study encompassing 3 training sessions with the Segway to correlate subjects' functional ability (e.g., cognition, balance, mobility, muscle strength) with their skill level on the device. [9] Participants were twenty-three subjects (age range, 19-65) with a wide range of disabilities (e.g., multiple sclerosis, spinal cord injury, amputation) who could walk at least 6m with or without assistance. Our Main Outcome Measures were the Berg Balance Scale, the Timed Up & Go test, and the Segway Task Assessment scale, developed by the investigators. No correlation was found because all participants successfully completed the final Segway Task Assessment, regardless of scores on functional assessments. We concluded that the Segway is a useful device for a broad range of populations with functional disabilities. Subjects found the Segway easy to use and were excited about its potential as an assistive device for use in their communities.

Phase 2: Meeting Mobility Goals

For therapists, selecting the appropriate mobility aid for someone requires individualized assessments to match the needs, abilities, and goals of the client with the properties of the device. The goal of Phase 2 was to determine how the Segway compares to clients' current methods for mobility at meeting specific mobility goals. This study included 10 subjects (aged 19–65 yrs) with a wide range of disabilities (e.g., multiple sclerosis, spinal cord injury amputee) who were able to walk at least 6 m with or without assistance. [10] Subjects navigated a 25 m obstacle course at our provincial adult rehabilitation center with their current mobility devices and then the Segway. The outcome measures used were the Wheelchair Outcome Measure score and the difference in the time required to complete the obstacle course.

We found a significant difference in Wheelchair Outcome Measure score between subjects' current mobility method and using the Segway for client specific goals (P < 0.01); however, there was no significant difference between obstacle course times. This study has shown that the Segway may be a good candidate for people with disabilities in choosing a mobility device as it allows for them to participate in social and functional activities in a manner that traditional mobility aids do not facilitate as well. However, it does have its limitations and should be considered as just one of the many mobility options offered to people with disabilities.

Phase 3: Physiologic Benefits?

Interestingly, during the previous studies, investigators received several anecdotal reports from subjects were of improvements in balance and reductions in spasticity immediately following Segway training. One subject who had severe hypertonicity in his left hand, and required assistance to open the hand in order to hold the Segway handle, could open and close it easily and independently after only 15 minutes on the Segway. In fact, most of the participants in the study commented that they were able to use the Segway for longer periods than were able to typically stand or experienced less pain immediately following their time on the Segway. Thus, the researchers postulated that perhaps consistent use of the Segway could also increase this stamina over time. The question then remains, why did participants experience decreases in spasticity and pain and are these changes measurable and significant?

Phase 3 of the research involves investigating a specific population (individuals with spinal cord injury) during a month long Segway training program. It is a pilot project which will attempt to determine what, if any, physiologic benefits such as spasticity and pain reduction can be derived from Segway training, and whether these potential benefits are short or long term in nature. Outcome measures include the Modified Ashworth Scale, the Spinal Cord Injury Spasticity Evaluation Tool, the Pain Outcomes Questionnaire- VA and the Fatigue Severity Scale. Volunteers participate in a program consisting of 3 sessions per week/30 minutes per session for 4 weeks. Testing occurs on the first day, at 2 weeks and at 4 weeks. Spasticity is measured both pre- and post-Segway training, and self-report questionnaires are completed subsequent to training. Due to the variable nature of spasticity, participants are also asked to keep a daily log which denotes activity levels, presence of infection, any changes in medication, et cetera. Expected completion date for this work is summer 2009.

References

[1]   Segway Inc. Segway Smart Motion™. The science behind the technology. Available at: http://www.segway.com/personaltransporter/ how_it_works.html. Accessed July 31, 2007.

[2]   Neebe M. Hands on: gear, gadgets & great ideas. First in the nation: Boston EMS integrates Segway human transporter into EMS operations. J Emerg Med Serv 2002;27(6):103-7.

[3]   Segway Inc. Personal transporters, concept centaur and robotics, all powered by Segway Smart Motion™.   Available   at: http://web.lesmielles.com/segway_channel_islands/segway_ci/products_page.htm. Accessed July 31, 2007.

[4] Road Access _ Disability Alliance. Articles, essays and support group items about Segway users who have mobility challenges. Nov. 1, 2004. Available at: http://www.digitalthreads.com/ segway/segdart1.html. Accessed July 31, 2007.

[5] Bricklin D. Segways and special needs. Apr 12, 2004. Available at: http://www.bricklin.com/segwayemail.htm. Accessed July 31, 2007.

[6] Sabatini J. With halfway to go, they're still standing. New York Times 2004;Oct 27. Available at: http://travel.nytimes.com/2004/10/27/automobiles/autospecial/27SEGW.html?ex_1186027200&en_b5a 473a80b193480&ei_5070. Accessed July 31, 2007.

[7] Mortenson WB, Miller WC, Boily J, et al. Perceptions of power mobility use and safety within residential facilities. *Can J Occup Ther.* 72(2005), 142-52.

[8] Hardy P. Powered wheelchair mobility: an occupational performance evaluation perspective. *Aust Occup Ther J.* 51(2004), 34-42.

[9] Sawatzky B, Denison I, Langrish S, Richardson S, Hiller K, Slobogean B. (2007). The Segway Personal Transporter as an Alternative Mobility Device for People with Disabilities: A Pilot Study. *Arch Phys Med Rehabil.* 88(2007), 1423-1428.

[10] Sawatzky B, Denison I, Tawashy A. The Segway for People with Disabilities: Meeting Clients' Mobility Needs. *Am J Phys Med Rehabil.* (2009) In Press.

Rehabilitation: Mobility, Exercise and Sports
L.H.V. van der Woude et al. (Eds.)
IOS Press, 2010
© 2010 The authors and IOS Press. All rights reserved.
doi:10.3233/978-1-60750-080-3-64

Adjustment of the subject-and-wheelchair fore-and-aft stability

P. VASLIN[a,1], A. FAUPIN[b], F.X. LEPOUTRE[b]
[a]*LIMOS, UMR 6158 CNRS – Université Blaise Pascal,*
ISIMA, B.P. 10125, 63173 Aubière Cédex, France
[b]*LAMIH, UMR 8530 CNRS – Université de Valenciennes et du Hainaut-Cambrésis,*
B.P. 311, Le Mont Houy, 59 304 Valenciennes Cédex, France

Abstract. A 2-D model has been designed for solving the problem of the subject-and-wheelchair fore-and-aft stability, and implemented into a simulation program, which computes the seat height and fore-and-aft position from the wheelchair dimensions, the subject's anthropometry, his sitting posture in the wheelchair, and a stability index chosen according to the subject's ability to control his equilibrium. This program should greatly help the medical staff for quickly and precisely choosing the wheelchair settings fitted to the patient's characteristics.

Keywords. wheelchair, adjustment, stability, simulation.

1. Introduction

Wheelchair settings and their respective outcomes on rolling resistance, propulsion efficiency or static stability have been described in several scientific studies [1, 2, 3]. However, the optimisation of some of these characteristics can lead to contradictory choices of a same adjustment: for instance, rolling resistance can be lowered by a rearward distribution of the total mass of the subject-and-wheelchair system [4], but this setting will also decrease the fore-and-aft stability of the system [2, 5], which may not be wished by some users (*e.g.* tetraplegic or old persons). For solving this tricky problem, a global mechanical approach was followed in order to adjust the system stability while taking into account both the subject's anthropometric features and the relevant wheelchair dimensions and settings.

2. Methods

Several wheelchair dimensions and settings may influence the subject's sitting posture and the system stability: the rear and front wheels diameters, the handrim diameter, the distance between rear and front wheels (wheelbase), the lengths of the seat, the backrest and the legrest, and their inclinations with respect to the horizontal or vertical directions, the mass of the wheelchair and the position of its centre of mass with respect to the rear wheels axle. The static position of the subject's centre of mass in the wheelchair reference frame can be computed from his weight and height using classical

---

[1]   Corresponding Author: Ph. Vaslin, LIMOS (UMR 6158 CNRS), Université Blaise Pascal, ISIMA, B.P. 10125, 63173 Aubière Cédex, France; E-mail: vaslin@isima.fr.

anthropometric tables [6], in a first approximation, and provided that his sitting posture in the wheelchair is known. This posture can be chosen according to either a "reference posture" [1, 2] or the subject's own wishes. At this stage, two settings remain to be defined: the height and the fore-and-aft position of the seat with respect to the rear wheel axle, or conversely. All other settings remaining unchanged, and provided that the hand position on the handrim is known, the seat height has a direct influence on the elbow flexion angle, whereas the seat advance mainly influences the system stability.

As a wheelchair has usually four wheels, various seat adjustments and subject's postures may be chosen, which satisfy the condition of the system stability but lead to different stability levels. A stability scale (0 – 5) was thus defined with continuous values between two realistic boundaries, whether the system weight is fully upon the rear wheels axle (0) or equally distributed between rear and front wheels (5). Finally, the system total weight and its fore-and-aft distribution were used for calculating the resultant braking force applied on the wheelchair in this particular setting [4, 7], using the results of drag-tests performed on three types of floor (linoleum, asphalt, carpet).

The geometrical and mechanical relations between all the above parameters were combined into a 2-D model, which solves the problem of the subject-and-wheelchair balance using Newton's classical equations of static equilibrium, and computes the seat height and fore-and-aft setting with respect to the wheelchair dimensions, the subject's anthropometry, his sitting posture in the wheelchair, and the stability index chosen according to the subject's ability to control his equilibrium. This model has been then implemented into a home-made simulation program, written with the free computing software Scilab (INRIA, France), and especially designed for presenting the results of the 2-D model on simple and pedagogic figures.

3. Results

Only a few results of this simulation program are presented below for the "reference posture" (Fig. 1), and an arbitrary sitting posture of the subject (Fig. 2). The seat height and advance were calculated for two stability indices corresponding to two current distributions of the system weight upon front wheels (2: 20% – 4: 40%). These distributions are shown on the figures by the vertical ground reaction forces applied on rear and front wheels, whereas the resultant braking force is drawn by the horizontal vector at the rear wheel axle. An accessory result calculated by the model is the footrest height, which is an issue for rolling on an uneven floor.

4. Conclusion

When compared to the empirical and time consuming adjustment of a wheelchair, based on successive trials and errors, this simulation program should greatly help the medical staff for quickly and precisely choosing the wheelchair settings fitted to the patient's characteristics. However, the mechanical model should still be improved by searching if some equations could be reversed in order to allow the user selecting the input and output variables relevant to his own method of adjusting a wheelchair.

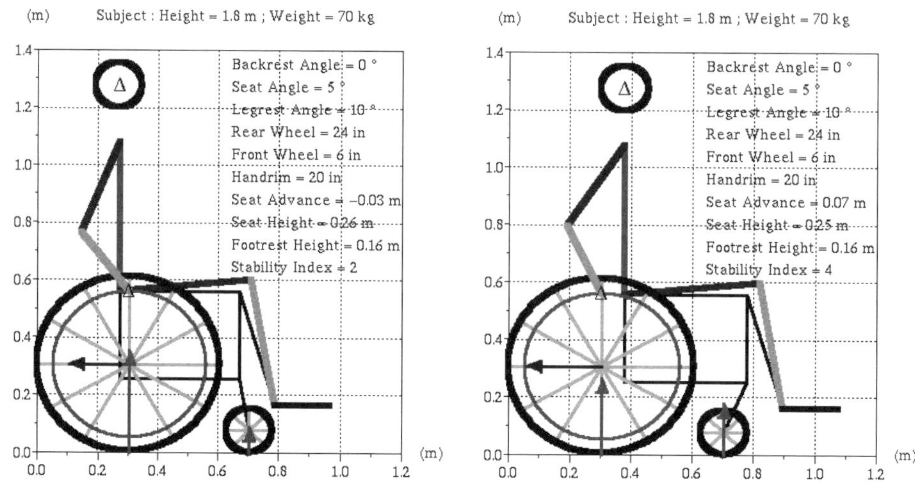

Figure 1. Simulated positions of the subject-and-wheelchair system computed for the « reference posture » of the subject (Trunk upright – Hands on handrims apexes – Elbow flexion angle: 120°).

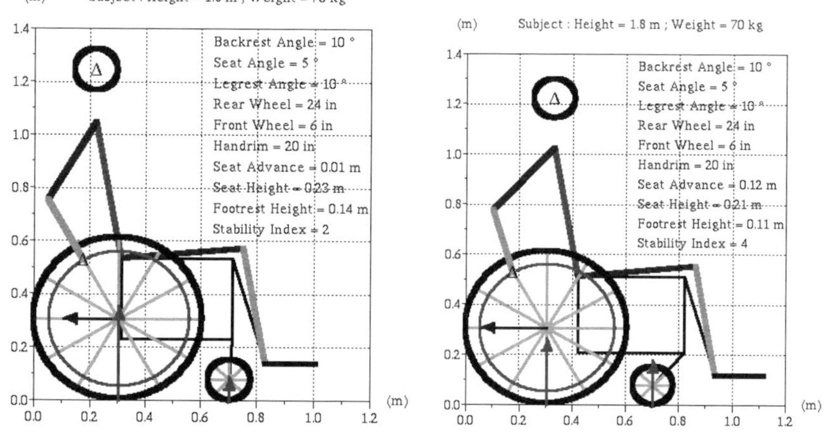

Figure 2. Simulated positions of the subject-and-wheelchair system computed for an arbitrary posture of the subject (Backrest angle: 10° – Hands 30° behind handrims apexes – Elbow flexion angle: 120°).

References

[1]   L.H.V. van der Woude, H.E.J. Veeger, R.H. Rozendal & T.J. Sargeant, Seat height in handrim wheelchair propulsion. *J. Rehab. Res. Dev.*, **26** (1989), 31-50.

[2]   C.E. Brubaker, Ergonometric considerations. *J. Rehab. Res. Dev.*, Clinical Suppl. 2 (1990), 37-48.

[3]   R.A. Cooper, *Wheelchair selection and configuration.* New York: Demos Medical Publishing, 1998.

[4]   N. de Saint Rémy, P. Vaslin, M. Dabonneville, L. Martel & A. Gavand, Dynamique de la locomotion en fauteuil roulant manuel : influences de la masse totale et de sa répartition antéro-postérieure sur la résultante des forces de freinage. *Science & Sports*, **18** (2003), 141-149.

[5]   J.D. Tomlinson, Managing maneuvrability and rear stability of adjustable manual wheelchairs: an update. *Physical Therapy*, **80** (2000), 904-911.

[6]   D.A. Winter, Anthropometry. In *Biomechanics and motor control of human movement.* New York: Wiley Interscience Publication, 1990, 51-74.

[7]   C. Sauret, P. Vaslin, M. Dabonneville & M. Cid, Drag force mechanical power during an actual propulsion cycle on a manual wheelchair. *Biomedical Engineering and Research*, **30** (2009), 3-9.

Rehabilitation: Mobility, Exercise and Sports
L.H.V. van der Woude et al. (Eds.)
IOS Press, 2010

doi:10.3233/978-1-60750-080-3-67

Evaluation of the external mechanical work produced during manual wheelchair locomotion on the field

N. DE SAINT REMY[a,1], P. VASLIN[a]
[a]*LIMOS, UMR 6158 CNRS, Université Blaise Pascal, ISIMA, B.P. 10125, 63173 Aubière Cédex, France*

Abstract. The physical capacity of wheelchair users is usually evaluated by their power output, which is generally calculated from the mechanical work of the resultant braking force only. This method does not take into account the kinetic energy variations of the subject-and-wheelchair system. The purpose of this study was to verify if these variations could be neglected for estimating the subject's mechanical work. Three young wheelchair users performed a straightforward displacement with a Wireless Wheelchair Ergometer. According to the subjects, their total estimated mechanical work could be 2 to 5 times higher than the mechanical work of the resultant braking force applied on the system. These results showed that the system's kinetic energy variations should not be neglected for estimating the subject's mechanical work in real conditions.

Keywords. manual wheelchair locomotion, mechanical work, braking force, kinetic energy variations.

1. Purpose

On wheelchair ergometers, the physical capacity of wheelchair users is usually evaluated by their power output, which is generally calculated from the mechanical work of the resultant braking force only. However, in real conditions, this method does not take into account the kinetic energy variations of the subject-and-wheelchair system. The purpose of this study was to verify if these variations could be neglected for estimating the subject's mechanical work.

2. Methods

Three young wheelchair users with different characteristics (Table 1) performed a 20-m straightforward displacement on the same horizontal floor with a Wireless Wheelchair Ergometer (WWE, Figure 1) equipped with several transducers [1]: a 3-D accelerometer fixed under the seat, between rear wheels axles; three six-component dynamometers: two are fixed on both rear wheels, which angular positions are measured by two angular potentiometers, and the third is fixed between the seat and the frame. The 23 signals are sampled at a rate of 500 Hz by a 16-bit A/D card, and sent through a wireless protocol to a remote computer.

---

[1] Corresponding Author: nicodsr@wanadoo.fr

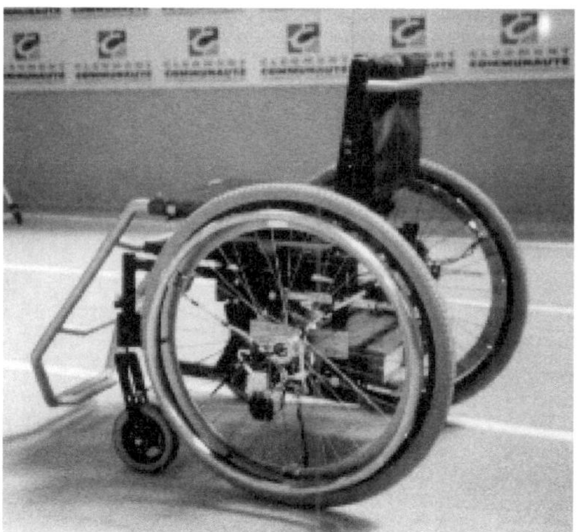

Figure 1. W.W.E. used in this study.

Table 1. Characteristics of the three young wheelchair users.

Wheelchair users	Sex	Age	Lesion level
1	F	21	T 12
2	F	21	T 6
3	M	33	T 4

The resultant braking force (F_B) during actual wheelchair propulsion was evaluated from a mathematical function that takes into account the two parameters which have a significant influence on F_B, the weight of the subject-and-wheelchair system (W) and its relative fore-and-aft distribution (D) on the front castors [2]:

$$FB = a \cdot W + b \cdot D + c \cdot W \cdot D \tag{1}$$

where F_B, W and the coefficient b are expressed in Newtons (N), D is a percentage (%), and the coefficients a and c have no unit. The three coefficients (a, b, c) have been calculated from four series of ten deceleration tests realised beforehand on the same floor than for the propulsion experiments.

The mechanical work of F_B ($W_{(\vec{F}_B)}$) has been calculated from the displacement of the wheelchair centre of mass ($\overrightarrow{OG}$), which was computed from the measurements of the angular potentiometers during the propulsion experiments:

$$W_{(\vec{F}_B)} = \overrightarrow{F}_B \cdot \overrightarrow{OG} \tag{2}$$

In this study, it was assumed that the centre of pressure (CoP) calculated from the measurements of the force-plate fixed under the seat could be assimilated to the vertical projection of the subject's centre of mass (CoM). The subject's velocity on the WWE was estimated from that hypothesis and used with the absolute wheelchair velocity for calculating the kinetic energy variations of the subject-and-wheelchair system (E_k) and then the subject's mechanical work ($W_{Subject}$) during the 20-m displacement:

$$W_{Subject} = \sum_{i=1}^{i=n} \left| \Delta E_{ki} - W_{(\vec{F}_B)i} \right| \tag{3}$$

3. Results

Whatever the lesion level of the subject, the kinetic energy variations of the system during a 20-m straightforward displacement were not negligible (Figure 2). Indeed, according to the subjects, their total mechanical work could be 2 to 5 times higher than only that of the resultant braking force applied on the subject-and-wheelchair system (Table 2).

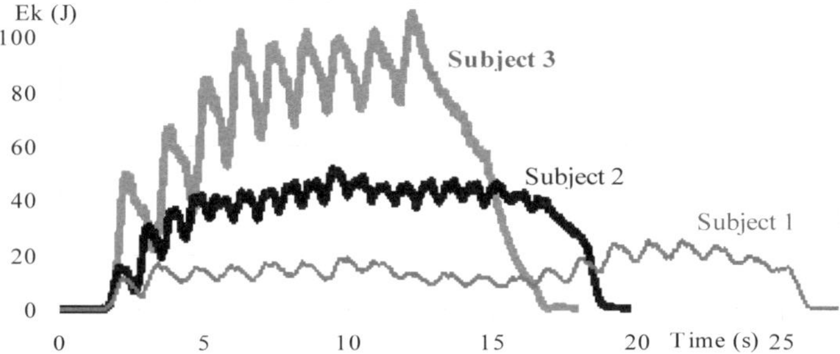

Figure 2. Time course of the system kinetic energy during a 20-m straightforward displacement performed by young wheelchair users.

Table 2. Velocities and mechanical works calculated during the 20-m straightforward displacement.

Wheelchair user	Velocity (m.s^{-1})	W_{BF} (J)	$W_{Subject}$ (J)	$W_{Subject}$ / W_{BF}
1	0,69	96	244	2,5
2	1,00	88	361	4,1
2	1,26	87	512	5,9

4. Conclusion

Provided that the the CoP calculated from the measurements of the force-plate fixed under the wheelchair seat could be assimilated to the vertical projection of the subject's CoM, these results showed that the system's kinetic energy variations should not be neglected for evaluating the mechanical work of wheelchair users in actual conditions. However, before drawing further conclusions of these results, some more experiments are needed with the WWE associated with a 3-D kinematic analysis system, in order to ascertain the main hypothesis used in this study.

References

[1] M. Dabonneville, Ph. Vaslin, Ph. Kauffmann, N. de Saint Rémy, Y. Couétard & M. Cid. A self-contained wireless wheelchair ergometer designed for biomechanical measures in real life conditions. *Technology and Disability* **17**, 2 (2005), 63–76.

[2] N. de Saint Rémy, Ph. Vaslin, M. Dabonneville & M. Cid. Computing wheelchair drag force from the system's total weight value and distribution. *Computer Methods in Biomechanics and Biomedical Engineering* **10**, suppl.1 (2007), 103–104.

Chapter 2

Handcycling

2.1

Oral Presentations

Rehabilitation: Mobility, Exercise and Sports
L.H.V. van der Woude et al. (Eds.)
IOS Press, 2010
© *2010 The authors and IOS Press. All rights reserved.*
doi:10.3233/978-1-60750-080-3-73

Shoulder joint moment contribution to movement during manual wheelchair propulsion

G. DESROCHES[a,1], N. LOUIS[b], R. DUMAS[a], P. VASLIN[c], P. GORCE[b], L. CHÈZE[a]
[a] *Université de Lyon, LBMC UMR_T 9406, UCBL-INRETS, Villeurbanne, France*
[b] *HANDIBIO-EA4322, Laboratoire de Bio-modélisation et d'ingénierie des Handicaps, Université du Sud Toulon-Var, La garde, France*
[c] *LIMOS UMR 6158, CNRS Université Blaise Pascal Clermont 2, Aubière, France*

Abstract. The purpose of this study was to establish the contribution (e.g. driving or stabilizing) of net shoulder joint moment to shoulder movement during manual wheelchair (MW) propulsion. Two male able-bodied propelled in a wireless wheelchair ergometer. Kinetics and kinematics of propulsion were recorded simultaneously bilaterally. An inverse dynamic method was used to compute net joint moment and angular velocity at shoulder level. The 3D angle between net shoulder joint moment and angular velocity was computed over the propulsive cycle to determine if net moment mainly drove (angle close to 0 or 180 degrees) or stabilized (angle close to 90 degrees) the shoulder joint. During the push phase, shoulder joint moments mainly propelled the joints but with an important combined stabilization action. Assuming that joint moments are mainly the result of muscle action, net shoulder joint moments for both subjects were mainly due to the dynamic stabilizers of the shoulder, the rotator cuff muscles. High and repetitive demand on the rotator cuff muscles could accelerate the onset of fatigue and increase risk of overuse injuries.

Keywords. angular velocity, joint moments, propulsion, shoulder, wheelchair

1. Introduction

To asses the impact of different experimental conditions on the load sustained by the shoulder during MW propulsion, inverse dynamic methods and net shoulder joint moments have been widely used [1]. Yet, no information is available on the actual contribution of the joint moment to the joint movement during MW propulsion. Joint power could provide insight on this contribution but its interpretation remains controversial in 3D [2]. Dumas et al. [2] proposed to compute the 3D angle between the direction of joint movement (i.e. joint angular velocity) and the equivalent joint actuator (i.e. joint moment). Depending on the orientation of the 3D moment direction with respect to 3D angular velocity direction, the moment can either drive the joint (aligned vectors) or stabilize the joint (orthogonal vectors).

Therefore, the purpose of this study was to establish the contribution (e.g. driving or stabilizing) of net shoulder joint moment to shoulder movement during MW

---

[1] Corresponding Author: Guillaume Desroches, Université Lyon 1, LBMC UMR_T 9406, Bâtiment Omega, 43 Bd du 11 novembre, 69 622 Villeurbanne, France ; E-mail : Guillaume.Desroches@univ-lyon1.fr

propulsion. This information could help to better understand biomechanics of MW propulsion and maybe the high incidence of shoulder pathologies.

2.   Methods

For this experiment, two male able-bodied were recruited (25 & 48 years old; 65 & 71 kg; 1.64 & 1.84 m). The measurements were made in a wireless wheelchair ergometer [3] which enabled to measure forces and moments applied by the hands bilaterally at the pushrim (500 Hz). Reflective markers were placed symmetrically on the right and left upper limbs and displacements were recorded by the Motion Analysis System (100 Hz). Both subjects propelled on a walking corridor of 4 m long at a comfortable speed for three trials (1.42 ± 0.07 m/s). The inverse dynamic method used was the one developed by Dumas et al. [4]. Outputs of the method were net joint moments and angular velocities at shoulder level in the laboratory coordinate system (LCS). The 3D angle ($\alpha_{M\omega}$) between the joint moment (M) and angular velocity (ω) vectors was computed [2]. The $\alpha_{M\omega}$ angle was computed bilaterally at the shoulder and normalized over the propulsive cycle (i.e. beginning of the push phase to the beginning of the next one) which was determined by the moment around the hub (Mz). Both subjects were averaged together.

The value of $\alpha_{M\omega}$ can vary between 0 and 180° over the push phase. These values can be separated into three distinct intervals which represent three different joint configurations [2]. In the range of 0 to 60°, the joint is primarily in a propulsion configuration while in the range of 120 to 180° the joint is primarily in a resistance configuration. In the range of 60 to 120° the joint is in a stabilization configuration. It is important to bear in mind that these intervals represent the evolution of $\alpha_{M\omega}$. A joint moment would purely propel or resist the movement when $\alpha_{M\omega}$ is equal to 0 or 180° respectively, while it would purely stabilize when $\alpha_{M\omega}$ equals 90°. Everything in between those values implies combined action but with a dominance depending in which interval $\alpha_{M\omega}$ lies.

3.   Results

At the beginning of the push phase (Figure 1; 0-10%) and for both shoulders, $\alpha_{M\omega}$ reveals that the joint is mainly in stabilization configuration when the hands make contact with the pushrims. In the middle of the push phase (Figure 1; 10-25%), both shoulders are in a propulsion configuration, even if the left one is closer to stabilization. At the end of the push phase (Figure 1; 25-35%), the right and left joint shift from a propulsion configuration to almost a resistance configuration.

During the recovery phase (Figure 1; 35-100%), both joints are in a propulsion configuration and, at the end of the recovery phase, the joints shift to a resistance configuration.

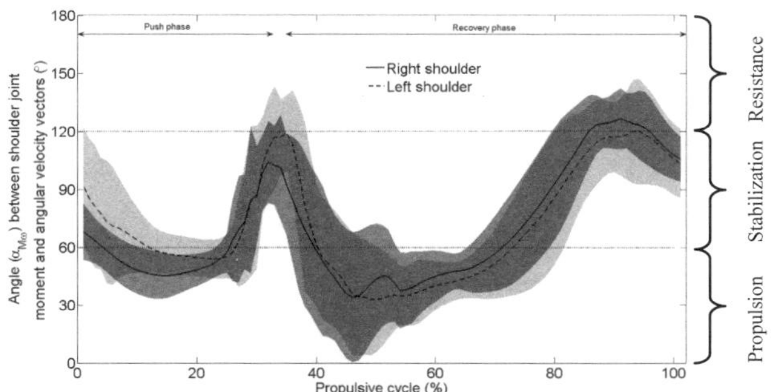

Figure 1. Evolution over the propulsive cycle of the 3D angle between shoulder joint moment and angular velocity vectors

4. Discussion

Although during the push phase of two able-bodied subjects the shoulder joints were mainly in a propulsion configuration, the values were very close to the stabilization configuration. This suggests that an important amount of the joint moment did not contribute directly to the movement but actively stabilized the joint. Assuming that joint moments are mainly the result of muscle action, net shoulder joint moments for both subjects were mainly due to the dynamic stabilizers of the shoulder, the rotator cuff muscles which concur with EMG studies of the shoulder during propulsion [5]. High and repetitive demand on the rotator cuff muscles could accelerate the onset of fatigue and increase risk of overuse injuries.

The $\alpha_{M\omega}$ could yield valuable information while comparing different propulsion conditions. Moreover, an advantage of $\alpha_{M\omega}$ is that it is dimensionless; thus, no normalization is needed when comparing among subjects.

5. Conclusion

During the push phase of two able-bodied subjects, shoulder joint moments mainly propelled the joints but with an important combined stabilization action. Conversely, in the recovery phase, shoulder joints were mainly in propulsion configuration.

References

[1]   G. Desroches, R. Aissaoui and D. Bourbonnais, Effect of system tilt and seat-to-backrest angles on load sustained by shoulder during wheelchair propulsion, *J Rehabil Res Dev*, **43** (2006), 871-82

[2]   R. Dumas and L. Cheze, Hip and knee joints are more stabilized than driven during the stance phase of gait: an analysis of the 3D angle between joint moment and joint angular velocity, *Gait Posture*, **28** (2008), 243-50

[3]   M. Dabonneville, P. Kauffmann, P. Vaslin, et al., A self-contained wireless wheelchair ergometer designed for biomechanical measures in real life conditions *Technology and Disability*, **17** (2005), 63-76

[4]   R. Dumas, R. Aissaoui and J.A. de Guise, A 3D generic inverse dynamic method using wrench notation and quaternion algebra, *Comput Methods Biomech Biomed Engin*, **7** (2004), 159-166

[5]   S.J. Mulroy, S. Farrokhi, C.J. Newsam, et al., Effects of spinal cord injury level on the activity of shoulder muscles during wheelchair propulsion: an electromyographic study, *Arch Phys Med Rehabil*, **85** (2004), 925-34

Rehabilitation: Mobility, Exercise and Sports
L.H.V. van der Woude et al. (Eds.)
IOS Press, 2010

doi:10.3233/978-1-60750-080-3-76

Perception of effort during incremental upper body exercise in able-bodied and paraplegic athletes

M. PRICE[a,1], C.D. THAKE, I.G. CAMPBELL[b]
[a] *Faculty of Health and Life Sciences, Coventry University, Coventry, UK*
[b] *Department of Sports Sciences, Brunel University, Uxbridge, UK*

Abstract. Purpose: To examine the relationship between ratings of perceived exertion (RPE) and physiological variables in able bodied and paraplegic athletes during arm crank ergometry (ACE). Methods: Eight male upper body trained able-bodied athletes (AB) and eight male paraplegic athletes (PA; T3 – L1) undertook an incremental ACE test to volitional exhaustion (35W every 2 min, 70 rev.min[-1]). Expired gas was collected via the Douglas bag technique in the final minute of each stage and analysed for minute ventilation (V_E) and oxygen consumption (VO_2). Heart rate and RPE were recorded during the last 15 seconds of each stage. Differences between groups for workloads of 35, 70 and 105W were analysed by two-way analysis of variance. Relationships between variables were analysed via Pearsons' correlation. Results: Heart rate was greater for PA when compared to AB between 35 and 105W (main effect; P<0.05) whereas VO_2 was lower. No differences were observed for V_E or RPE (P>0.05). Significant correlations (r=0.73 – 0.87; P<0.05) were observed between RPE and; VO_2, %VO_2peak, HR and %HRpeak for both groups. V_E vs. RPE was best expressed as a curvilinear function. Conclusions: The relationship between RPE and physiological variables in AB and PA athletes during incremental submaximal ACE appears similar.

Keywords. effort perception, exercise intensity.

1. Introduction

Ratings of perceived exertion (RPE) have been used within a wide range of studies examining responses of wheelchair users such as wheelchair propulsion strategies[1] and wheelchair design in relation to shoulder pain.[2] In addition, RPE has been routinely monitored in wheelchair athletes during performance based and prolonged exercise studies.[3, 4] Surprisingly, there are few studies specifically examining the use of RPE in wheelchair user populations and how it may differ when compared to able-bodied individuals. This may be of importance for the interpretation of effort perception during exercise as the original RPE scale was validated using able-bodied persons. As persons with a spinal cord injury have a reduced recruitable muscle mass for exercise and generally less ability to stabilize the lower body RPE may be accentuated for a given exercise intensity. The aim of this study was to examine the

---

[1] Corresponding Author: Michael J. Price, Faculty of Health and Life Sciences, James Starley Building, Coventry University, Coventry, CV1 5FB; mike.price@coventry.ac.uk.

relationship between RPE and conventional markers of exercise intensity in able-bodied and wheelchair athletes during incremental arm exercise.

2. Method

Eight male upper body trained athletes (AB) and eight male wheelchair athletes with paraplegia (PA; T3 – L1) volunteered to participate in this study which had received University Ethics Committee approval. All undertook an incremental exercise text to volitional exhaustion on a cycle ergometer (Monark 814E) modified for arm exercise. The protocol began with an initial exercise intensity of 35W and increasing by 25W every two minutes (70 rev.min^{-1}). Expired gas was collected via the Douglas bag technique in the final minute of each stage and analysed for minute ventilation ($\dot{V}_E$) and oxygen consumption ($\dot{V}O_2$). Heart rate (HR; Polar monitor) and RPE (Borg Scale, 6-20) were recorded during the last 15 seconds of each stage. Regression equations for RPE against $\dot{V}O_2$, % peak $\dot{V}O_2$ ($\dot{V}O_{2peak}$), HR and % peak HR (HR$_{peak}$) were determined for each athlete. HR at given levels of RPE (11, 13, 15 and 17) were determined for each athlete. Differences between peak responses were analysed by independent t-tests. Differences between groups at power outputs of 35, 70 and 105W were analysed by two-way analysis of variance with repeated measures (group × power output) as were heart rates at given values of RPE (group × RPE). Relationships between variables were analysed via Pearsons' correlation.

3. Results

$\dot{V}O_{2peak}$ (2.34 ±0.24 vs. 3.57 ±0.40 L.min^{-1}) and peak power output (121 ±21 vs. 201 ±36 Watts) were lower for the PA athletes when compared to the AB athletes, respectively (P<0.05) whereas as HRpeak was similar (176 ±20 vs. 183 ±10 beats.min^{-1}, respectively; P>0.05). When compared across power outputs $\dot{V}O_2$ was greater for the AB athletes (main effect for group; P<0.05) whereas % $\dot{V}O_{2peak}$, heart rate and %HR$_{peak}$ were greater for the PA athletes (main effects for group; P<0.05). There were no difference between PA and AB for RPE across workloads (35W: 11.3 vs. 11.1; 70W: 14.5 vs. 13.5; 105W: 17.1 vs. 16.0, respectively; P>0.05).

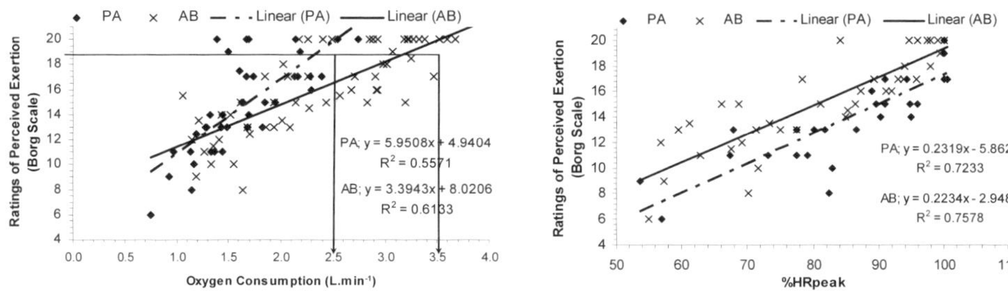

Figure 1. Relationship between ratings of perceived exertion and oxygen consumption (left panel) and %heart rate peak (right panel). Arrows represent oxygen uptake at RPE of 20.

The individual relationships between RPE and $\dot{V}$ O_2 demonstrated steeper gradients for the PA athletes than for the AB athletes (P<0.05). Group data is shown in Figure 1. When expressed as RPE vs. % $\dot{V}$ O_{2peak} no differences were evident (P>0.05). V_E vs. RPE demonstrated a curvilinear function. Relationships between RPE and HR showed similar gradients for PA and AB athletes but with PA athlete values being approximately 1.5 RPE units higher for a given HR than the AB. Similarly, when heart rates at specific RPE values were determined for each athlete values were greater for PA than AB (main effect for group; P<0.05). Values for %HR_{peak} at a given RPE were ~10% greater for PA when compared to AB.

4. Discussion

Oxygen consumption was higher for the AB athletes when compared to the PA athletes at 35, 70 and 105Watts. This is most likely due to a greater muscle mass and muscle activity within the lower body contributing to stabilization and force production. When % $\dot{V}$ O_{2peak} was considered the PA athletes utilized a greater proportion of their functional capacity at each power output. The PA athletes also demonstrated a steeper gradient for the relationship between RPE and oxygen consumption indicating greater perceptions of effort at a given metabolic rate. These responses are consistent with the lower peak power output and $\dot{V}$ O_{2peak} values of PA athletes and reduced functional range. When values were normalized to peak oxygen consumption there were no differences between groups. The use of RPE in PA athletes for exercise intensities based upon relative oxygen consumption would therefore appear valid.

Although representing oxygen consumption relative to peak values normalized the RPE responses this did not occur for the heart rate response. Here a given RPE demonstrated %HR_{peak} values ~10% higher for the PA athletes than for the AB athletes. As none of the PA athletes tested had significantly reduced peak heart rate values or demonstrated autonomic dysreflexia this most likely reflects the reduced ability to redistribute blood from the lower body resulting in a lower stroke volume and elevated heart rate for a given cardiac output.[5]

The present study has shown that for given overall RPE values heart rates are greater for PA than AB athletes. Future work should examine more specific localized RPE values between PA and AB athletes and differences between specific and non-specific exercise modes.

References

[1]   J.P. Lenton, N.E. Fowler, L. van der Woude, V.L. Goosey-Tolfrey, Wheelchair propulsion: effects of experiences and push strategy on efficiency and perceived exertion, *Applied Physiology Nutrition and Metabolism* **33** (2008), 870–879.

[2]   M.E. Nash, D. Koppens, M. Van Haaren, A.L. Sherman, J.P. Lippiatt, J.E. Lewis, Power-assisted wheels ease energy costs and perceptual responses to wheelchair propulsion in persons with shoulder pain and spinal cord injury, *Archives of Physical Medicine and Rehabilitation* **89** (2008), 2080-2085.

[3]   C. Perret, G. Mueller, H. Knecht, Influence of creatine supplementation on 800 m wheelchair performance: a pilot study, *Spinal Cord* **44** (2006), 275-279.

[4]   M.J. Price, I.G. Campbell, Thermoregulatory responses of paraplegic and able-bodied athletes at rest and during prolonged exercise and passive recovery, *European Journal of Applied Physiology* **76** (1997), 552-570.

[5]   M.T. Hopman, Circulatory responses during exercise in individuals with spinal cord injury. *International Journal of Sports Medicine* **15** (1994), 126-131.

Rehabilitation: Mobility, Exercise and Sports
L.H.V. van der Woude et al. (Eds.)
IOS Press, 2010

doi:10.3233/978-1-60750-080-3-79

Effects of hand cycle training on wheelchair capacity during clinical rehabilitation in persons with a spinal cord injury

L.J.M. VALENT[a,c,1], A.J. DALLMEIJER[b], J.H.P. HOUDIJK [a,c], J.R. SLOOTMAN[a],
T.W.J. JANSSEN[c,d], L.H.V. VAN DER WOUDE[e]

[a]*Heliomare Rehabilitation Research and Development, Wijk aan Zee*
[b]*Department of Rehabilitation Medicine, VU University Medical Center,
Amsterdam*
[c]*Research Institute MOVE, Institute for Fundamental and Clinical Human
Movement Sciences, Faculty of Human Movement Sciences, VU University Amsterdam*
[d]*Rehabilitation Center Amsterdam, Amsterdam*
[e]*Centre for Human Movement Sciences, University Medical Centre Groningen,
University of Groningen, Groningen, The Netherlands*

Abstract. In the past decade, the add-on hand cycle has become popular for mobility in the Netherlands. Consequently hand cycling (HC) has become an integrated part of the rehabilitation program. The purpose of the current study was to evaluate the effects of a structured HC training program on physical capacity in subjects with spinal cord injury (SCI). Twenty subjects who followed HC training in addition to usual clinical rehabilitation were compared with matched control subjects. Primary outcome was hand rim wheelchair capacity: peak power output (PO_{peak}), peak oxygen uptake (VO_{2peak}) and oxygen pulse. Secondary outcomes were arm muscle strength, pulmonary function and hand cycle capacity. Strong tendencies for improvement attributed to HC training were found in wheelchair capacity, reflected by PO_{peak} and oxygen pulse. Shoulder exo- and endo-rotation and unilateral elbow flexion strength improved but not pulmonary function. Hand cycle capacity (PO_{peak}) improved comparing pre and post test results. Additional HC training during clinical rehabilitation seems to show similar or slightly favourable results on fitness and muscle strength compared with regular care.

Keywords. clinical rehabilitation, spinal cord injury, peak oxygen uptake, peak power output, muscle strength, pulmonary function, hand cycling.

1. Introduction

During clinical rehabilitation, various aerobic exercise modes are available to improve the physical capacity of patients with SCI. Compared with hand rim wheelchair propulsion, HC is found to be less straining and more efficient [1] and is assumed to be a suitable exercise mode. The following hypothesis was tested: When compared to

---

[1] Corresponding Author: Linda Valent, Heliomare research & development, Relweg 51, 1949 EC Wijk aan Zee, The Netherlands; E-mail: l.valent@heliomare.nl

regular care, structured HC training has a positive effect on wheelchair (and hand cycle) exercise capacity in subjects with SCI during clinical rehabilitation.

2. Methods

Subjects

Patients with an acute SCI, prognosis of 'remaining mainly wheelchair-bound', able to propel a hand cycle and aged between 18 and 65 years participated on a voluntary basis and after signing an informed consent. The study was approved by the local ethical committee. The controls were selected from a previously studied cohort, matched on age, gender, level and completeness of lesion [2].

Design and statistical analysis

Experimental subjects received HC training (twice a week, 45 minutes) in addition to regular care, while controls received regular care only. The first measurement occasion [3] was in the week before the start of active rehabilitation/HC training and the second occasion was in the week before discharge. The pre- and post-test outcomes of the experimental subjects were compared with the controls using ANOVA for repeated measures analyzing the interaction of measurement (pre/post test) and group (training/control) ($p \leq 0.05$).

Testing procedure

Wheelchair exercise capacity (PO_{peak}, VO_{2peak}), was determined in a graded wheelchair exercise test on a treadmill [4]. Strength of arm muscle groups (shoulder abduction, exo- and endo-rotation and elbow flexion and extension) were tested with hand-held dynamometer [5]. Pulmonary function was determined (forced vital capacity, peak expiratory flow). HC capacity (PO_{peak}, VO_{2peak}) was determined in a graded exercise test again on a motor driven treadmill [6].

3. Results

Training

Three subjects dropped out due to medical conditions such as the flu, urinary tract infections, autonomic dysregulation and pressure sores. Results were available for 10 subjects with paraplegia (n=10) and tetraplegia (n=7). Non-compliance was 13±3% of all training sessions. No overuse injuries were reported associated to HC training. During the training period, subjects reported a perceived exertion between 4-7 on the 10-point Borg-scale [7].The training period (17±8 weeks) and total number of training sessions (32±16) varied substantially between subjects.

Outcome

Positive trends of additional HC training were found for PO_{peak} (p=0.079) and oxygen pulse (0.052) but no significant effect was found for VO_{2peak} (Figure 1). Significant training effects were found for muscle strength of elbow flexion (only left), shoulder exo-rotation and shoulder endo-rotation (both left and right) only. No training effect was found for pulmonary function. Comparing pre- with post-test results on HC cycle capacity (Figure 1) only, a significant improvement in PO_{peak} was found (p=0.00) but again only a trend for improvement in VO_{2peak} (p=0.07).

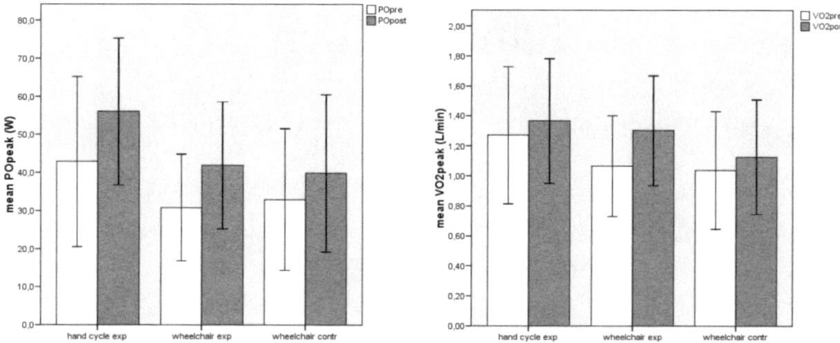

Figure 1a and 1b. Mean PO_{peak} and VO_{2peak} pre-test (white bars) and post-test (grey bars) for the hand cycle test (experimental group only) and the wheelchair test experimental (exp) and control (contr) group.

4.   Conclusions

Compared with usual rehabilitation care, HC seems to be a safe exercise mode for persons with SCI to build up fitness and muscle strength, showing similar or favourable results. The small heterogeneous subject group and large variation in length of the training period may have affected statistical power of this study. Future research on hand cycle training protocols is recommended.

References

[1]   Dallmeijer AJ, Submaximal physical strain and peak performance in handcycling versus handrim wheelchair propulsion. *Spinal Cord* **42** (2004):91-8.
[2]   Haisma JA, Changes in physical capacity during and after inpatient rehabilitation in subjects with a spinal cord injury. *Arch Phys Med Rehabil* **87** (2006):741-8.
[3]   Dallmeijer AJ, Hand-rim wheelchair propulsion capacity during rehabilitation of persons with spinal cord injury. *J Rehabil Res Dev* **42**(3 Suppl 1) (2005):55-63.
[4]   Kilkens OJ, The longitudinal relation between physical capacity and wheelchair skill performance during inpatient rehabilitation of people with spinal cord injury. *Arch Phys Med Rehabil* **86** (2005):1575-81.
[5]   Andrews AW, Normative values for isometric muscle force measurements obtained with hand-held dynamometers. *Phys Ther* **76**(1996):248-59.
[6]   Valent LJ, The individual relationship between heart rate and oxygen uptake in people with a tetraplegia during exercise. *Spinal Cord* **45** (2007):104-11.
[7]   Noble BJ, A category-ratio perceived exertion scale: relationship to blood and muscle lactates and heart rate. *Med Sci Sports Exerc* (1983)**15**:523-8.

Rehabilitation: Mobility, Exercise and Sports
L.H.V. van der Woude et al. (Eds.)
IOS Press, 2010
© 2010 The authors and IOS Press. All rights reserved.
doi:10.3233/978-1-60750-080-3-82

Propulsion effectiveness of synchronous handcycling

S. VAN DRONGELEN[a,1], U. ARNET[a], L.H.V. VAN DER WOUDE[b],
H.E.J. VEEGER[c]

[a] *Swiss Paraplegic Research, Nottwil, Switzerland*
[b] *Centre for Human Movement Sciences, University Medical Centre Groningen,
Groningen, The Netherlands*
[c] *Research Institute MOVE, IFKB, VU University, Amsterdam, The Netherlands*

Abstract. The purpose of this study was to evaluate the effectiveness of force application during submaximal handcycling. In a laboratory subjects propelled a kinetics-instrumented handcycle on a treadmill at 3 different speeds, while power output was kept constant at 35 W by a pulley system. Mean fraction of effective force (FEF) was between 79 and 83 % and significantly influenced by the velocity. For 6 subjects a pattern of FEF was found showing an average FEF above 80 % between -7° and 100° and between 205° and 310° of the crank rotation, where at 0° the crank is pointing towards the subject. It still has to be studied whether FEF and mechanical efficiency are related. A linked segment model analysis will be necessary to study the effect of gravity on the applied forces and joint torques.

Keywords. handcycling, force production, effectiveness, able-bodied.

1. Introduction

In addition to the mechanical load on the upper extremities and the mechanical efficiency of handbike propulsion, the effectiveness of force application is a significant factor to evaluate the benefits of the handbike. Veeger et al. introduced the fraction of effective force (FEF) to describe how effective the forces are applied to the handrim in wheelchair propulsion [1]. During wheelchair propulsion, there is only a small period of time (20-40% of the cycle) in which force is applied to the rim, which is within the push angle. The force is directed more downwards and not in the mechanically optimal tangential direction. This downward directed force is associated with functional-anatomical constraints of the upper body segments in the guided hand rim propulsion motion [2].

From previous research it is known that during cycling an effective force is applied only for a limited time [3]. Only the downward phase is effective, in the upward phase the leg is moved by the contra lateral leg. Handcycling is also a cyclic movement but little to nothing is known about the force application. It is likely that force is produced over the major part of the cycle, although initial research in asynchronous handcycling shows that the FEF may again be low [4].

The purpose of this study was to evaluate the effectiveness of force application during submaximal synchronous handcycling.

---

[1] Corresponding Author: Stefan van Drongelen, Swiss Paraplegic Research, Guido A. Zächstrasse 4, CH-6207, Nottwil, Switzerland. E-mail: stefan.vandrongelen@paranet.ch

2.　Methods

Subjects and protocol

Ten able-bodied male subjects participated in this study after having given written informed consent. The subjects had the following characteristics (mean ± SD): age 30 ± 4 years, height 1.77 ± 0.06 m and body mass 75 ± 9 kg. All subjects were non-experienced handbike users. The study protocol was approved by the local medical ethics committee.

The subjects were asked to propel a kinetics-instrumented handbike on a level treadmill at a velocity of 1.39, 1.67 and 1.94 ms^{-1} for one minute. Power output was kept constant at 35 W by means of a pulley system for all conditions [5]. The applied forces were measured during the last 30 seconds of each exercise bout.

Data analysis and statistical analysis

Forces were corrected for the orientation of the handgrip and expressed as radial and tangential force. Fraction of effective force (FEF) was calculated per cycle as the ratio between the mean tangential force and the mean total force. Variables were calculated as mean over all the complete cycles in the last 30 seconds of the exercise bout.

A one-factor repeated measures ANOVA was performed to evaluate the effect of velocity on forces and FEF. Level of significance was set at $p < 0.05$.

3.　Results

When propelling at 1.94 ms^{-1}, the resistance was sometimes not high enough, causing the crank to slip. The data were therefore not reliable and not used in the data analysis.

Mean calculated power output was 31.7 ± 2.4 W. The mean FEF was 83.0 ± 4.8 % for 1.39 ms^{-1} and 79.2 ± 5.8 % for propelling at 1.67 ms^{-1}. Velocity had a significant effect on total force, effective force and FEF ($p < 0.001$).

Preliminary analysis of the data showed that six of the ten subjects showed a consistent pattern of FEF over the 2 speeds. In this pattern the FEF was on average higher than 80 % between -7° and 100° and between 205° and 310° where at 0° the crank is pointing towards the subject (Figures 1 and 2).

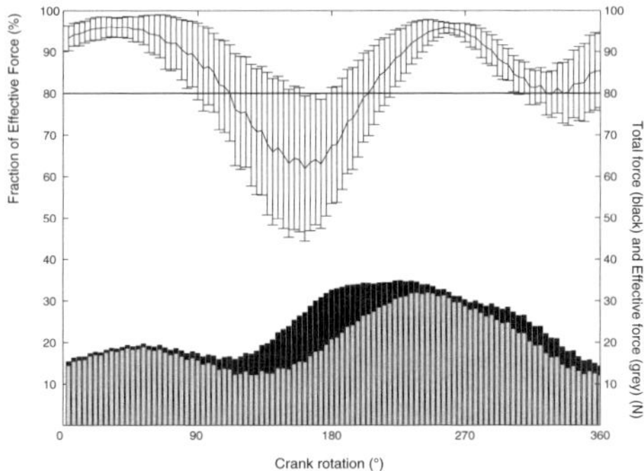

Figure 1. Mean pattern (n=6) plus standard deviation of the fraction of effective force for handbiking at 1.39 ms^{-1}. Mean patterns of the total force and effective force (= tangential force) are plotted at the bottom.

4.   Discussion and conclusion

The decline of FEF with velocity was also found in wheelchair propulsion [6] and might be related to the less optimal coordination and direction of forces with higher velocities.

The FEF values were in the range of the FEF values found for able-bodied subjects propelling a wheelchair. However in wheelchair propulsion there is less time to exert force (only 20-40% of the cycle), besides force has to be applied to a moving handrim. It is suggested that in part therefore the mechanical efficiency (ME) is low in wheelchair propulsion. The relationship between FEF and ME in handbiking has to be studied.

The pattern of FEF for the 6 subjects showed an expected pattern with an effective push and pull phase and transitions from pushing to pulling around 0° and 145°. The overall FEF of approximately 80% appears relatively high, compared to wheelchair propulsion. The effect of gravity should, however, be taken into account to be able to judge the applied forces and joint torques. To this end a linked segment model analysis will be necessary.

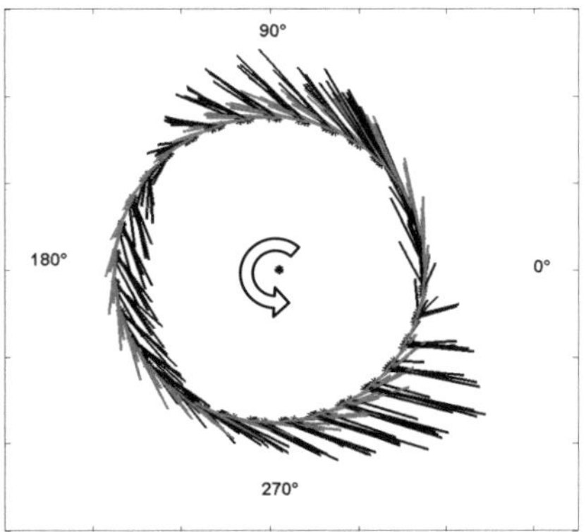

Figure 2. Total force (black) and effective force (grey) around the crank. The arrow indicates the direction of rotation. Subject sitting at the right, at 0° the crank is pointing towards the subject.

References

[1]   H.E.J. Veeger et al., Load on the upper extremity in manual wheelchair propulsion, *J Electromyogr Kinesiol* **1** (1991), 270-2 80.
[2]   L.A. Rozendaal et al., The push force pattern in manual wheelchair propulsion as a balance between cost and effect, *J Biomech* **36** (2003), 239-247.
[3]   M.O. Ericson et al., Efficiency of pedal forces during ergometer cycling, *Int J Sports Med* **9** (1988), 118-122.
[4]   H. Abbasi Bafghi et al., Biophysical aspects of submaximal hand cycling, *Int J Sports Med* **29** (2008), 630-638.
[5]   L.H.V. van der Woude, Peak power production in wheelchair propulsion, *Clin J Sport Med* **4** (1994), 14-24.
[6]   H.E.J. Veeger et al., Effect of handrim velocity on mechanical efficiency in wheelchair propulsion, *Med Sci Sports Exerc* **24** (1992), 100-7.

Rehabilitation: Mobility, Exercise and Sports
L.H.V. van der Woude et al. (Eds.)
IOS Press, 2010

doi:10.3233/978-1-60750-080-3-85

The power balance model: Useful in the study of elite handcycling performance

W.G. GROEN, L.H.V. VAN DER WOUDE[b], J.J. DE KONING[a]

[a] *Faculty of Human Movement Sciences, Research Institute MOVE, VU University, Amsterdam, The Netherlands*
[b] *Centre for Human Movement Sciences, University Medical Centre Groningen, University of Groningen, The Netherlands*

Abstract. Purpose: To apply the power balance model to elite handcycling, to obtain realistic values for power output and power losses on a range of regular velocities on a treadmill and on a track in association to the physiological responses under these conditions. Methods: Four elite Dutch handcyclists rode at three intensities (~70, 85 and 100% of estimated peak race-power output) in a standardized instrumented handcycle, both on a treadmill and on an indoor cycling track (250m). Biomechanical and physiological data were obtained. Results: VO_2 on the treadmill ranged from 1661 to 2825 mL·min^{-1} at 98 and 167 W respectively. VO_2 on the track ranged from 1356 to 2555 mL·min^{-1} at 102 and 168 W respectively. The empirically derived relationship between velocity and power output on the track was: $PO=0.20v^3+2.90v$ ($R^2=0.95$). Mean gross mechanical efficiency during submaximal performance was 16.0 ± 2.1 on the treadmill and 18.8 ± 2.6 on the track ($p=0.12$). Conclusion: Handcycling is a relatively efficient mode of propulsion with associated high metabolic demand at race velocities. The power balance model enabled simulation of realistic power conditions on a treadmill. In addition, it gained insight into the magnitude of power dissipation during elite handcycling.

Keywords. handcycling, power balance model, mechanical efficiency

1. Introduction

One way to study cyclic human (sports) performance is with the use of a Power Balance Model (PBM) as proposed by Van Ingen Schenau [1]. This model has proven to allow predictions of performance in various cyclic activities such as cycling, running and speed skating. Furthermore, the model has proven to be an effective tool to uncover the performance determining factors in speed skating [2] as well as finding optimal pacing strategies in track cycling [3]. The approach of the PBM appears to be highly appropriate in the study of hand rim wheelchair propulsion [4], although limited data specific to the applicability of the PBM to handcycling are available.

The aim of this study was to model performance in elite handcyclists under lab as well as track conditions using the PBM. This would provide indicators of mechanical constraints (air friction, rolling friction) of submaximal as well as peak performance handcycling, generate a better understanding of the concomitant metabolic cost and mechanical efficiency in elite handcycling, and demonstrate the applicability of the PBM to handcycling.

2.   Methods

Four elite Dutch subjects rode five minutes at ~70, 85 and 100% of estimated race-power output in a standardized instrumented handcycle, both on a treadmill (Bonte, The Netherlands) and an indoor cycling track (250m).

The PBM was used to calculate power output (PO) for each treadmill trial. Three input parameters for these calculations were required: 1) self reported race velocity, 2) empirically derived frontal area, and 3) rolling frictional force. Consequently 70 and 85% of race PO could be calculated.

Treadmill speed was limited for safety reasons. Therefore, drag force on the treadmill was limited to rolling friction and internal friction. The difference in calculated PO and actual PO on the treadmill was accounted for by applying an extra pulling force by a pulley system [5]. For the track sessions, predicted PO was calculated back to real world velocities by using the PBM.

PO, velocity (v) and heart rate (HR) were measured with a special hub (Powertap). Metabolic (VO_2, VCO_2 and RER) and respiratory data (VE) were measured continuously with a portable system (Cosmed K4b^2, Italy). Mean values of minutes 3 to 5 of each exercise level (steady-state) were used for analysis.

Gross mechanical efficiency (GME) for submaximal intensities was calculated by dividing the external power by the metabolic power.

3.   Results

VO_2 on the treadmill ranged from 1661 to 2825 mL·min^{-1} at a PO of 98 and 167 W respectively. VO_2 on the track ranged from 1356 to 2555 mL·min^{-1} at 102 and 168 W respectively. HR on the treadmill ranged from 107 to 163 b·min^{-1} at 98 and 167 W respectively. HR on the track ranged from 113 to 182 b·min^{-1} at 105 and 168 W respectively. HR showed a linear increase with increasing PO and did not differ significantly between track and treadmill.

VE on the treadmill ranged from 45 to 100 L·min^{-1} at 80 and 167 W respectively. VE on the track ranged from 48 to 144 L·min^{-1} at 87 and 168 W respectively. VE shows a non-linear increase with increasing PO and did not differ significantly between track and treadmill.

RER on the treadmill ranged from 0.88 to 1.06 at 96 and 132 W   respectively. RER on the track ranged from 0.94 to 1.22 at 105 and 131 W respectively. RER increases linear with increasing PO and did not differ significantly between track and treadmill.

The empirically derived relationship between PO and velocity on the track was: $PO=0.20v^3+2.90v$ ($R^2=0.95$). Furthermore mean GME during submaximal performance was 16.0 ± 2.1 on the treadmill and 18.8 ± 2.6 on the track (p=0.12).

4.   Discussion and conclusion

Based on the results from this investigation, the PBM for handcycling can be described as: $PO = 0.20v^3+2.90v$, in which 0.20 represents the air friction constant and 2.90 represents the rolling friction force. The estimated PO by the model was replicated nicely on the treadmill with the help of a pulley system that provided an external force. This is illustrated by the linear regression $y=0.97x-2.4$ ($R^2=0.85$). The relationship between velocity and PO in elite handcycling has to our knowledge, never been reported before.

Handcycling is a relatively efficient mode of upper body propulsion with associated high metabolic demand at race velocities. The PBM enabled simulation of realistic power conditions on a treadmill. In addition, it gained insight into the magnitude of power dissipation during elite handcycling.

References

[1]   G. J. van Ingen Schenau, P.R. Cavanagh. Power equations in endurance sports. *J Biomech.* **23** (1990), 865-881.

[2]   J.J. de Koning, C. Foster, J. Lampen, F. Hettinga, M.F. Bobbert. Experimental evaluation of the power balance model of speed skating. *Journal of Applied Physiology* **98** (1) (2005), 227-33.

[3]   J. J. de Koning, M.F. Bobbert, C. Foster. Determination of optimal pacing strategy in track cycling with an energy flow model. *J Sci Med Sport.* **2** (1999), 266-277

[4]   L.H.V. van der Woude, A..J. Dallmeijer, T.W.J. Janssen, D. Veeger. Alternative modes of manual wheelchair ambulation: an overview. *Am J Phys Med Rehabil.* **80** (2001), 765-777

[5]   D. Veeger, , L. H. V. van der Woude, R.H. Rozendal. The effect of rear wheel camber in manual wheelchair propulsion. *J Rehabil Res Dev.* **26** (1989), 37-46.

2.2

Poster Presentations

Rehabilitation: Mobility, Exercise and Sports
L.H.V. van der Woude et al. (Eds.)
IOS Press, 2010
© 2010 The authors and IOS Press. All rights reserved.
doi:10.3233/978-1-60750-080-3-91

The Figure Eight Drive: A two-speed drivetrain for handcycles in the developing world

M. BOLLINI[a,1]

[a]*Department of Mechanical Engineering, Massachusetts Institute of Technology,
Cambridge, MA 02142*

Abstract. The Figure-Eight Drive is a novel handcycle drivetrain designed
specifically for the developing world. Utilizing a retro-direct chain configuration,
the system offers users two forward motion gear ratios that can be switched
between by changing the direction of pedaling. Movement in the reverse direction
can be achieved by rotating the steering column 180 degrees. The drivetrain was
designed at the Massachusetts of Institute of Technology and was successfully
implemented and tested during the summer of 2007 at the Association for the
Physically Disabled of Kenya in Nairobi, Kenya, where it is now in production.
The Figure-Eight Drive can be constructed entirely out of conventional bicycle
components already found on handcycles across the developing world. It has been
well received by handcycle users and manufacturers because of its simplicity, low-
cost, and significant improvement in mobility and usability compared to current
single speed and derailleur handcycles currently in production.

Keywords. handcycles, developing countries, mobility.

1. Introduction

While wheelchairs are ubiquitous in the western world, they are biomechanically
inefficient [1] and are difficult to operate over rough terrain and long distances. Instead
of wheelchairs, the disabled in developing countries frequently use locally designed
and manufactured handcycles as their primary means of ambulation. While these
handcycles offer a significant biomechanical advantage over wheelchairs, they are
frequently available only in single-speed configurations. This single gear makes it
impossible for users to navigate hilly terrain. While multi-geared systems that make use
of bicycle derailleurs are available, these systems are uncommon because they are
expensive, fragile, and difficult to use while using the arms to pedal and steer. The
Figure-Eight Drive is an implementation of a retro-direct bicycle drivetrain that allows
users to change between two gears, one high and one low, simply by changing the
direction of their pedaling. Both directions result in forward motion, providing users
with a simple and robust two-speed drivetrain.

---

[1] Corresponding Author: Mario Bollini, mbollini@mit.edu

2. Design

The Figure-Eight Drive was designed during the spring of 2007 at the Massachusetts Institute of Technology by the biomechanics group of the class Wheelchair Design for Developing Countries. The system utilizes two bicycle chains, one in a loop such as a chain found on standard single speed handcycles and another in a figure-eight loop on the opposite side of the steering column. The chain in the standard loop (henceforth to be referred to as the O-side chain) is looped around a bicycle crank at the top of drivetrain, and around a standard freewheel at the bottom wheel hub. The figure-eight chain (henceforth to be referred to as the 8-side chain) is looped around a reverse-mounted freewheel at the top of the drivetrain near the pedals, and around a forwards-mounted freewheel at the bottom wheel hub. The slack side of the 8-side chain is passed through a steel tube to prevent it from grinding against the return chain. Figure 1 shows the chain and freewheel configurations.

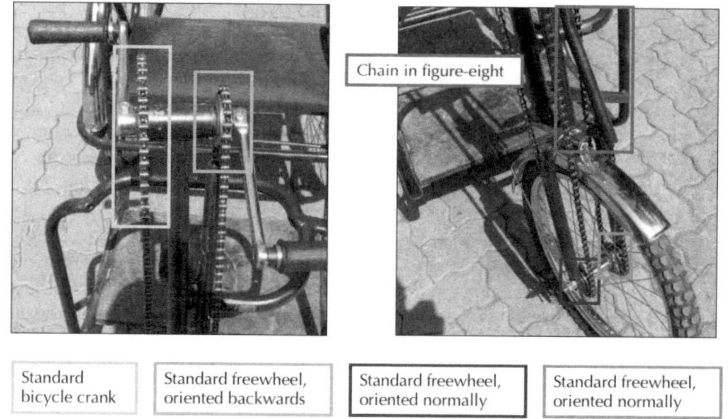

Figure 1. The freewheel mounted at the top of the 8-side chain near the pedals is in the reverse direction, while both freewheels near the wheel are in the forwards direction. The chain on the right hand side of the image, the 8-side chain, is in a figure-eight loop.

When pedaling forwards, the O-side chain engages, driving the tricycle forwards just as it would on a single-speed handcycle. The freewheel at the top of the 8-side chain ratchets and does not engage, leaving the 8-side chain stationary. This is the high gear of the Figure-Eight Drive. When pedaling backwards, the O-side chain freewheels, just as one's bicycle chain freewheels when one pedals backwards on bicycle. The freewheel on the top of the 8-side chain, however, engages and drives the 8-side chain backwards. Because this chain is in a figure-eight loop, the backwards motion of the chain drives the handcycle forwards. This is the low gear of the Figure-Eight Drive. Thus the drivetrain offers users one high and one low gear, switch able between simply by changing the direction of pedaling.

While the two chain solution allows users to ambulate and coast in the forward direction, the chains lock when the drive wheel rotates backwards, meaning that users cannot move in the reverse direction. Though this is convenient in that one can remove one's hands from the pedals while climbing without fear of rolling backwards down the hill, it dramatically reduces the mobility of the handcycle. In order to allow users to move their handcycles in reverse, the fork was designed to allow the steering column to be rotated 180 degrees, allowing users to both freewheel and ambulate backwards.

3. Development and testing

A proof-of-concept prototype was constructed at MIT in order to validate the design. During the summer of 2007, the author traveled to Nairobi, Kenya to implement and test the drivetrain at the Association of the Physically Disabled of Kenya (APDK). The prototype was developed through four generations. The final version of the prototype was constructed entirely out of stock bicycle components and required no machined parts, adding approximately $3 to the $200 cost APDK's existing single-speed handcycle.

The prototype was tested by numerous handcycle users on and around the APDK campus. It was preferred over existing single and multiple speed derailleur based handcycles for its ease of use and its wide gear ratio range, which allowed users to both travel quickly over flat terrain and to climb hills easily. The ability of the handcycle to move in reverse via the pedal-drivetrain was also appreciated by handcycle users. In addition on on-site testing, four models of the final Figure Eight Drive prototype were constructed and given to handcycle users for long duration usability and durability testing. After over six months of use, no negative feedback was received.

4. Results and conclusion

In September of 2007, APDK presented the Figure-Eight Drive at the Pan African Wheelchair Congress in Arusha, Tanzania. It was extremely well received; over 100 compact disks containing manufacturing instructions were distributed to interested African wheelchair and handcycle manufacturers. The Figure-Eight Drive has also been manufactured locally Tanzania and the Philippines. The Figure-Eight Drive is currently being produced and sold in Kenya by APDK.

The Figure-Eight Drive has proven to be an effective replacement for both single and multi geared handcycle systems. It allows users to travel over terrain that is impossible to traverse with single speed handcycles. It is cheaper to manufacture, easier to use, and significantly more robust than current derailleur based handcycles. User feedback continues to be extremely positive, demonstrating the system's ability to meet user needs better than current systems. The Figure-Eight Drive is constructed using materials and manufacturing techniques that are ubiquitous across the developing world, making it an accessible mobility solution for handcycle users worldwide.

References

[1]   L.H.V. van der Woude et al., Wheelchair ergonomics and physiological testing of prototypes, *Ergonomics* **12** (1986), 1561-1573.

Rehabilitation: Mobility, Exercise and Sports
L.H.V. van der Woude et al. (Eds.)
IOS Press, 2010
© 2010 The authors and IOS Press. All rights reserved.
doi:10.3233/978-1-60750-080-3-94

Lower limb skin blood flow and calf volume changes during continuous and intermittent upper body exercise

M. PRICE[a,1], R. BHOGAL[a], C.D. THAKE[a], L.M. BOTTOMS[b]
[a] *Faculty of Health and Life Sciences, Coventry University, Coventry, UK*
[b] *Faculty of Science and Technology, University of Central Lancashire, Preston, UK*

Abstract. Purpose: To determine the changes in thigh and calf skin blood flow during continuous and intermittent upper body exercise. Methods: Eight healthy able-bodied males undertook a preliminary incremental arm crank ergometry (ACE) test to volitional exhaustion and two experimental trials. Experimental trials consisted of either 28 min of continuous ACE at 50% peak power (CON) or 28 min intermittent exercise (INT) involving alternating 2 min bouts of ACE at 25% and 75% peak power. Changes in skin blood flow were measured by Laser Doppler techniques. Changes in calf volume were measured by strain gauge plethysmography. Heart rate and expired gas were continuously monitored. Aural and skin temperatures were measured. Results: Calf volume decreased in both trials, decreasing to a greater extent during INT (P<0.05). Changes in skin blood flow of the thigh and calf demonstrated intensity dependent increases during INT whereas a more steady state increase was observed during CON. There were no differences in aural temperature between trials. Calf skin temperature decreased in both trials and to a greater extent during INT. Conclusions: Increases in skin blood flow occur concurrently with a decrease in calf volume. Additionally, changes in skin blood flow appear to change rapidly with changes in exercise intensity.

Keywords. calf blood flow, aural temperature.

1. Introduction

Calf volume has been shown to decrease during continuous steady state arm crank ergometry in able-bodied individuals.[1] However, this response is much reduced in persons with paraplegia due to the loss of sympathetic nervous system induced vasoconstriction and blood redistribution from the lower limb.[1] The cause of this residual vasconstriction may possibly include humoral agents and muscle metaboreflexes. This is consistent with Sinoway et al. [2] and Seals [3] who suggested that vasoconstriction in non exercising muscles was a result of muscle metaboreflexes. For example, Sinoway et al.[2] observed a correlation between calf muscle pH and vasoconstriction following isometric hand grip exercise.

Lower body intermittent exercise demonstrates greater blood lactate concentrations when compared to continuous lower body exercise matched for energy expenditure. [4] It is likely, but not yet reported, that this would also occur for upper body exercise.

---

[1] Corresponding Author: Michael J. Price, Faculty of Health and Life Sciences, James Starley Building, Coventry University, Coventry, CV1 5FB; mike.price@coventry.ac.uk.

Greater acidosis of the circulating blood during intermittent arm exercise may subsequently affect pH and blood flow in non exercising muscle contributing to the stimulus for muscle metaboreflexes. This may result in greater lower limb vasoconstriction during intermittent when compared to continuous upper body exercise. Therefore the aim of this study was to determine skin blood flow responses and volume changes of the calf during intermittent and continuous upper body exercise.

2.　Method

Eight healthy able-bodied males (age: 22.8 ±1.8 yrs; body mass: 75.5 ±11.2 kg) undertook a preliminary incremental arm crank ergometry (ACE) test to volitional exhaustion (initial intensity 50W, followed by 20W. 2 min^{-1}, 70 $rev.min^{-1}$) and two experimental trials. Experimental trials consisted of either 28 min of continuous ACE at 50% peak power (CON) or 28 min intermittent ACE (INT) involving alternating 2 min bouts of 25% and 75% peak power. Changes in skin blood flow at the thigh (SBF_{Thigh}) and calf (SBF_{Calf}) were measured by Laser Doppler techniques (Moor Instruments). Changes in calf volume were measured by strain gauge plethysmography (Hokanssen). Heart rate (HR; Polar monitor) and expired gas (Cosmed K4) were continuously monitored. Blood lactate (Biosen) was measured from an earlobe at rest and 5, 13 and 25 min of exercise. Laser doppler, plethysmography, HR and expired gas data were averaged over the last 15 s of each 2 min exercise bout. Aural and skin (arm, chest, thigh, calf) temperatures were recorded every minute (Grant Instruments). All data were analysed via two-way ANOVA with repeated measures (trial × time).

3.　Results

Peak oxygen uptake and peak power output for the group were 2.30 ±0.40 $L.min^{-1}$ and peak power output; 144 ±13W, respectively. Significant differences were observed for heart rate and oxygen consumption during each trial. Heart rate fluctuated with exercise intensity during INT (146 ±13 to 174 ±11 $beats.min^{-1}$) as did oxygen consumption (1.29 ±0.15 to 1.89 ±0.23 $L.min^{-1}$). Both variables reached steady state during CON (153 ±15 $beats.min^{-1}$ and 1.47 ±0.24 $L.min^{-1}$ at 28 min, respectively). A significant interaction was observed for blood lactate with greater values during INT (8.1 ±1.7 $mmol.L^{-1}$) than CON (5.5 ±1.8 $mmol.L^{-1}$) at 25 min (P<0.05). Aural temperature increased by similar, although significantly different, amounts during CON (0.74 ±0.34°C) than INT (0.60 ±0.37°C; P<0.05). Arm skin temperature was greater during INT (main effect for group; P<0.05) and calf skin temperature decreased to a greater extent during INT than CON (P<0.05). No other thermoregulatory differences were observed. A significant interaction was observed for changes in calf volume with both trials demonstrating a decrease in volume during exercise. A greater decrease was observed during INT (-1.96 ±1.03 %) than CON (-1.50 ±0.60 % at 28 min; P<0.05). Significant main effects for trial were observed for SBF_{Thigh} and SBF_{Calf} (Figure 1; P<0.05) with greater increases during CON for SBF_{Calf} and greater values during INT for SBF_{Thigh}. Values for both sites fluctuated with intensity during INT.

4.　Discussion

All physiological variables, except aural temperature, indicate the INT trial elicited a greater physiological strain than CON for the same total external work done. This most likely represents differences in exercise intensity and subsequent fuel utilization and predominant energy systems during INT as observed for lower body exercise.[4]

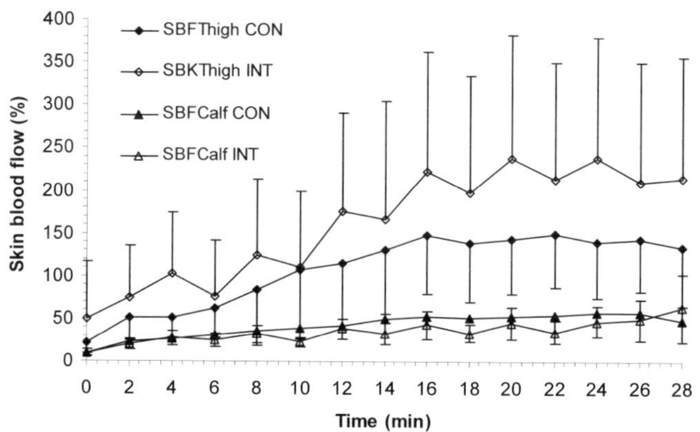

Figure 1. Changes in skin blood flow during continuous and intermittent upper body exercise.

The decrease in calf volume is similar to that observed previously for 10 minutes of exercise at 50% maximal power output and reflects sympathetically induced vasoconstriction in the lower limb.[1] However, the decrease in calf volume was greater during INT for the last half of the exercise protocol when compared to CON suggesting that changes may somehow be related to the greater intensities encountered during INT. This was also reflected in the calf skin temperature values being cooler during INT than CON. It is possible that greater acidosis of the circulating blood during INT may have contributed to and accentuated metaboreflexes within the non exercising muscle of the leg.

Skin blood flow for the thigh and calf demonstrated intensity dependent changes with exercise intensity. However, in contrast to the calf volume changes skin blood flow changes demonstrated increases rather than decreases throughout exercise. The calf volume decrease may therefore be due to blood redistribution away from non exercising muscle to aid cardiovascular stability during exercise which is greater than the increase in SBF_{Calf} resulting in calf volume remaining at a reduced level.

These results have provided an able-bodied model of calf haemodynamics which may have important implications for populations with reduced vascular control in the lower limb during upper body exercise.

References

[1] M.T. Hopman, P.H. Verheijrn, R.A. Binkhorst, Volume changes in the legs of paraplegic subjects during arm exercise, *Journal of Applied Physiology* **75** (1993), 2079–2083.

[2] L. Sinoway, S. Prophet, I. Gorman, T. Mosher, J. Shenberger, M. Dolecki, R. Briggs, R. Zelis, Muscle acidosis during static exercise is associated with calf vasoconstriction, *Journal of Applied Physiology* **66** (1989), 428-436.

[3] D.R. Seals, Sympathetic neural discharge and vascular resistance during exercise in humans, *Journal of Applied Physiology* **66** (1989), 2472-2478.

[4] M.A. Christmass, B. Dawson, P. Passeretto, P.G. Arthur, A comparison of skeletal muscle oxygenation and fuel use in sustained intermittent and continuous exercise, *European Journal of Applied Physiology* **80** (1999), 423-435.

Chapter 3

Prosthetics and Orthotics Gait

3.1

Keynote

Rehabilitation: Mobility, Exercise and Sports
L.H.V. van der Woude et al. (Eds.)
IOS Press, 2010
© *2010 The authors and IOS Press. All rights reserved.*
doi:10.3233/978-1-60750-080-3-99

Roll-over shape as a tool for design, alignment, and evaluation of ankle-foot prostheses and orthoses

A.H. HANSEN[a,b,1], D.S. CHILDRESS[b]
[a] *Jesse Brown VA Medical Center, Chicago, Illinois USA*
[b] *Northwestern University Prosthetics Research Laboratory and
Rehabilitation Engineering Research Program, Chicago, Illinois USA*

Abstract. The effective rocker shapes created by able-bodied (human) lower limb systems (roll-over shapes) have been useful for understanding lower limb function in walking. This paper describes the effects of walking speed, shoe heel height, added weight attached to the trunk, and shoe rocker radius on the characteristics of the physiologically produced roll-over shapes. In general, we have found that the able-bodied human responds to various conditions of level walking to maintain the same invariant roll-over shape. Able-bodied lower limb roll-over shapes measured during ramp walking are rotated in ways that could be mimicked using changes in equilibrium point (alignment) of prosthetic and orthotic components. New systems are becoming available and others are being developed to automatically adapt to different ramp surfaces. More research is needed to demonstrate the likely biomechanical benefits of these adaptable systems to their users.

Keywords. rocker, cam, artificial limb, prosthetics, orthotics, ramp walking.

1. Introduction

Rockers have been used by many investigators to describe aspects of walking. Perry [1] described the actions of the foot and ankle during walking as a series of three rockers. Others have used rockers in mathematical and physical models of walking [2-6]. The rocker is an attractive model because of its simplicity and close similarity to actual function during a large period of the gait cycle (namely foot contact to opposite foot contact). In this short paper, we describe the results of many studies involving direct measurement of physiologic effective rockers, or ***roll-over shapes***, used by able-bodied persons during walking. We also describe the clinical uses of these results to date, including design, alignment, and evaluation of prosthetic and orthotic systems.

Roll-over shapes are measured by transforming the center of pressure (CoP) of the ground reaction force into a shank- or leg-based coordinate system. CoP data transformed into the shank-based coordinates are called ankle-foot roll-over shapes, while those transformed into leg-based coordinates are called knee-ankle-foot roll-over shapes [7]. Generally speaking, these two shapes are similar for level walking and both are closely approximated using a circular arc model. Results described in this paper refer mainly to the knee-ankle-foot roll-over shapes.

---

[1] Corresponding Author.

2. Invariance of roll-over shapes for level walking conditions

We have conducted a series of experiments on able-bodied persons to gain an understanding of the roll-over shape under clinically relevant conditions. In general, we have found that the roll-over shape does not change appreciably as persons walk faster or slower [7], as they walk carrying weight attached to their trunk [8], or as they wear shoes of different heel heights [9]. Additionally, we are currently conducting a study that illustrates a significant response of the human ankle to different shoe rockers in order to keep the ankle-foot-shoe roll-over shape invariant. The invariance of the roll-over shape suggests that this shape may provide some biomechanical benefit during walking. Additionally, the invariant roll-over shape serves as a convenient constraint for design, alignment, and evaluation of prosthetic and orthotic components.

3. Clinical uses of roll-over shape invariance

We have utilized the invariant roll-over shape to design an inexpensive yet highly functional prosthetic foot called the Shape&Roll Prosthetic Foot [10]. This foot deforms to the appropriate (biomimetic) roll-over shape for its user via a series of flexural hinges that are created by simple saw cuts in the component's forefoot section.

The invariant roll-over shape appears to be a goal of the transtibial prosthesis alignment process in the sagittal plane. Prosthetic feet with widely different mechanical characteristics are aligned by skilled prosthetists in a way that "nests" their individual shapes closely together [11]. This finding may explain why many gait studies of different kinds of prosthetic feet have not found many consistent differences between feet. Prosthetists may have "aligned away" the differences between the prosthetic feet used in many of these studies.

Roll-over shape arc length has been shown to be an important feature of prosthetic feet, particularly when persons walk at normal and fast speeds. Prosthetic feet with short arc lengths tend to provide their user with a "drop-off" effect in late stance phase, which leads to an increase in initial contralateral limb loading. This finding also appears to explain the results of previous studies that have reported increases in initial contralateral limb loading [12]. Lastly, ankle-foot orthoses have been shown to improve the roll-over shape characteristics of persons with hemiplegia [13].

4. Rotated roll-over shapes for ramp walking

The knee-ankle-foot roll-over shape changes orientation on up- and down-hill slopes compared with the invariant level roll-over shape [14]. On up-hill grades, the roll-over shape "dorsiflexes," while on down-hill grades, the roll-over shape "plantarflexes." These changes are logical and necessary for providing the body an upright and balanced posture on these surfaces. However, they also indicate a major area in which current prosthetic and orthotic components are lacking. The rotated roll-over shapes for ramp walking could be mimicked by automatic changes in prosthesis or orthosis alignment. Few commercially available systems have achieved this function in the past. The Mauch and Habermann ankles used damping control to roughly mimic a changing equilibrium point. Although both designs were ahead of their time, neither system became a successful commercial product.

5.　Automatically adapting prosthetic components

Many currently available ankle-foot systems are flexible, but not adaptable. Only a few commercially available systems claim to adapt to different slopes. Research studies of these components are needed to investigate the effectiveness and clinical impact of their different approaches to adaptability. Our group has also worked on this problem, developing a design concept and prototypes for an ankle-foot system that automatically adapts to different surface inclination on each and every step using two stiffness modes and a floating equilibrium point [15]. In early stance, prior to foot flat, our system is in a low stiffness mode and allows the foot to "find" the walking surface. At foot flat, the system changes into a higher stiffness mode and sets the equilibrium point of the ankle. The switching of stiffness modes at foot flat allows for a more "dorsiflexed" alignment during uphill walking and a more "plantarflexed" alignment during downhill walking. A strength of the current system is its completely passive nature (i.e., no motors are batteries are needed). However, more work is needed to make this system more robust.

Significant design challenges exist to transfer our growing understanding of ankle-foot biomechanics into simple and practical devices for persons with disabilities. Designs should address the specific needs of persons with disabilities at various functional levels. For example, lightweight and inherently stable devices may be best for prosthesis users in the lowest functional levels, while automatically adapting and/or powered ankle-foot systems [16] may be best for more active prosthesis users.

References

[1]　J. Perry, *Gait Analysis: Normal and Pathological Function*, Slack Inc., Thorofare, 1992.

[2]　J. Morawski and I. Wojcieszak, Miniwalker – a resonant model of human locomotion, Biomechanics VIA, E. Asmussen, K. Jorgensen, University Park Press, Baltimore, 2A (1978), 445-451.

[3]　T. McGeer, Passive dynamic walking, *International Journal of Robotics Research* **9** (1990), 62-82.

[4]　S. Collins et al., Efficient bipedal robots based on passive-dynamic walkers, *Science* **307** (2005), 1082-1085.

[5]　M. Ju, The modeling and simulation of constrained dynamical systems with application to human gait, PhD thesis, Case Western Reserve University, Cleveland, 1986.

[6]　B. Koopman, The three-dimensional analysis and prediction of human walking, PhD thesis, University of Twente, The Netherlands, 1989.

[7]　A.H. Hansen et al., Roll-over shapes of human locomotor systems: effects of walking speed, *Clinical Biomechanics* **19** (2004), 407-414.

[8]　A.H. Hansen and D.S. Childress, Effects of adding weight to the torso on roll-over characteristics of walking, *Journal of Rehabilitation Research and Development* **42** (2005), 381-390.

[9]　A.H. Hansen and D.S. Childress, Effects of shoe heel height on biologic roll-over characteristics during walking, *Journal of Rehabilitation Research and Development* **41** (2004), 547-554.

[10]　M. Sam et al., The Shape&Roll prosthetic foot (part I): Design and development of appropriate technology for low-income countries, *Medicine Conflict and Survival* **20** (2004), 294-306.

[11]　A.H. Hansen et al., Alignmentn of transtibial prostheses based on roll-over shape, *Prosthetics and Orthotics International* **27** (2003), 89-99.

[12]　C.M. Powers et al., Influence of prosthetic foot design on sound limb loading in adults with unilateral below-knee amputations, *Archives of Physical Medicine and Rehabilitation* **75** (1994), 825-829.

[13]　S. Fatone and A.H. Hansen, Effect of an ankle foot orthosis on roll-over shape in adults with hemiplegia, *Journal of Rehabilitation Research and Development* **44** (2007), 11-20.

[14]　A.H. Hansen et al., Roll-over characteristics of human walking on inclined surfaces, *Human Movement Science* **23** (2004), 807-821.

[15]　R.J. Williams et al. Prosthetic ankle-foot mechanism capable of automatic adaptation to the walking surface, *Journal of Biomechanical Engineering* **131** (2009), 035002:1-7.

[16]　S. Au et al., Powered ankle-foot prosthesis to assist level-ground and stair-descent gaits, *Neural Networks* **21** (2008), 654-666.

3.2

Oral Presentations

Rehabilitation: Mobility, Exercise and Sports
L.H.V. van der Woude et al. (Eds.)
IOS Press, 2010

doi:10.3233/978-1-60750-080-3-105

Stance-time asymmetry: comparison between C-leg users and able-body subjects

M. RAGGI[a], A.G. CUTTI[a], S. LIPPI[a], A. DAVALLI[a]
[a]*INAIL Prostheses Centre, Vigorso di Budrio, Italy*

Abstract. The stance time symmetry has been assessed on a population of monolateral transfemoral amputees (all C-Leg users) and control subjects through baropodometric insoles. Subjects walked at three self-selected speeds on a daily-living environment for 80m. Results were compared by speed and population, showing both higher asymmetry and variability for the amputees. No relation was found between speed and symmetry.

Keywords. transfemoral amputees, gait symmetry, baropodometric insoles.

1. Introduction

It is well known in clinics that unilateral above knee amputees (AKA) present temporal walking asymmetries, e.g. they tend to spend more time on their sound side, compared to the prosthetic side (stance time symmetry, STS) [1].

Being related to important comorbidities such as low-back pain [2], knee ostheoarthritis and fall-risk [3], the restoration of a physiologic STS is a primary goal of the AKA rehabilitation. Despite the relevance of this topic, only few quantitative data are currently available regarding the AKA temporal asymmetries and their range of variation compared with control subjects; moreover, the populations included in those studies are generally small and do not include C-Leg users. The aim of this study was to start filling this gap of knowledge.

2. Material and Methods

Twenty-six AKA (age: 42±12) were recruited at our institution to participate in the experiment; 15 healthy able-bodied subjects (CTRL, age: 27±2) were also included as control group. All subjects gave their informed consent. All AKA: 1) were fitted with a C-Leg (Otto-Bock, D) 2) had the same mobility level (K3); 3) had completed their training period under the same rehabilitation team; 4) had been using their current prosthesis by at least one month by the time of test; 5) were using energy-storing feet.

Each subject was asked to walk at his/her self-selected comfortable, slow and fast speed (CS, SS, FS) along a 80m straight corridor, wearing baropodometric insoles (PedarX – Novel, D) inside the usual shoes. This experimental setup allowed the measurement of a large number of consecutive gait cycles (generally about 40 per side) in an environment close to the subject's daily life. To assess the mean trial speed, the walking time was measured with a stopwatch. Heel-strikes (toe-offs) were determined when the vertical ground reaction force fell above (below) the 10% of the subject's body weight. For each couple of consecutive gait cycles, indices of symmetry (IoSs) [4] for step, stance and stride times were calculated between the sound and affected side (right and left, for CTRL), as reported below:

- Step IoS = Step time$_{SOUND}$ / Step time$_{AFFECTED}$
- Stance IoS = Stance time$_{SOUND}$ / Stance time$_{AFFECTED}$
- Stride IoS = Stride time$_{SOUND}$ / Stride time$_{AFFECTED}$

For each subject and for each speed, the median values of the three IoSs were calculated (MIoSs) and aggregated by speed and population in box & whiskers plots with notches. Within each population, statistically significant differences between step, stance and stride MIoSs were investigated with a non-parametric Kruskal-Wallis test. The Pearson's correlation coefficient was calculated between step and stance MIoSs on the whole dataset.

3. Results and Discussion

The speed ranges for the two populations' trials are shown in Table 1. Step and stance MIoSs are reported in Figure 1 and Table 2, aggregated by trial speed.

Stride MIoS did not differ among the two populations, among the three speeds (all median values and whiskers were equal to 1). Step and stance MIoSs were statistically different between the two populations, for all the three speeds, with AKAs MIoS showing both higher median values and higher variability. Within the same population, MIoSs did not show statistically significant differences among the three speeds. On the whole dataset, step and stance MIoSs did not show statistically significant differences and were found significantly correlated (r = 0.92, CI 95% = 0.89 - 0.95).

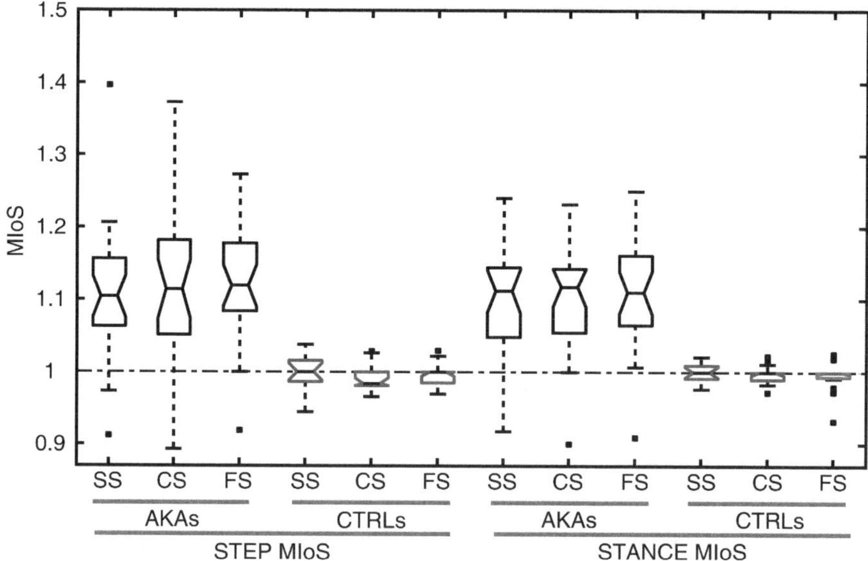

Figure 1: step and stance MIoSs for the AKA and CTRL groups, aggregated by trial speed

Table 1. AKA and CTRL trial speeds' ranges.

Trial speed	AKA speeds range [Km/h]	CTRL speeds range [Km/h]
SS	2.9 - 4.1	3.0 - 4.4
CS	3.3 - 5.4	4.1 - 5.7
FS	4.4 - 6.7	5.5 - 7.2

Table 2. AKA's step and stance MIoSs: median value, 1st and 3rd quartiles, whiskers.

	Trial speed	Median	Q_{1-3}	Whiskers
STEP	SS	1.104	1.063 - 1.157	0.973 - 1.125
	CS	1.114	1.051 - 1.182	0.893 - 1.373
	FS	1.119	1.083 - 1.178	1.000 - 1.273
STANCE	SS	1.112	1.048 - 1.145	0.917 - 1.241
	CS	1.117	1.054 - 1.143	1.000 - 1.232
	FS	1.110	1.065 - 1.161	1.007 - 1.250

4. Conclusion

The AKA and CTRL populations were different in terms of step and stance symmetry; even comparing two speed-matched groups (AKA SS and CTRL SS; AKA FS and CTRL NS) step and stance MIoSs were statistically different. Within the same population, the MIoSs did not significantly change with speed. Inside each population, step and stance MIoSs were found both correlated and not statistically different; this suggests that only one of these two parameters could be monitored in order to assess an amputee's temporal symmetry. In conclusion, despite of the high activity level and the high-end prosthetic components, this AKA population showed a step and stance temporal asymmetry higher than the able-bodied subjects; this suggests that further studies are required to assess which should be the optimal degree of symmetry for each transfemoral amputee.

References

[1] Nolan L, et al., Adjustments in gait symmetry with walking speed in trans-femoral and trans-tibial amputees, *Gait & Posture* **17** *(2003)*. 142-151.

[2] Ehde DM, et al., Back pain as a secondary disability in persons with lower limb amputations, *Arch. Phys. Med. Rehab* **82** (2001), 731-734.

[3] Miller WC, et al., The prevalence and risk factors of falling and fear of falling among lower extremity amputees, *Arch. Phys. Med. Rehab* **82** (2001), 1031-1037.

[4] Andres RO, et al., Prosthetic alignment effects on gait symmetry: a case study, *Clin Biomech.* **5** (1990), 88-96.

Rehabilitation: Mobility, Exercise and Sports
L.H.V. van der Woude et al. (Eds.)
IOS Press, 2010

doi:10.3233/978-1-60750-080-3-108

Walking with above knee prosthesis

T. ERJAVEC[a], M. PREŠERN[a], J. ŠTRUKEL[a]
[a] *Institute for rehabilitation, republic of Slovenia*

Abstract. The paper discusses metabolic and cardiovascular parameters during walking with above-knee prosthesis in patients after amputation due to vascular causes. According to the measured parameters, walking is ranged at the level of moderate physical activities. During walking, non-malignant arrhythmia, asymptomatic ECG criteria for coronary ischemia and especially highly increased blood pressure are frequently observed. Due to long periods of low physical activity before and after the surgery as well as comorbid heart diseases, the risk of proximate cardiac events during gait training and walking with above-knee prosthesis is high. Therefore, accurate evaluation of cardiovascular ability is necessary before prosthetic fitting. At the Institute for Rehabilitation, Republic of Slovenia (IRRS), submaximal stress testing on an. arm ergometer The difference between the calculated oxygen consumption during stress testing and during the 6-minute walk test is not statistically significant.

Keywords. above knee amputation, ambulation, energy cost, heart diseases.

1. Introduction

Amputation is a severe physical and psychical disability. Undoubtedly, every individual having undergone amputation wishes to be fitted and walk with prosthesis as soon as possible. In persons after amputation due to vascular diseases, a number of questions arise. That is especially true of patients with above-knee amputation. Below-knee prosthetic fitting is performed regularly even in very old persons. The energy cost of walking is low, the prosthesis offers support and decreases the risk of fall.

In above-knee prosthetic fitting of vascular patients, special consideration should be given to their cardio-respiratory endurance.

Patients with PAD are usually regarded as a group that is at a particularly high risk of proximate cardiac ischemic events so it is very important to know the cardiac condition before training and fitting with prosthesis.

At the IRRS, all patients are tested by means of submaximal exercise stress testing on a manual bicycle before starting rehabilitation programs. In that manner, arrhythmia, coronary ischemia and hypertensive reaction to exertion are identified. The results serve as a basis for prescription of physical therapy and as an important criterion in the decision for fitting with above-knee prosthesis.

It has been proven that walking with above-knee prosthesis demands much more effort than regular walking. However, the most significant piece of information for individual patients is the level of stress induced by their walking and the status of their heart. Based on those data, safe gait training can be performed also at the patient's home.

2. Aim of the study

The aim of the study was to determine the level of effort required by walking, subjective experiencing of exertion during walking, monitoring of the subjects' heart activity and identifying increased blood pressure during the 6-minute walk test with above-knee prosthesis.

The subjects' gait performance at the end of rehabilitation programs was compared to their physical ability assessed with exercise stress testing at the admission.

3. Methods of work

The study included 70 patients after above-knee amputation due to vascular causes at their first rehabilitation treatment at the IRRS. The patients had been fitted with above-knee skeletal single axis prosthesis. Seven patients walked with a walker, the rest walked with crutches.

In the last days before their discharge, the 6-minute walk test was performed. The patient walked on level ground at their individually selected speed. They walked with crutches or reciprocal walker. The prostheses were donned optimally by the patients themselves and/or with the assistance of physical therapists.

By means of a closed system, metabolic parameters were measured telemetrically (VO2, VCo2, VE, BF, RER, oxygen pulse, VE/Vo2). The device "Oxicon mobile-Jaeger" was used. The ECG curves were monitored continuously by means of 12 electrodes. Blood pressure was measured before and immediately after walking, in standing position, with a quicksilver manometer.

Exercise stress testing was carried out at the admission on an arm ergometer with adjusted protocol. The oxygen consumption was calculated with arm ergometer equation.

The level of achieved stress and the calculated oxygen consumption were compared to the length of walking and the measured oxygen consumption during walking.

4. Patients

The study included 70 patients, 44 men and 36 women, average age 70.4 ± 6.9.

24.3 % patients were treated for ischemic heart disease, 8.6 % for cerebrovascular disease, 12.8 % of them had cardiac arrhytmias, the same percent hypertensive heart disease and 21.4 % obstructive lung disease.

5. Results

The average distance covered was 84.2. ±16.1 m. The speed and distance of walking depended mostly on the patients' age and sex. Among the male patients, aged 53 to 60, the average distance covered was 125.4m. There were no female patients in that age group. In the age group 61 to 70, the average distance covered by the male patients was 111m and the by female patients 85m. In the group aged 71 and above, the average walked distance was practically the same in both sexes (men 74.4m and women 74.2m).

The average length of the distance covered was proportional to the level of achieved stress on the arm ergometer at the admission.

The average VO2 was 10.9 ±2.6 ml/kg/min (54.2 ±13.1 maximal predicted)

The heart frequency was 77±11.9 % of the expected maximal, VE 27.6±7.8 l, oxygen pulse 6.7±1.6 ml , RER 0.88±0.07.

The difference between the measured oxygen consumption during walking (average 10,97 ml/kg/min) and the calculated oxygen consumption at the achieved level of stress (11.5 ml/kg/min) was not statistically significant (p = 0,06).

Heart rhythm disorders were detected in 20 % of the patients. In three cases, the rhythm disorders were hemodinamically important (paroxysmal ventricular tachycardia, two paroxysmal AF). In 10 % of the patients, criteria for coronary ischemia were observed. Two of them had clinical symptoms.

At the end of walking, 18 % of the patients had systolic blood pressure over 200 mmHg .

6. Conclusion

According to the measured parameters, walking with above-knee prosthesis was ranged at the level of moderate physical activities.

The length of walking is proportionally opposite to the age of the patients and proportional to the level of achieved stress in exercise stress testing on a manual bicycle. The oxygen consumption at the 6-minute walk test and the consumption at the submaximal stress testing on a arm ergometer do not differ statistically.

During walking, frequent hemodynamically insignificant heart rhythm disorders were observed. Even in patients with IHS, symptomatic angina pectoris was rare, while ECG criteria for it were more frequently detected.

At the end of walking, the levels of blood pressure were high. Apart for irregular basal values, the high levels can be ascribed to the still insecure and unrelaxed manner of walking.

The 6-minute walk test is useful in evaluating the economy and safety of walking with above-knee prosthesis. It can serve as a basis for the prescription of programmed gait training for improving physical ability after the discharge of patients to their home environment.

References

[1] A. Cristian, H. George, M.S. Kraft, S. Robert, P.T. Galley, Predictive Outcome Measures Versus Functional Outcome Measures in the Lower Limb Amputee. *JPO* **18 (01S)** (2006), 51- 58.

[2] M. Vestering, T. Schoppen, R. Dekker, J. Wempe, J. Geertzen, Development of an exercise testing protocol for patients with lower limb amputation:result of a pilot study, *Int J Rehabil Res* **28 (3)** (2005), 237-244.

[3] H. Linde, J.H.B. Geertzen, C.J. Hofstad, J. Limbeek, K. Postema, Prosthetic prescription in the Netherlands: an observation study, *Prosthetic and Orthotics International* **27** (2003), 170-178.

[4] M.C. Munin, M.C.E. Guzman, M.L. Boninger, S.G. Fitzgerald, L.E. Penrod, J. Singh, Predictive factors for succesfull early prosthetic ambulation among lower- limb amputees, *JRRD* **38 (4)** (2001), 379-384.

[5] T. Erjavec, M. Prešern-Štrukelj, H. Burger, The diagnostic importance of exercise testing in developing appropiate rehabilitation programmes for patients following transfemoral amputation. *Eur Phys Rehabil Med* **44(** 2008), 133-9.

Rehabilitation: Mobility, Exercise and Sports
L.H.V. van der Woude et al. (Eds.)
IOS Press, 2010
© 2010 The authors and IOS Press. All rights reserved.
doi:10.3233/978-1-60750-080-3-111

Metabolic energy cost and external mechanical work of level walking after ankle arthrodesis using different types of footwear

S.J.P.M. VAN ENGELEN[*][a], Q.E. WAJER[*][a], L.W. VAN DER PLAAT[b],
C.N. VAN DIJK[b], J.H.P. HOUDIJK[a1]

[a] *Research Institute MOVE, Faculty of Human Movement Sciences, VU University Amsterdam*
[b] *Orthopedic Research Centre Amsterdam, Academic Medical Centre, Amsterdam*
Authors equally contributed

Abstract. The purpose of this study was to evaluate metabolic energy cost and external mechanical work for step-tot-step transitions during level walking after tibiotalar arthrodesis and to examine if curve-shaped shoes reduce external mechanical work and metabolic energy cost of level walking. Oxygen uptake, forceplate data and kinematic data were recorded in 18 controls and 15 patients while walking at a fixed speed of 1.25m/s. Subjects were offered three walking conditions: barefoot, normal walking shoes and curve-shaped shoes. The results showed that patients with a tibiotalar arthrodesis had a 11.8% higher metabolic energy cost. During step-to-step transitions positive work during push-off with the fused ankle was decreased but negative work during collision of the unaffected leading leg was not increased. Total absolute external mechanical work over a complete stride was not different between groups and therefore could not explain the increased metabolic energy cost in patients. Both in patients and controls curve-shaped shoes led to decreased push-off and increased collision and higher metabolic energy cost. From the results it was concluded that metabolic energy cost increases after ankle arthrodesis, but external mechanical work for step-to-step transitions cannot account for this increase. Curve-shaped shoes did not reduce metabolic energy cost of walking.

Keywords. metabolic energy cost, external mechanical work, ankle arthrodesis.

1. Introduction

Ankle arthrodesis is a surgically achieved bony fusion of the tibiotalar joint which immobilizes the ankle [1]. Walking with an ankle arthrodesis is suggested to lead to an increase of 10% in oxygen consumption compared to healthy gait [2]. The increased oxygen consumption might be explained by the double-inverted-pendulum model of level walking [3]. According to this model energy cost of walking is for substantial part

---

[1] Corresponding author: Han Houdijk, Faculty of Human Movement Sciences, VU University Amsterdam, Van der Boechorststraat 9, 1081 BT Amsterdam. Email address: h.houdijk@fbw.vu.nl

determined by the amount of work needed for step-to-step transitions [4]. At heel-strike of the leading leg energy is dissipated which most efficiently is regenerated by a push-off using a powerful plantar flexion in the trailing leg during or just prior to heel-strike. The model predicts that more energy is dissipated during heel-strike when push-off power during double support is reduced and when the roll-over shape of the foot-ankle-complex is deteriorated [4-6].

The purpose of this study was to evaluate metabolic energy cost and external mechanical work for step-to-step transitions during level walking after ankle arthrodesis and to examine if curve-shaped shoes reduce external mechanical work and metabolic energy cost of level walking.

2. Methods

18 Controls and 15 patients participated in this study. Oxygen uptake was measured continuously for five minutes while subjects walked on a motorized treadmill using a breath-by-breath volume and gas analyzer (Oxycon Alpha, Jaeger, Germany). Forceplate data (ground reaction force and centre of pressure) was collected while subjects walked on a walkway in which a set of two forceplates were incorporated in series. In patients both the healthy and affected leg were successively used as the leading leg. In controls only the step in which the right leg was leading was measured. During the trials on the walkway kinematic data was recorded with an opto-electronic system (OPTOTRAK, Northern Digital, Ontario, Canada). Infrared LED's were attached to the lateral femoral condyles, lateral malleoli and the fifth metatarsal heads on both legs. Subjects were offered three walking conditions: barefoot, normal walking shoes and curved-shaped shoes. Walking speed for all trails was fixed at 1.25m/s.

From the collected data we calculated (1) metabolic energy cost (J/kg/m) from oxygen uptake and walking speed, (2) external mechanical work (J/kg/m) of each leg during double and single support and total absolute work over a stride from ground reaction forces (GRF) according to the individual limb method described by Donelan et al. [4] and (3) the roll-over shape of the ankle-foot-complex from kinematic data using the method described by Hansen et al. [6]. Differences in outcome measures between groups and between shoe conditions were tested for statistical significance by means of a two way repeated measures ANOVA. Significance level was set at $p<0.05$.

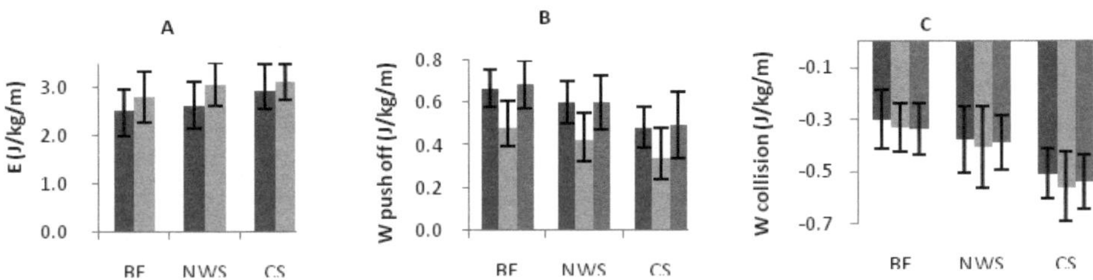

Figure 1: (A) Metabolic energy cost, left bar representing controls, right bar patients. (B) External mechanical work during push-off and (C) collision, left bar representing controls, middle bar patients with their fused ankle, right bar patients with their healthy ankle. All panels show patients and controls in three shoe conditions (BF, barefoot; NWS, normal walking shoes; CS, curve-shaped shoes).

3. Results

Metabolic energy cost during walking was significantly higher in patients than in controls (p=0.037). On average metabolic energy cost in patients was 11.8% higher (figure 1A). In double support, positive external mechanical work was significantly lower in patients performing push-off with their fused ankle than in controls (p<0.001). When push-off was performed with the healthy ankle, no significant difference in positive work was found (figure 1B). Collision was not significantly different between patients and controls, whether patients landed on their healthy or fused ankle (figure 1C). Total absolute external mechanical work was not different between the groups.

Surprisingly, the roll-over shape of patients and controls was not significantly different whichever leg patients used. Perhaps, the roll-over shape in patients is not altered due to compensatory movements of other joints of the foot or patients use a different roll-over strategy. Walking on curved-shaped shoes had no influence on the roll-over shape. In both patients and controls the roll-over shape was similar for all walking conditions. However, both in patients and controls curve-shaped shoes led to decreased push-off (p<0.001, figure 1B) and increased collision (p<0.003, figure 1C). In concert, walking on curve-shaped shoes required significant more metabolic energy than walking barefoot (p<0.001) and walking on normal walking shoes (p=0.013, figure 1A).

4. Conclusion

Based on the results of this study it can be concluded that ankle arthrodesis has no effect on external mechanical work required for step-to-step transitions, but the metabolic energy cost in level walking is higher after an ankle arthrodesis. Although the range of motion of the immobilized leg is decreased, the roll-over shape does not seem to be affected. Both in patients and controls, walking on curve-shaped shoes decreases push-off and increases collision. Consequently, metabolic energy cost is higher when walking on curve-shaped shoes.

References

[1]   R.L. Waters, G. Barnes, T. Husserl, L. Silver, R. Liss, Comparable energy expenditure after arthrodesis of the hip and ankle. *J Bone Joint Surg Am.* **70(7)** (1988), 1032-7.

[2]   A.D. Kuo, Energetics of actively powered locomotion using the simplest walking model. *J Biomech Eng,* **124(1)** (2002), p.113-20.

[3]   J.M. Donelan, R. Kram, A.D. Kuo (a). Mechanical work for step-to-step transitions is a major determinant of the metabolic cost of human walking. *J Exp Biol.* **205(Pt 23)** (2002), p.3717-27.

[4]   J.M. Donelan, R. Kram, A.D. Kuo (b). Simultaneous positive and negative external mechanical work in human walking. *J Biomech.* **35(1)** (2002), p.117-24.

[5]   P.G. Adamczyk, S.H. Collins, A.D. Kuo, The advantages of a rolling foot in human walking. *J Exp Biol,* **209**(Pt 20) (2006), p.3953-63.

[6]   A.H. Hansen, D.S. Childress, E.H. Knox, Roll-over shapes of human locomotor systems: effects of walking speed. *Clin Biomech (Bristol, Avon).* **19(4)** (2004), p.407-14.

Rehabilitation: Mobility, Exercise and Sports
L.H.V. van der Woude et al. (Eds.)
IOS Press, 2010

doi:10.3233/978-1-60750-080-3-114

Pedaling forces normalized to body weight in cyclists with a uni-lateral transtibial amputation

W.L. CHILDERS[a,1], K.L. PERELL-GERSON[b], R. KISTENBERG[a], R.J. GREGOR[a]

[a]*School of Applied Physiology, Georgia Institute of Technology , Atlanta, GA USA*
[b]*Dept. of Kinesiology, California State University, Fullerton, Fullerton, CA, USA*

Abstract. Persons with lower limb amputation may be on weight-bearing restrictions following amputation. Cycling provides a method for rehabilitation within a limited body weight environment. Pedal force data obtained from studies on intact cyclists and cyclists with uni-lateral trans-tibial amputation were used to calculate forces normalized to body weight on the shank or residual limb segment and then related to power output. Linear regression was used to develop models describing this relationship. Results show that patients operating within power outputs typical in rehabilitation will experience compressive forces below 30% body weight. Therefore, we conclude that cycling may be safely utilized as a rehabilitation modality for patients on weight-bearing restrictions.

Keywords. cycling, amputee, rehabilitation, prosthesis, body weight.

1. Introduction

While movement is encouraged early in the rehabilitation plan to improve patient outcomes, weight-bearing restrictions may be necessary to reduce the forces imposed on the healing residual limb [1, 2]. Cycling serves as a rehabilitation modality within a limited weight-bearing environment that encourages rhythmic, reciprocal movement [3] and may provide an intermediate step to encourage neuromuscular learning and weight bearing on the residual limb before the patient can progress to standing balance and gait training. While much is known about the forces produced during intact cycling [4], the relationship between power outputs and forces imposed on the lower limb relative to body weight has not been published. The purpose of this study was to discuss the relationship between different power outputs and forces experienced by the residual limb relative to body weight with comparison to intact cyclists.

2. Methods

Regression analysis was performed on 42 datasets from ten CTA (eight males and two females; average age 38.8 +/- 13.1 yrs, height 1.76 +/- 0.08 m, and mass 82.5 +/- 13.5 kg) and 28 datasets from twelve intact cyclists (eleven males and one female; average

---

[1] Corresponding Author. W. Lee Childers, School of Applied Physiology, Georgia Institute of Technology, 281 Ferst Ave., Atlanta, GA 30332, USA. lee@gatech.edu. +001-404-894-7658

age 39.5 +/- 11.8 yrs, height 1.81 +/- 0.06 m, and mass 73.8 +/- 6.4 kg). These datasets were derived from previous studies [5, 6]. All subjects signed separate written consent for IRB approval. The subjects rode on a stationary bicycle adjusted to their preferred position with a centripetal resistance unit (1-UP USA Inc.) and adapted with dual piezoelectric element force pedals [7]. The subject's personal prosthesis was modified by removing the pylon and foot section and replacing it a stiff aluminum pylon/foot section (STIFF) for all ten CTAs [5, 6]or a flexible carbon fiber pylon/foot section (FLEX) for eight CTAs [5].

One study [5] utilized eight CTA subjects and nine intact subjects pedaled for six minutes at loads corresponding to 70 and 90% of their age-predicted maximum heart rate at preferred cadence. The CTA group pedaled at both intensities with a stiff and flexible prosthetic foot. An additional eight CTA datasets and were obtained from a separate study [6] where two CTA and two intact cyclists pedaled at 100 watts at 60 and 90 rpm as well as loads corresponding to 70 and 90% of their age-predicted maximum heart rate. The remaining two CTA and two intact datasets were obtained during pilot testing at 200 watts and 90 rpm.

Both orthogonal and shear components of the pedal reaction force [7] were recorded over the final one minute at each randomly selected load condition. Five complete pedal cycles from each trial were averaged together for analysis. The maximum orthogonal component of force was normalized to the subject's body weight (%BW) for each limb. The maximum orthogonal component of force occurs at approximately 90 degrees of crank rotation [4]. Linear regression formulas were employed relating power output to %BW of the limb. Pearson's product moment correlation coefficient was used to test whether %BW was significantly correlated to power output. Fischer's Z-Transformation was used to test if relationships between limbs or groups were significantly different. Significance was defined as $p < 0.05$.

3. Results

Percent BW versus power outputs are plotted as linear regression lines for both dominant (DOM) and nondominant (nonDOM) limbs in each group (Fig 1). The relationship between %BW and power was not significantly different between the DOM and nonDOM limbs of the intact group, therefore, those limbs were combined into one dataset (n = 56). Power correlated significantly with %BW for all groups and both limbs within each group (p <0.001) (Fig. 1). The relationship between %BW and power for the intact group was significantly different from the sound limb but not the amputated limb of the CTA group.

4. Discussion

There is a strong, positive relationship between %BW and power output during cycling for intact cyclists and CTA. This relationship is not different between the amputated limb of CTA and the intact group indicating that the clinician may use the same linear model to predict %BW for both groups. The y-intercepts for all linear models were greater than zero and averaged 21.5% (Fig. 1). A non-zero %BW measurement when power output is low may be explained by inertial forces developed at the foot/pedal interface due solely to the reciprocal movement of the limbs. Orthogonal pedal forces remained below 30% body weight for power outputs similar to those selected by cyclists with lower limb impairment (20 – 75 watts) [8].

In conclusion, these findings suggest that cycling may serve as a rehabilitation modality, even within the confines of post-surgical weight bearing restrictions, to promote cardiovascular conditioning, range of motion, and strength gains for an individual with lower limb loss. The models presented here may also be used to describe the lower limb weight bearing forces achieved by a patient prior to progression into balance or gait training activities.

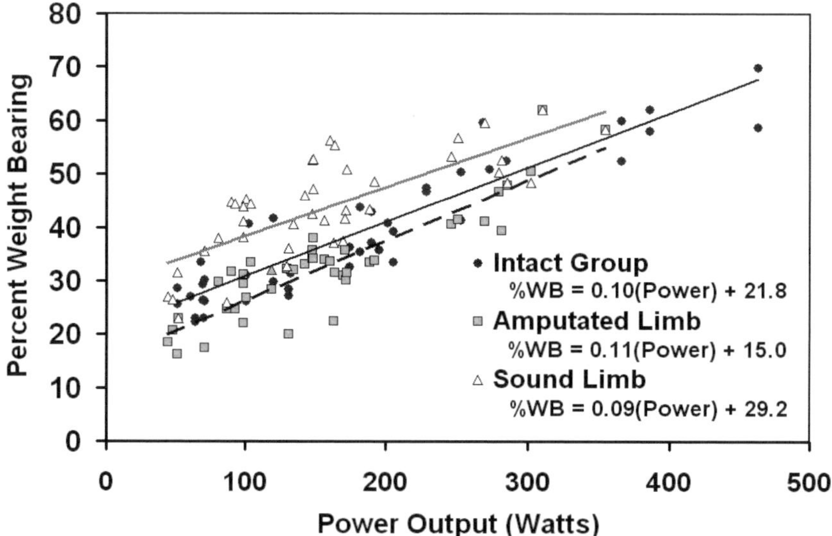

Figure 1. Percent body weight for the shank vs. power output for both limbs combined in the intact group (solid line), amputated (dashed) and sound (grey) limb for the CTA group. Equations for the linear model are given below the respective group. The linear model for the intact group and the amputated limb of the CTA group was not significantly different.

The authors gratefully acknowledge Beth Brown and Kate McDonald for their review and edits of the manuscript, and Laura Jones for her help with data collection. We would also like to thank Ossur, Prosthetic Design Inc. and Serotta Bicycles for their donations.

References

[1]	D.G. Smith, J.W. Michael, J.H. Bowker, *Atlas of Amputation and Limb Deficiencies; Surgical, Prosthetic, and Rehabilitation Principles, Third ed.*, American Academy of Orthopaedic Surgeons, Rosemont, 2004.

[2]	M.M. Lusardi, C.C. Nielsen, *Orthotics and Prosthetics in Rehabilitation*, Butterworth Heinemann, Boston, 2000.

[3]	J. Zachazewski, D. Magee, W. Quillen, *Athletic injuries and rehabilitation*. First ed., WB Saunders Co., Philadelphia, 1996.

[4]	R.J. Gregor, J.P. Broker, M.M. Ryan, The biomechanics of cycling, *Exer Sports Sci Rev*, **19** (1991) 127-169.

[5]	T. Chin, S. Sawamura, H. Fujita, S. Nakajima, I. Ojima, H. Oyabu, Y. Nagakura, H. Otsuka, A. Nakagawa, Effect of endurance training program based on anaerobic threshold (AT) for lower limb Amputees, *J Rehab Res Dev* **38** (2001), 7-11.

[6]	L. Jones, R.J. Gregor, Lower limb joint forces in transtibial amputees during cycling, Unpublished Masters Final Project, Georgia Institute of Technology, (2008).

[7]	J.P. Broker, R.J. Gregor, A dual piezoelectric element force pedal for kinetic analysis of cycling, *Int J Sport Biomech*, **6** (1990), 394-403.

[8]	K.L. Perell, R.J. Gregor, A.M.E. Scremin, Lower limb cycling mechanics in subjects with unilateral cerebrovascular accidents, *J Appl Biomech*, **14** (1998), 158-179.

3.3

Poster Presentations

Rehabilitation: Mobility, Exercise and Sports
L.H.V. van der Woude et al. (Eds.)
IOS Press, 2010

doi:10.3233/978-1-60750-080-3-119

The impact of an actuated ankle/foot on the walking performance in healthy subjects and following neurologic injuries: a systematic review

S. DUERINCK[1], E. SWINNEN, P. VAES, P. VAN ROY, R. MEEUSEN
Faculty of Physical Education and Physiotherapy, ARTS (Advanced Rehabilitation, Technology and Science)
ALTACRO (Automated Locomotor Training using an Actuated Compliant Robotic Orthosis)
Vrije Universiteit Brussel, Brussels, Belgium

Abstract. This systematic review summarizes scientific papers concerning the impact of actuation of the ankle/foot on biomechanical function of the ankle/foot in the lower extremity during gait in healthy subjects and spinal cord injured patients (SCI). The results show significant changes in 3D joint angles, joint moments and muscular activity for the different designs in actuated ankle/foot orthosis (AFO).

Keywords. locomotion, ankle, exoskeleton, gait, rehabilitation, actuation.

1. Introduction

The restoration of gait is an integral part of rehabilitation in patients with impairments of the central nervous system [1]. Excess ankle plantar flexion during swing (76%) and impaired initial foot contact (52%) [2] are amongst the most frequently observed and most relevant impairments for functional locomotion in spinal cord injured patients. In addition, the rehabilitation of the biomechanical ankle function contributes to the improvement of gait performance, represented by 3D kinematics (3D joint angles and angular velocity of ankle, knee and hip), kinetics (joint moments) and muscular activity pattern in the lower limb, in people suffering from ankle paralysis as a consequence from a stroke [3][4], SCI [2][4] or multiple sclerosis.
Modern concepts of motor learning favor a task specific training based on the principle of repetition [5]. The technological evolution in robotics has enabled the construction of powered exoskeletons and the application of task specific training. Ever since the introduction of robotic gait training, a variety of driven gait orthotics have been applied [6],[7].

---

[1] Corresponding Author: Saartje Duerinck, Vrije Universiteit Brussel, Laarbeeklaan 103, 1090 Brussels, Belgium; E-mail: sduerinc@vub.ac.be

The aim of this study is to present a systematic review of scientific publications concerning the alteration in muscle activity, 3D kinematics and kinetics of the lower limb with two types of ankle/foot actuation, isolated versus as part of a driven gait orthosis, during gait in healthy subjects and neurologic patients. Furthermore, the aim is to provide an answer to the question: "how do different control methods for AFO and AFO with different degrees of freedom perform in obtaining a "normal" gait pattern?".

2.　Methods

A bibliographic survey of the English, German, French literature was conducted through Medline, ISI Web of Knowledge, PEDro and Cochrane Controlled Trails Register (1985 to 2009), using 'actuation', 'ankle', 'robotics' and 'orthotics' as most relevant keywords.

The inclusion of appropriate studies was performed in three stages. Firstly, a selection of the articles was made based on the presence of keywords in the title. Secondly, the abstracts of the relevant publications were scanned by two independent observers, using in- and exclusion criteria. Thirdly, an evaluation of the methodological quality of the selected studies was performed by two independent reviewers.

3.　Results

A total of 26911 titles were yielded based on the introduction of several keyword combinations in different databases. After screening by title, removing duplicates and an evaluation based on a set of in- and exclusion criteri, 31 studies met the inclusion criteria and were subjected to a methodological evaluation of the full text. Ultimately 12 surveys satisfied the sever selection criteria.

Two forms of orthotic devices, designed for actuation of the ankle/foot, were could be distinguished. Only one survey compared the influence of a unilateral AFO load, rigidly attached to the Lokomat. Both control and patients showed an increase in peak hip extension and a select increase in muscle activation (healty subjects M. soleus, M. gastrocnemius, M. vastus lateralis, M. vastus medialis during stance phase) due to additional weight at ankle/foot. Eleven papers report the changes in gait performance for healthy subjects and SCI patients in terms of biomechanical parameters in the lower limb, due to the application of an isolated AFO. Three different actuation methods were assessed independently in healthy subjects: series elastic actuators for the actuation of plantar and dorsiflexion, a spring parallel with a pneumatic artificial muscle for the simultaneous actuation in the sagittal and frontal pane. Nine studies applied pneumatic artificial muscles for plantar and dorsiflexion actuation, what resulted in an increase in dorsiflexion ankle angle during heel strike and swing phase. Three studies reported an increase in peak plantar flexion angle during stance phase and no changes in hip and knee angles as compared to the non plantar flexion actuated condition. The activity of the M. soleus decreases significantly during actuation of the ankle/foot. The initial minutes of walking in a AFO are characterized by the M. soleus and M. gastrocnemius showing a constant EMG activity throughout the entire gait cycle, after adaptation the M. soleus activity alters to a two burst pattern. Sawicki et al. (2006) applied bilateral dorsiflexion AFO actuated by pneumatic artificial muscles in SCI patients in combination with body weight support and resulted in an increase in ankle dorsiflexion angle at push-off and a decrease in M. soleus activity through the entire gait cycle.

Only two studies compared different controllers for the dorsiflexion actuation of the ankle/foot during gait. Kao & Ferris (2009) compared the influence of actuating the ankle/foot using continuous control versus swing control. Changes in 3D kinematics, EMG and kinetic variables were assessed using a footswitch control with proportional myoelectrical control.

The systematic search of the literature did not reveale studies comparing AFO characterized by different degrees of freedom in healthy subjects nor in patients following neurological injuries.

4. Discussion

Our results indicate an increase in dorsiflexion ankle angle at heel strike and swing phase due to actuation of the ankle dorsiflexion in healthy subjects. Plantar flexion actuation increases peak plantar flexion angle during stance phase and shows no changes in hip and knee angles as compared to the non plantar flexion actuated condition. The activity of the M. soleus decreases significantly during actuation and evolves from continuous to a burst-like. In combination with body weight support AFO results in an increase in ankle dorsiflexion angle at push-off and a decrease in M. soleus activity throughout the entire gait cycle.

When drawing final conclusions concerning therapeutic strategies in patients, based on these results, one should be careful, due to a few methodological flaws (i.e. methods for measuring changes in 3D kinematics) and the little evidence concerning the application of an actuated AFO in SCI, stroke and multiple sclerosis patients.

References

[1] SCHMIDT H, WERNER C, BERNARDT R, HESSE S, KRUGER J, Gait rehabilitation machines based on programmable footplates, Journal of neuroengeneering and rehabilitation, 2007, 4(2), 1-7

[2] VAN DER SALM A, NENE AV, MAXWELL DJ, VELTINK PH, HERMENS HJ, IJZERMAN MJ, Gait impairements in a group of patients with incomplete spinal cord injury and their relevance regarding therapeutic approaches using functional electrical stimulation, Artificial organs, 2005, 29(1), 8 – 14.

[3] INTISO D, SANTILLI V, GRASSO MG, ROSSI R, CARUSO I, Rehabilitation or walking with electromyographic biofeedback in dropfoot after stroke, Stroke, 1994, 25(6), 1189 -1192

[4] BURRIDGE JH, WOOD DE, TAYLOR PN, MCLELLAN DL, Indices to describe different muscle activation patterns, identified during treadmill walking, in people with spastic drop-foot, Med Eng Phys., 2001, 427 – 434

[5] ASANUMA H, KELLER A, Neurobiological basis of motor learning and memory, Concepts neuroscience,1991, 2, 1 - 30

[6] HESSE S, UHLENBROCK D, A mechanized gait trainer for restoration of gait, Journal of rehabilitation research and development, 2000, 37(6), 701-708.

[7] VAN DER KOOIJ H, VENEMAN J, EKKELENKAMP R, Design of a compliantly actuated exoskeleton for an impedance controlled gait trainer robot, Conf Proc IEEE Eng Med Biol Soc, 2006, 1,189-193.

[8] LAW EA, Evidence-based rehabilitation: a guide to practice, SLACK Incorporated (2008).

[9] SAWICKI GS, DOMINGO A, FERRIS DP, The effects of powered ankle-foot orthoses on joint kinematics and muscle activation during walking in individuals with incomplete spinal cord injury, Journal of neuroengineering and rehabilitation, 2006, 3(3), 1 – 17

[10] KAO P-C, FERRIS DP, Motor adaptation during dorsiflexion-assisted walking with a powered orthosis, Gait and posture, 2009, 29, 230 – 236

Rehabilitation: Mobility, Exercise and Sports
L.H.V. van der Woude et al. (Eds.)
IOS Press, 2010

doi:10.3233/978-1-60750-080-3-122

Security aspects of gait on stairs for transtibial amputees

L. FRADET[1] M. ALIMUSAJ, F. BRAATZ, S.I. WOLF
Department of Orthopaedic Surgery, University of Heidelberg, Germany

Abstracts. This study proposed to investigate security aspects of gait on stairs for transtibial amputees (TTAs) and proposed to assess the effects of a new adaptive prosthetic ankle on these specific aspects. 11 TTAs and 12 controls underwent a traditional 3D gait analysis on an instrumented staircase. TTAs walked with the prosthetic ankle set in: a) the adapted mode that provides dorsiflexion during stair walking; b) a neutral position. The position of the CoP and of the foot relative to the stairs, the toe-clearance, and the coefficients of friction were computed. During stair ascent, data imply an equivalent or safer gait strategy for TTAs than for controls, especially on the involved side. No modifications were noticed between adapted and neutral modes. During stair descent, TTAs placed their prosthetic foot closer to the stair edge. The coefficient of friction was also higher during loading response on TTAs' sound side compared to controls. Both phenomena were reduced in adapted mode. For TTAs, stair descent was then less safe than stair ascent but safety was improved when walking in adapted mode.

Keywords. transtibial amputee, stairs, safety.

1. Introduction

Transtibial amputees (TTAs) suffer from loss of muscle strength, joint mobility, balance, or proprioception, increasing their risk of falling compared to age-matched, able-bodied individuals [1]. This risk is amplified during stair ambulation since this walking condition increases the kinetic demand compared with level walking [2] and then emphasizes motor deficits. However, the origin of the falls is not well identified in TTAs during stair walking. Moreover, it is well-known that populations being prone to risk of falling modify their gait in order to reduce the risk.

The present study proposes to analyse different aspects characterizing gait security during stair walking. In addition, the effects on these security aspects of a new prosthetic ankle, the Proprio-Foot® (Össur), will be analysed. This new prosthetic ankle aims indeed to reduce risk of falling by increasing dorsiflexion during stair walking.

2. Method

Patients came a first time to the laboratory to be provided with the new prosthetic ankle (Proprio-Foot®, Össur) and to be instructed to its different features. After at least 14 days of adaptation, patients returned to the laboratory to undergo a conventional 3D gait analysis (12 cameras of 120Hz, Vicon, Oxford) while walking on stairs equipped

---

[1] Corresponding Author; Email: Laetitia.Fradet@ok.uni-heidelberg.de

with 2 force-plates (Kistler, Winterthur). TTAs walked with the new prosthetic ankle, which provided 4° dorsiflexion during stair walking, and with the same adaptive prosthetic ankle fixed at neutral position to simulate a conventional prosthetic ankle. These two modes will be further referred to as "adapted" and "neutral" modes, respectively. 12 healthy controls followed the same protocol.

During stair ascent, toe-clearance was computed as the distance separating the two stairs edges to avoid during swing phase and the tip of the toe. During stair ascent and descent, the positions of the foot and of the centre of pressure (CoP) were computed relative to the stair edge and the required coefficient of friction was obtained by dividing the shear forces by the force that is normal to the slope of the ramp [3].

A t-test was used for comparisons between TTAs and control subjects whereas a paired t-test was used for comparisons between conditions (adapted vs neutral mode).

3. Results

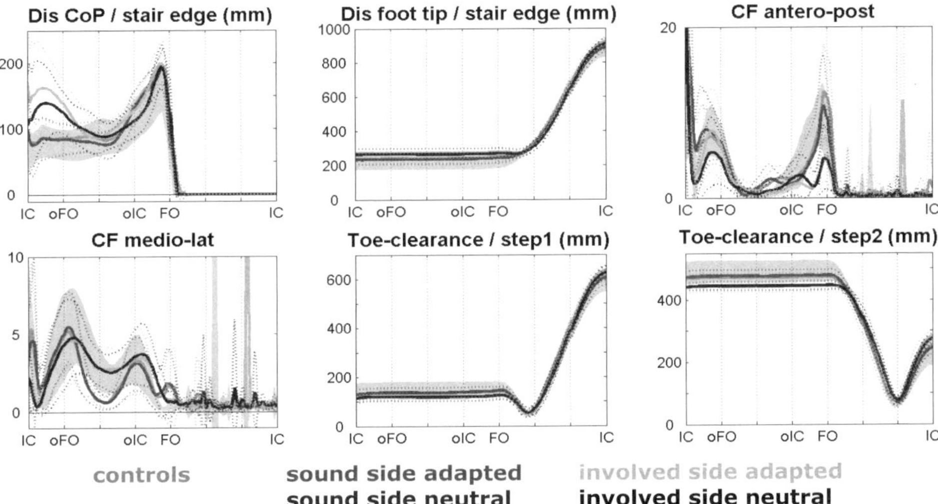

Figure 1. Distance between the CoP/ foot tip and the stair edge, coefficient of friction (CF) along the antero-posterior and the medio-lateral axes, and toe-clearance (TC) during stair ascent. Diagrams are normalized to gait subphases. For patients, means and standard deviations are given, for controls, only standard deviations.

IC: Initial Contact; oIC: opposite Initial Contact; FO: foot-off; oFO: opposite Foot-off.

Stair ascent

Figure 1 illustrates the variation of the data during stair ascent and Table 1 provides the statistical results. The foot tip and the CoP on the TTAs' involved side were positioned deeper on the stair compared to controls. The antero-posterior coefficient of friction was smaller at the end of single-limb stance phase for the TTAs' involved side than for controls. No significant difference was noticed for toe-clearance.

When comparing adapted with neutral mode, only the antero-posterior coefficient of friction was significantly different, this later being smaller for adapted than for neutral mode.

Stair descent

The foot tip of TTAs' involved side were placed more forwards on the stair (Table 1) in order to use the stair edge to perform the roll-over of the foot, which is difficult to realize when lacking dorsiflexion. The coefficient of friction was doubled on the TTAs' sound side compared to controls on the antero-posterior axis during loading response but was smaller on the medio-lateral axis during single limb stance. This later was also greater for the TTAs' involved side than for controls, even though not significantly.

In adapted mode, the position of the CoP was less forward on the stairs, since foot contact was realized with the heel and not with a flat foot as in neutral mode. The increase on the sound side of the medio-lateral coefficient of friction was also reduced.

Table 1. Mean ± sd for the distance between the CoP/ foot tip and the stair edge, for the coefficient of friction (CF) along the antero-posterior and medio-lateral axes, and for toe-clearance (TC).

	Controls	Patients' sound side		Patients' involved side	
Stair ascent		Neutral	Adapted	Neutral	Adapted
Dis CoP/stair edge loading response	140 ± 21	142 ± 23	141 ± 24	181 ± 20***	179 ± 24**
Dis foot tip/stair edge stand phase	243 ± 22	245 ± 14	240 ± 22	276 ± 23***	273 ± 17**
CF antero-post loading response	7.6 ± 0.9	8.9 ± 3.7	10.8 ± 5.8	7.4 ± 1.8	5.0 ± 1.1*,°
CF antero-post pre-swing	12.5 ± 3.1	15.7 ± 6.3	12.3 ± 7.0	5.0 ± 2.6***	4.9 ± 2.9**
CF medio-lat loading response	5.0 ± 1.9	6.1 ± 2.1	6.5 ± 1.7	5.4 ± 2.6	5.7 ± 2.2
CF medio-lat pre-swing	3.9 ± 1.1	5.0 ± 2.8	4.7 ± 2.1	4.2 ± 1.8	4.6 ± 2.0
TC 1st Stairp swing phase	48 ± 14	45 ± 8	43 ± 18	44 ± 14	47 ± 11
TC 2nd Stairp swing phase	67 ± 10	66 ± 10	65 ± 19	73 ± 13	64 ± 10
Stair descent					
Dis CoP/stair edge loading response	65 ± 22	74 ± 24	76 ± 21	80 ± 38	109 ± 43**,°°
Dis foot tip/stair edge stand phase	-34 ± 25	-27 ± 27	-27 ± 18	-72 ± 53*	-57 ± 40*
CF antero-post loading response	11 ± 4	22 ± 7***	22 ± 8***	5 ± 2***	4 ± 2***,°
CF antero-post pre-swing	28 ± 9	24 ± 8	21 ± 10°	14 ± 6*	14 ± 4***
CF medio-lat single-limb stance	4.3 ± 1.7	2.6 ± 0.9*	2.6 ± 1.0*	4.8 ± 1.9	4.4 ± 1.8

*: $p<0.05$; **: $p<0.01$; ***: $p<0.001$ significance of the *t*-test during the comparison with controls.
°: $p<0.05$; °°: $p<0.01$; °°°: $p<0.001$ significance of the *t*-test during the comparison with the neutral ankle.

4. Discussion/Conclusion

During stair ascent, the strategy used by TTAs resulted in a greater security. Conversely, during stair descent, the lack of dorsiflexion compromised the TTAs' safety as attested by the greater coefficients of friction found for TTAs compared to controls and the position of the prosthetic foot placed more forward on the stair edge.

The dorsiflexion brought by the new prosthetic ankle during stair walking reduces the risk of sliding or falling as attested by the decrease of the coefficients of friction and the position of the foot placed less forward on the stair edge during stair descent.

References

[1] W.C. Miller, M. Speechley, B. Deathe, The prevalence and risk factors of falling and fear of falling among lower extremity amputees, *Arch Phys Med Rehabil* **82** (2001), 1031–1036.

[2] T. Schmalz, S. Blumentritt, B. Marx, Biomechanical analysis of stair ambulation in lower limb amputees, *Gait Posture* **25** (2007), 267-278.

[3] J.P. Hanson, M.S. Redfern, M. Mazumdar, Predicting slips and falls considering required and available friction, *Ergonomics* **42** (1999), 1619-33.

Chapter 4

Aging, Mobility and Chronic Diseases

4.1

Keynote

Rehabilitation: Mobility, Exercise and Sports
L.H.V. van der Woude et al. (Eds.)
IOS Press, 2010

doi:10.3233/978-1-60750-080-3-127

Exercise in rehabilitation and chronic disease

W.R. Frontera
Dean, Faculty of Medicine, University of Puerto Rico
and
Lecturer
Department of Physical Medicine and Rehabilitation
Harvard Medical School

Abstract. Exercise is an effective rehabilitation intervention. Abundant scientific research during the last two decades shows that exercise can also be effective in the prevention or treatment of chronic diseases. Physical inactivity has been identified as one of the most important causes of morbidity and mortality. The programs that promote physical activity should become higher priorities in national health care systems. The relationship between the level of physical activity and chronic disease was first studied in the context of heart and cardiovascular disease. The level of exercise and physical fitness correlates with all cause mortality. This relationship is independent of the presence of all other risk factors for cardiovascular disease. The incidence and morbidity associated with several chronic diseases such as obesity, diabetes, hypertension, and cancer have been shown to correlate with the level of physical activity of the population under study. Although the optimal exercise intervention has not been defined, it has been suggested that at least 30 minutes of moderate intensive physical activity on most, preferably all days of the week is a reasonable recommendation. This level of physical activity is effective in the primary prevention of chronic diseases mentioned above.

4.2

Oral Presentations

Rehabilitation: Mobility, Exercise and Sports
L.H.V. van der Woude et al. (Eds.)
IOS Press, 2010

doi:10.3233/978-1-60750-080-3-131

131

Quantifying effects of dual task performance and cognition on gait coordination in elderly geriatric patients

C.J.C. LAMOTH[a,1], F.J.A. VAN DEUDEKOM[b], J.P. VAN CAMPEN[b], O.J. DE VRIES[c], M. PIJNAPPELS[d]

[a] *Center for Human Movement Sciences, University Medical Centre Groningen, University of Groningen, the Netherlands*
[b] *Department of Geriatric Medicine, Slotervaart Hospital, Amsterdam, the Netherlands*
[c] *Department of Internal Medicine, VU Medical Center, Amsterdam, the Netherlands*
[d] *Research Institute MOVE, Faculty of Human Movement Sciences, VU University, Amsterdam, the Netherlands*

Abstract. The effects of a cognitive dual task on gait coordination in 24 older geriatric day clinic patients while walking at self-selected speed was studied and related to cognitive function. Trunk accelerations were registered (DynaPort®; McRoberts) and used to calculate gait and trunk parameters. The Mini Mental State Examination and the Seven Minute Screen were administered. With dual task, walking speed was significantly lower, while variability of stride time increased and stability and regularity of lateral trunk accelerations decreased. These results provide support that changes in cognitive functions are likely to contribute to an increased fall risk.

Keywords. elderly walking; gait coordination; dual task; cognitive impairment.

1. Introduction

One in three community-dwelling persons over 65 years of age falls at least once a year and this rate increases with age and frailty. Major risk factors for falling are: gait and balance disorders, impaired vision and physical condition, cognitive impairment, gender and age[1]. Normal daily life activities often challenges to maintain balance and walking while performing concurrent (cognitive) dual tasks. Changes in gait characteristics during aging such as lower walking speed, reduced step length, increased step time have been interpreted as a more cautions gait pattern, adopted to decrease fall risk. A more conscious walking, however, may imply that walking requires more attention. Particularly in the frail elderly, changes in cognitive functions have been suggest to increase fall risk [2,3].

The aim of the present study was to examine the effect of a cognitive dual task in frail elderly on gait coordination and assess if such dual task effects on gait correlate with cognitive function. Specifically, stride variability and trunk accelerations patterns were studied as indicators of dynamic balance ability during walking.

---

[1] Corresponding Author.

2. Methods

Twenty four elderly persons (age=80.9±3.6 years, men/women 9/15) were recruited from the geriatric day clinic of the Slotervaart hospital in Amsterdam. In all participants the Mini Mental State Examination (MMSE) and the Seven Minute Screen (SMS) were administered to evaluate cognitive functions. The MMSE was used to divide participants into two groups: people with an indication of cognitive impairment (CI; MMSE<23; N=12) and people without cognitive impairment (CNI; MMSE>26; N=12).

Participants walked 100 meter at self-selected speed, once without and once while performing a verbal dual task: citing words starting with the letter "R" or "G". The verbal dual task was also performed during sitting. When walking, trunk accelerations in 3 orthogonal directions were measured with a tri-axial piezo-capacitive accelerometer (DynaPort®MiniMod, McRoberts BV, The Hague, the Netherlands), fixed with an elastic belt at the level of lumbar segment L3. Data were sampled at 100 Hz.

Data and statistical analyses

Anterior-posterior (AP) and medio-lateral (ML) acceleration time-series were analyzed. Outcome measures during walking with and without dual task were:
- Gait parameters: walking speed, stride frequency (SF), mean and coefficient of variation (CV) of stride times, the scaling-exponent α to examine the time dependent variability of stride times, and the phase variability index (PVI) as a measure of the variability of the coordination between right and left steps.
- Trunk ML and AP acceleration parameters[4]: the root mean squares (RMS), the harmonicity ratio (HR) as an index of smoothness of the accelerations, the scaling-exponent α to assess time dependent variations in accelerations, and the maximum Lyapunov exponent (λ_{max}) to index local stability.
- The performance on the DT, the MMSE and the SMS tests.

Wilcoxon-signed rank test was applied to examine the effect of dual tasking on stride and trunk acceleration parameters. Differences between the CI group and CNI group were analysed with the Mann-Whitney U-test. To examine the relation between cognitive function, MMSE scores and gait and trunk parameters, Spearman correlations were calculated.

3. Results

Under dual task conditions, walking speed and SF decreased significantly ($P < 0.01$), while the scaling-exponent α of stride times and the PVI increased significantly ($P < 0.01$). Dual tasking significantly decreased the RMS, the scaling exponent α, λ_{max} and the HR of AP and ML trunk accelerations (all $P <0 .01$), indicating a lower amplitude, loss of local stability and decreased smoothness of accelerations, respectively.

A significant group effect was found on the RMS (P = 0.03), scaling-exponent α of ML accelerations (P < 0.01), the scaling-exponent α of stride times (P = 0.03),.and the PVI (P = 0.04) (see Figure 1).

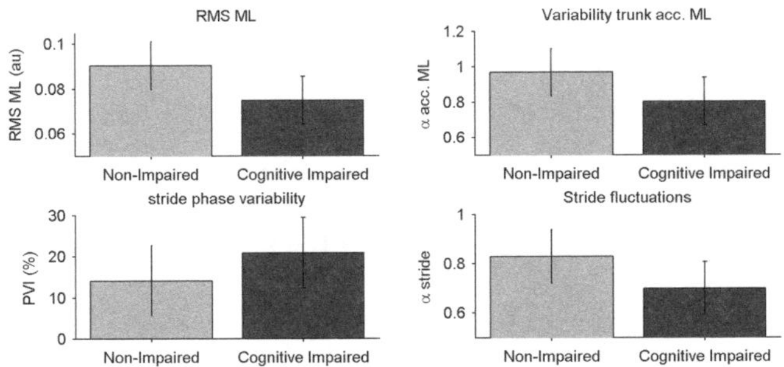

Figure 1. Differential effects of dual tasking on gait and trunk variables on both groups

Overall, correlations between MMSE, SMS scores and gait and trunk acceleration measures were low (r<0.3). Variability (α) of trunk accelerations correlated significantly, but moderately with SMS (α ML, r=0.51, α AP, r=-0.35) and MMSE values (α ML, r=0.36). Within the CI group, the associations were higher for several measures (Table 1).

Table 1: Spearman correlation values between SMS test scores, the MMSE values and gait and trunk acceleration parameters within the CI group (N=12). ** P <0.01; * P <0.05

	SMS	Speed	Stride			RMS	HR	λmax acc.
			Mean	CV	PVI	AP	AP	AP
SMS		.62**	.52*	.36*	-.66**	-.46*	.63*	-35
MMSE	.70**	.71**	.68**	.71**	.68**	.61**	-.68**	.69**

4. Conclusion

Despite the reduced walking speed during dual tasking, trunk accelerations patterns were more irregular and variable, especially in cognitive impaired subjects. For the cognitive impaired group, an association between cognitive function and several gait parameters was observed. Although the slowing of gait while performing a dual task could reflect an adaptation to more difficult circumstances, the resulting trunk adaptations were a significant consistent instability factor, suggesting an increased fall risk. The results of the present study provide further support that changes in cognitive functions are likely to contribute to an increased fall risk, especially when combining balance or walking tasks with concurrent (cognitive) tasks. Fall management should consist of a combination of identification and treatment of the underlying causes of physiological and cognitive impairments.

MP was financially supported by NWO grant # 916.76.077.

References

[1]   Ganz, A Bao, Y.Shekelle, PG., Rubenstein, LZ,.Will My Patient Fall? JAMA. 2007;297(1):77-86.
[2]   Beauchet O, Najafi B, Dubost V, Aminian K, Mourey F, Kressing RW. Age-related decline of gait control under dual task condition. *Journal of the American Geriatrics Society,* 2003;51:1187-1188
[3]   Yogev-Seligmann G, Hausdorff JM, Galidi N. The role of executive function and attention in gait. *Movement Disorders,* 2008;23(3):329-342
[4]   Lamoth CJC, van Lummel RC, Beek PJ. Athletic skill level is reflected in body sway: A test case for accelerometry in combination with stochastic dynamics. *Gait Posture,* 2009;29:546-551

Rehabilitation: Mobility, Exercise and Sports
L.H.V. van der Woude et al. (Eds.)
IOS Press, 2010

doi:10.3233/978-1-60750-080-3-134

Prospective study on physical activity levels after spinal cord injury during inpatient rehabilitation and the year after discharge

R.J. VAN DEN BERG-EMONS[a], J.B. BUSSMANN[a], J.A. HAISMA[a], T.A. SLUIS[b], L.H.V. VAN DER WOUDE[c], M.P. BERGEN[b], H.J. STAM[a]

[a] *Department of Rehabilitation Medicine, Erasmus Medical Center, Rotterdam, The Netherlands*
[b] *Rijndam Rehabilitation Center, Rotterdam, The Netherlands*
[c] *Research Institute MOVE, Institute for Fundamental & Clinical Human Movement Sciences, Faculty of Human Movement Sciences, Vrije Universiteit, Amsterdam, The Netherlands*

Abstract. Purpose: To assess change over time in physical activity level (PAL) after spinal cord injury (SCI), to explore its determinants, and to compare PAL 1 year after discharge from the rehabilitation center with able-bodied level. Methods: PAL, as indicated by duration of dynamic activities per day and intensity of everyday activity, was measured in 40 persons with SCI with an accelerometry-based activity monitor during 2 consecutive weekdays. Measurements were obtained at start of active rehabilitation, 3 months later, at discharge, 2 months after discharge, and 1 year after discharge. Results: Random coefficient analyses demonstrated that duration of dynamic activities and intensity of everyday activity increased during inpatient rehabilitation at rates of 41% and 19%, respectively ($P<.01$). Shortly after discharge, there was a strong decline (33%; $P<.001$) in duration of dynamic activities. One year after discharge, this decline was restored to discharge level, but was low in comparison with able-bodied level. Level and completeness of lesion were determinants of change in PAL after discharge. Conclusion: PAL increased during inpatient rehabilitation, but this increase did not continue after discharge and level 1 year after discharge was distinctly lower than able-bodied level. Subpopulations had a different change over time in PAL after discharge.

Keywords. activities of daily living, rehabilitation, spinal cord injury.

1. Introduction

Because of loss of motor, sensory, and autonomic innervation below the lesion level, persons with a spinal cord injury (SCI) are often restricted in their performance of everyday physical activities. As a consequence, persons with SCI are, more than the able-bodied population, at risk of developing a hypoactive lifestyle, with possible detrimental effects on physical fitness, social participation, and quality of life [1]. Furthermore, a hypoactive lifestyle can increase the risk of developing secondary health problems later in life, such as cardiovascular disease and diabetes [2]. Despite the possible detrimental effects of a hypoactive lifestyle, few studies have objectively investigated the impact of SCI on the physical activity level (PAL). Aim of the study was to objectively, and in detail in persons with SCI, (1) determine the change in PAL during inpatient rehabilitation and in the year after discharge from the rehabilitation center; (2) explore the association between (the change in) PAL, personal characteristics (ie, age and sex), and lesion characteristics (ie, level and completeness); and (3) determine PAL 1 year after discharge in comparison with the level in able-bodied persons.

2. Methods

This prospective cohort study was part of a national research program [3]. We collected data at 5 standardized test occasions: at the start of active inpatient rehabilitation (T1), 3 months later (T2), at discharge from inpatient rehabilitation (T3), and 2 months (T4) and 1 year (T5) after discharge. From the SCI department of Rijndam Rehabilitation Center in Rotterdam, The Netherlands, we recruited 40 persons with SCI who were in their initial inpatient rehabilitation from 2001 until 2005 (mean age 42.1±14.7 yrs; 78% male; 44% tetraplegia; 69% complete lesion). We objectively measured PAL during 2 consecutive weekdays using an activity monitor. The activity monitor is based on long-term (>24h) ambulatory monitoring of signals from body-fixed accelerometers [4]. From the accelerometer signals, the duration, rate, and moment of occurrence of activities associated with mobility (the stationary activities, lying, sitting, and standing; the dynamic activities walking [ie, climbing/descending stairs and running], cycling, manual wheelchair driving [including hand biking], and general non-cyclic movement), and transitions between postures can be automatically detected with a 1 second resolution. Furthermore, from each measured signal, information on the variability of the acceleration signal (motility, which is related to the intensity of everyday physical activity) can be obtained. For statistical analysis we used random coefficient analyses and *t*-tests.

3. Results

Random coefficient analyses demonstrated that duration of dynamic activities (composite measure of walking, manual wheelchair driving, general non-cyclic movement) and intensity of everyday activity increased during inpatient rehabilitation at rates of 41% and 19%, respectively (P<.01). Shortly after discharge, there was a strong decline (33%; P<.001) in duration of dynamic activities (Figure 1). One year after discharge, this decline was restored to the discharge level, but was low (34% of level in able-bodied persons). Level of lesion and completeness of lesion were determinants of the change in PAL after discharge in that persons with paraplegia and persons with an incomplete lesion showed significantly more improvement in the duration of dynamic activities in the year after discharge than did persons with tetraplegia and persons with a complete lesion, respectively.

4. Conclusion

PAL increased during inpatient rehabilitation, but this increase did not continue after discharge and level 1 year after discharge was distinctly lower than able-bodied level. Subpopulations had a different change over time in PAL after discharge.

5. Implications for treatment

We suggest that rehabilitation should be aimed at increasing PAL in persons with SCI. Treatment should make persons more aware of the possible consequences of their low PAL and should focus on stimulating persons to develop and maintain a more active lifestyle, particularly after discharge from the rehabilitation center and particularly in persons with tetraplegia and persons with complete lesions. Since PAL showed a (nonsignificant) deterioration after the early phase of inpatient rehabilitation (T3 vs T2) (see Figure 1), behavioral strategies preferably should start as early as possible in the rehabilitation process. To improve activity patterns throughout life, these strategies should continue to be used after discharge from the rehabilitation center.

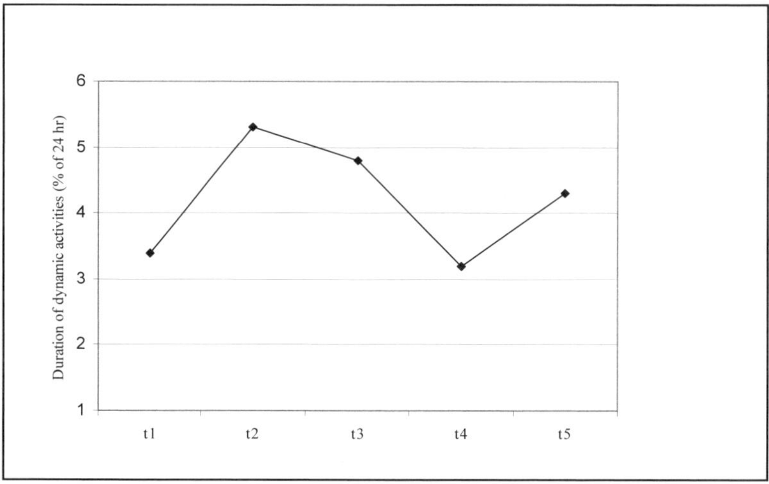

Figure 1. Change over time in duration of dynamic activities (as percentage of a 24h period) as estimated with random coefficient analyses. The duration of dynamic activities at T3 was significantly different from T1 ($P<.001$) and from T4 ($P<.001$).

References

[1]   A.L. Stewart, R.D. Hays, K.B. Wells, W.H. Rogers, K.L. Spritzer, S. Greenfield, Long-term functioning and well-being outcomes associated with physical activity and exercise in patients with chronic conditions in the Medical Outcomes Study, *J Clin Epidemiol* **27** (1994), 719-30.
[2]   J.W. Twisk, H.C. Kemper, W. van Mechelen, G.B. Post, F.J. van Lenthe. Body fatness: longitudinal relationship of body mass index and the sum of skinfolds with other risk factors for coronary heart disease. *Int J Obes Relat Metab Disord* **22** (1998), 915-22.
[3]   S. de Groot, A.J. Dallmeijer, M.W. Post et al. Demographics of the Dutch multicenter prospective cohort study 'Restoration of mobility in spinal cord injury rehabilitation'. *Spinal Cord* **44** (2006), 668-75.
[4]   J.B. Bussmann, W.L. Martens, J.H. Tulen, F.C. Schasfoort, H.J. van den Berg-Emons, H.J. Stam. Measuring daily behavior using ambulatory accelerometry: the Activity Monitor. Behav Res Methods *Instrum Comput* **33** (2001), 349-56

Rehabilitation: Mobility, Exercise and Sports
L.H.V. van der Woude et al. (Eds.)
IOS Press, 2010

doi:10.3233/978-1-60750-080-3-137

137

Muscle strength and mobility in diabetic patients with and without polyneuropathy

T.H. IJZERMAN[a], T. MELAI[a,b], K. MEIJER[a], N.C. SCHAPER[c],
P.J.B. WILLEMS[a], A.L.H. DE LANGE[b], H.H.C.M. SAVELBERG[a]
[a] *Nutrition and Toxicology Research Institute Maastricht, Dept. Health, Medicine
and Life Sciences, University Maastricht*
[b] *Fontys University of Applied Sciences, Eindhoven, The Netherlands*
[c] *Cardiovascular Research Institute Maastricht, Academic Hospital*

Abstract. The purpose of this study was to investigate the effect of diabetic polyneuropathie (DPN) on muscle strength of the lower limb and mobility. Based on previous studies we expect that diabetes leads to a loss in muscle strength and that this process will be enhanced by neuropathy. Moreover, it has been hypothesized that muscle weakness is a main factor in limitations of the mobility. The study enrolled 62 subjects: 27 DPN patients, 16 age matched diabetic type 2 patients (DM2) without DPN (DC) and 19 healthy subjects (C). They performed isometric knee and ankle strength tests on a dynamometer. Mobility was determined from a timed 'get up and go test', a six minute walk test and the PASE (physical activity scale for the elderly) questionnaire. Healthy elderly had significantly higher muscle strength compared to the DC and DPN groups ($p<0.01$). No significant differences were found between DC and DPN. For both groups DC en DPN muscle weakness strongly correlates with the level of mobility in daily life ($p<0.05$ for all outcome parameters).Muscle weakness itself seems to be a strongly predictor for the decline in mobility. Moreover, DPN does not lead to a larger decrease of muscle weakness compared to DM2 patients.

Keywords. type 2 diabetes mellitus, polyneuropathy, muscle strength, mobility.

1. Introduction

Impaired mobility is a major health problem affecting many subjects with diabetes mellitus (DM). It is associated with loss of quality of life and it is a strong predictor for poor health outcomes. Reduced lower extremity muscle function, as a consequence of diabetic polyneuropathy (DPN), is a major cause of impaired mobility. The loss of motor and sensory nerve functions can lead to loss of muscle mass and strength.

The purpose of the present study was to compare mobility and muscle strength in the lower extrimities in DPN and type 2 diabetes mellitus (DM2) patients and to investigate whether mobility and muscle strength are related. The disablement process in DM patients is often progressive and results in worsening of the impairments. Based on previous studies [1,2] we expect that DM2 causes a decline of muscle strengh and that due to motor and sensory nerve damage DPN will enhance this process. It has been hypothesized that muscle weakness is an important factor in the limitation of mobility.

2. Subjects and Methods

Subjects

DPN patients (n=27), age matched DM2 patients without DPN (DC) (n=16) and healthy age matched subjects (C) (n=19) performed maximal, voluntary, isometric knee-joint extensor and flexor and ankle plantar and dorsal flexor strength tests in a dynamometer. The diagnosis of DPN was based on a standardized clinical neurological examination. [3]

Methods

Mobility tests
Mobility was determined from a timed 'get up and go' test (TGUG), a six minute walk test (6MWT) and the physical activity scale for the elderly questionnaire (PASE).
Isometric knee and ankle tests
The subjects were instructed to develop subsequently a maximal extending and a maximal flexing knee joint moment in 5 different angles of the right leg; 100°, 90°, 70°, 50° and 30° were 0° is a fully extended leg. The hip angle was constantly at 90°. The maximal dorsal and plantar ankle joint moments were determined in five different angles; maximal dorsal flexion, 90°, 110°, 130° and maximal plantar flexion. The maximal joint moment were normalized for body weight. Optimal angles were determined by meaning of a second degree polynomial regression through the normalized strength data.

3. Results

With respect to mobility a decreasing trend from C to DC and from DC to DPN was found (Table 1).

Table 1. Differences in mobility and maximal torques and optimal angles of the ankle and knee

Mobility	DPN	DC	C
6MWT (m)	455 (+/- 117) *#	555 (+/- 89) *	660 (+/- 68)
TGUG (s)	9.86 (+/- 3.17) *	8.35 (+/- 1.03)	7.16 (+/- 0.93)
PASE	136.6 (+/-79.4)	155.0 (+/- 116)	191.5 (+/- 72)
Maximal Torque			
Dorsal flexion (Nm/kg)	0.42 (+/- 0.13) *	0.47 (+/- 0.12) *	0.62 (+/- 0.11)
Plantar flexion (Nm/kg)	0.58 (+/- 0.21) *	0.64 (+/- 0.23) *	0.93 (+/- 0.35)
Knee extension (Nm/kg)	0.91 (+/- 0.24) *	0.95 (+/- 0.36) *	1.27 (+/- 0.32)
Knee flexion (Nm/kg)	1.58 (+/- 0.32) *	1.69 (+/- 0.50) *	2.07 (+/- 0.35)
Optimal angle			
Dorsal flexion (°)	115 (+/- 13)	111 (+/- 13)	110 (+/- 6)
Plantar flexion (°)	89 (+/- 19)	86 (+/- 20)	86 (+/- 16)
Knee extension (°)	72 (+/- 11)	76 (+/- 10)	74 (+/- 11)
Knee flexion (°)	89 (+/- 19)	91 (+/- 12)	87 (+/- 15)

*Different from Control (p≤0.05). #Different from DM (p<0.01)

The 6MWT showed significant differences between every single group (p<0.01). The TGUG test resulted in significant difference between the DPN and C group (p≤0.05); no significant differences were found between the three groups regarding to the PASE questionnaire. A clear tendency in decreased mobility was observed in the DC and DPN group, where DPN showed the lowest mobility scores (Table 1).

Overall muscle strength was significantly higher in healthy elderly than in the DC and DPN group (p<0.01)(table 1). No significant differences were found between the DC and DPN group. No significant differences were found with respect to the optimal knee and ankle angles (table 1). The degree of muscle weakness correlated strongly with the level of mobility (figure 1).

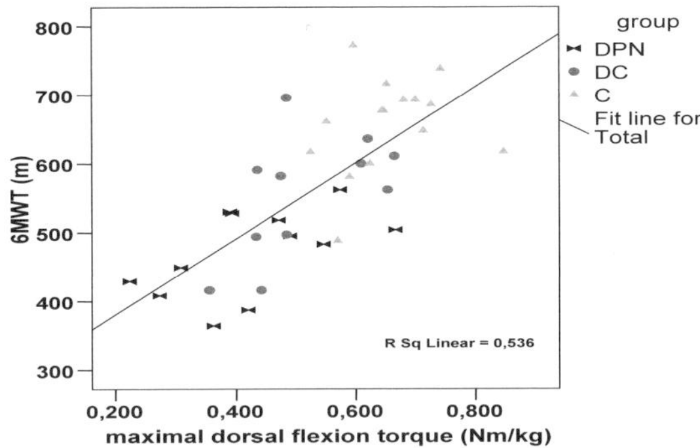

Figure 1. Correlation between maximal dorsal ankle torque and 6MWT.

4. Discussion

We hypothesized that muscle strength and mobility in DM2 patients is impaired and that DPN aggravates his impairment. We have shown that DM2 patients have decreased muscle strength compared to healthy age matched elderly. Nevertheless, the presented data suggest that DPN has no additional effect on muscle strength above diabetes itself. In other words, the diminished nerve function in the lower extremities does not cause decreased muscle strength. But yet, patients with DPN walk less far in spite of relative similar muscle strength. These data suggest that the decreased mobility in DPN patients, compared to DM2 patients, is not due to muscle weakness but to other features like diminished sensory and motor nerve functions.[1]

5. Conclusion

Muscle weakness itself is associated to the decline in mobility. Moreover it seems that DPN does not lead to a larger decrease of muscle strength compared to patients with DM2. More research is needed to determine the influence of nerve damage in DPN patients on muscle strength and to find an explanation for a reduced mobility in DPN subjects compared to DM.

References

[1]	C.S. Andreassen et al, Muscle weakness: a progressive late complication in diabetic distal symmetric polyneuropathy, *Diabetes* **55** (2006), 806-12.
[2]	A.A. Sayer et al, Type 2 diabetes, muscle strength, and impaired physical function: the tip of the iceberg?, *Diabetes Care* **28** (2005), 2541-2.
[3]	G.D. Valk et al, The assessment of diabetic polyneuropathy in daily clinical practice: reproducibility and validity of Semmes Weinstein monofilaments examination and clinical neurological examination, *Muscle Nerve* **20** (1997), 116-8.

Rehabilitation: Mobility, Exercise and Sports
L.H.V. van der Woude et al. (Eds.)
IOS Press, 2010
© *2010 The authors and IOS Press. All rights reserved.*
doi:10.3233/978-1-60750-080-3-140

Determination of overweight in Spinal Cord Injury: comparison of different methods

I. ERIKS-HOOGLAND[a,1], R. HILFIKER[a], S. BALK[b], M. BAUMBERGER[b], C. PERRET[b]

[a] *Swiss Paraplegic Research, Nottwil, Switzerland*
[b] *Swiss Paraplegic Centre, Nottwil, Switzerland*

Abstract. Obesity has become a major health problem in persons with a spinal cord injury (SCI). An in SCI persons validated measure of fat mass is the use of single frequency bio-impedance with a for the SCI population specific equation (BIA+ equation). Conversely, clinical management relies on measures which are both valid and practical in day-to-day practice. Lacking an alternative, BMI is still in clinical management although it is shown to be not valid in SCI populations. Potential alternatives for clinical practice are the simple measurement of waist circumference (WC) or the calculation of an anthropometric index integrating using waist circumference, calf circumference, chest diameter and measurement of subscapular skin fold (AI). To examine the validity of WC and an AI in comparison to BIA + equation we studied these measurments in 23 adult male persons with motor complete paraplegia (duration > 1 year). An estimation of obesity using WC and AI and comparing them with BIA+equation using Bland and Altman plots and statistics and Pearson's correlation coefficients was made. Good agreement between BIA+equation and AI with a small systematic difference (mean difference: -0.28) was found. The correlation (Pearson's r) between WC and the BIA+equation % FM was very high (0.83). Concluded can be that using an AI is suited to determine obesity in adult male SCI persons. WC measurment is promising, but needs further validation.

Keywords. spinal cord injuries, overweight, anthropometrics, body mass index, bio-impedance.

1. Introduction

Obesity has become a major health problem in persons with a spinal cord injury (SCI) because of its relation to, among others, cardiovascular diseases, metabolic diseases and musculoskeletal disorders [1-4]. An in SCI persons validated measure of fat mass is the use of single frequency bio-impedance with a for the SCI population specific equation (BIA+ equation) [5]. Conversely, clinical management relies on measures which are both valid and practical in day-to-day practice.

Lacking an alternative, BMI is still used in research and clinical management although it is shown to be not valid in SCI populations [5-8].

---

[1] Corresponding Author: Inge Eriks-Hoogland, Swiss Paraplegic Research, Guido A. Zächstrasse 4, CH-6207, Nottwil, Switzerland. E-mail: inge.eriks@paranet.ch

Potential alternatives for clinical practice are the simple measurements of waist circumference (WC) [9] or the calculation of an anthropometric index integrating waist circumference, calf circumference, chest diameter and measurement of subscapular skin fold (AI) [10].

2.   Objective

To examine the validity of WC and an AI in comparison to BIA + equation.

3.   Methods

Patients

A convenience sample of 23 adult male persons with motor complete paraplegia, with duration of longer than 1 year was included in the study. All subjects gave their informed consent prior to the study.

Study design

All subjects were measured by the same researcher, using a standardized protocol. Subjects omitted caffeine, alcohol and energy rich nutrition 24 hours before measurement and did not perform straining exercises 12 hours before measurement.
   Of all subjects the following outcomes were measured:
- WC: measured at minimal waist after normal expiration
- Calf circumference: in supine position, heels on knee roll
- Subscapular skin fold: Right subscapular skin fold in lying position
- Chest diameter: supine position, at nipple level during mid expiration

4.   Statistics

Estimation of obesity using WC and AI and comparing them with BIA+equation using Bland and Altman plots and statistics and Pearson's correlation coefficients.

5.   Results

Of the 23 included subjects, 22 were classified AIS A, 1 AIS B. Lesion level varied between Th2 and L1.
   Good agreement between BIA+equation and AI with a small systematic difference (mean difference: -0.28) was found (Fig1). The correlation (Pearson's r) between WC and the BIA+equation % FM was very high (0.83).

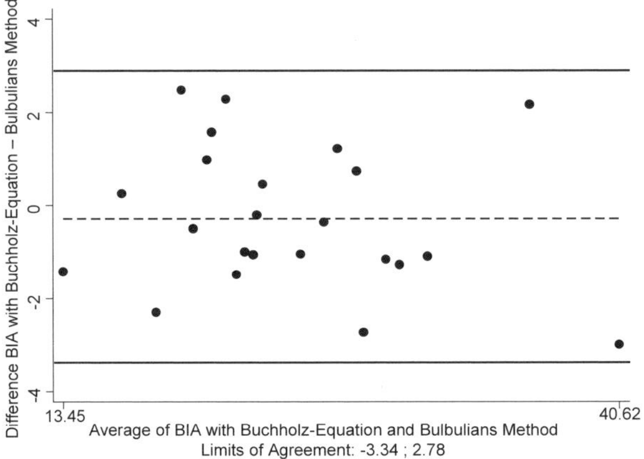

Figure 1: Measured percentage body fat: Difference of the measurement with the BIA/ with the Buchholz-Equation correction, and the AI index (Bulbulians method) versus the average of values measured by both methods with 95% limits of agreement (-3.34 to 2.78).

6.   Conclusion

Using an AI is suited to determine obesity in adult male SCI persons. WC is promising, but needs further validation.

References

[1]   Strauss DJ, Devivo MJ, Paculdo DR, Shavelle RM. Trends in life expectancy after spinal cord injury. *Archives of physical medicine and rehabilitation* 2006; 87: 1079-85.

[2]   Garshick E, Kelley A, Cohen SA, Garrison A, Tun CG, Gagnon D et al. A prospective assessment of mortality in chronic spinal cord injury. *Spinal Cord* 2005; 43: 408-16.

[3]   Maruyama Y, Mizuguchi M, Yaginuma T, Kusaka M, Yoshida H, Yokoyama K et al. Serum leptin, abdominal obesity and the metabolic syndrome in individuals with chronic spinal cord injury. *Spinal Cord* 2008; 46: 494-9.

[4]   Mercer JL, Boninger M, Koontz A, Ren D, Dyson-Hudson T, Cooper R. Shoulder joint kinetics and pathology in manual wheelchair users. *Clin Biomech (Bristol, Avon)* 2006; 21: 781-9.

[5]   Buchholz AC, McGillivray CF, Pencharz PB. The use of bioelectric impedance analysis to measure fluid compartments in subjects with chronic paraplegia. *Archives of physical medicine and rehabilitation* 2003; 84: 854-61.

[6]   Buchholz AC, Bugaresti JM. A review of body mass index and waist circumference as markers of obesity and coronary heart disease risk in persons with chronic spinal cord injury. *Spinal Cord* 2005; 43: 513-8.

[7]   Jones LM, Legge M, Goulding A. Healthy body mass index values often underestimate body fat in men with spinal cord injury. *Archives of physical medicine and rehabilitation* 2003; 84: 1068-71.

[8]   Spungen AM, Bauman WA, Wang J, Pierson RN, Jr. Measurement of body fat in individuals with tetraplegia: a comparison of eight clinical methods. *Paraplegia* 1995; 33: 402-8.

[9]   Ross R, Berentzen T, Bradshaw AJ, Janssen I, Kahn HS, Katzmarzyk PT et al. Does the relationship between waist circumference, morbidity and mortality depend on measurement protocol for waist circumference? *Obes Rev* 2008; 9: 312-25.

[10]   Bulbulian R, Johnson RE, Gruber JJ, Darabos B. Body composition in paraplegic male athletes. *Medicine and science in sports and exercise* 1987; 19: 195-201.

Rehabilitation: Mobility, Exercise and Sports
L.H.V. van der Woude et al. (Eds.)
IOS Press, 2010

doi:10.3233/978-1-60750-080-3-143

143

Relation between shoulder proprioception, kinematics and pain after stroke

M.H.M. NIESSEN[a,b,1], H.E.J. VEEGER[a], C.G. MESKERS[c], P.A. KOPPE[b],
M.H. KONIJNENBELT[b], T.W.J. JANSSEN[a,b]

[a] *Research Institute MOVE, Faculty of Human Movement Sciences, VU University Amsterdam*
[b] *Duyvensz-Nagel Research Laboratory, Rehabilitation Center Amsterdam, Amsterdam*
[c] *Department of Rehabilitation Medicine, Leiden University Medical Center, Leiden*

Abstract. Purpose: To identify a possible relationship between chronic Post-Stroke Shoulder Pain (PSSP), scapular resting pose and shoulder proprioception. Methods: A total of 21 inpatients with stroke and 10 healthy control subjects were included and kinematics and proprioception of both shoulders were measured. Results: The contralateral (i.e. paretic) shoulder of patients with PSSP showed more scapular lateral rotation and larger errors on proprioception tests compared to both patients without PSSP and control subjects. Additionally, the contralateral shoulder of patients with deteriorated proprioception showed more scapular lateral rotation compared to control subjects whereas their ipsilateral (i.e. unaffected) shoulder showed more scapular lateral rotation when compared to both control subjects and patients with good proprioception. Conclusions: A clear relation between affected shoulder kinematics, affected proprioception and PSSP was found. In determining the risk of developing PSSP, attention should be paid to a patients shoulder proprioception and kinematics. If both are altered after stroke, this could worsen the initial pathology or cause secondary pathologies and thus initiate a vicious circle of repetitive soft tissue damage leading to chronic PSSP. Additionally, more attention should be paid to the ipsilateralshoulder since it could be used in determining the risk of developing PSSP in the contralateral shoulder.

Keywords. stroke, pain, proprioception, kinematics, shoulder.

1. Introduction

In the development of Post-Stroke Shoulder Pain (PSSP), alterations to shoulder proprioception (i.e. afferent information arising from peripheral areas of the body that contributes to joint stability, postural control, and motor control) [1,2] as well as alterations in shoulder kinematics could play an important role [3].

We hypothesize that shoulder pain will be related to both a disturbed shoulder pose and a disturbed proprioception. Then, shoulder pain, whatever the initiating factor, may eventually be the consequence of a vicious circle of repetitive soft tissue damage caused by improper kinematics and deteriorated proprioception.

---

[1] Corresponding Author: Martijn H. Niessen, MSc, Research Institute MOVE, Faculty of Human Movement Sciences, VU University Amsterdam, Van der Boechorststraat 9,1081 BT Amsterdam, The Netherlands. E-Mail: m.niessen@fbw.vu.nl

2.　Methods

Twenty one patients in the subacute phase after stroke were recruited from the inpatient stroke unit of a general rehabilitation hospital. All patients had experienced their first stroke and had no history of shoulder complaints prior to the stroke. Only patients who were able to perform all the required physical, cognitive, and communicative tests for this study were included. Measurements were done on the contralateral side (relative to the affected hemisphere, i.e. paretic) as well as the ipsilateral side (relative to the affected hemisphere, i.e. non-paretic) since it has been shown that both shoulders could be affected after stroke. We included a control group (n=10), mainly consisting of employees from the rehabilitation center. The study was approved by the local institutional medical ethical review committee and all subjects signed an informed consent statement before the start of the measurements.

Shoulder proprioception

An isokinetic dynamometer was used to measure proprioception. During the tests, subjects were blindfolded to rule out visual clues. Subjects did not wear earphones because communication with the experimenter was necessary.

The threshold to detection of passive motion (TDPM) is a measure of an individual's kinaesthesia [1,2]. Subjects were seated next to the dynamometer. With the subject being instructed to relax, the dynamometer moved the subject's arm into two directions: internal or external rotation, and subjects had to indicate when they detected the motion.

Passive reproduction of joint position (PRJP) tests gives a measure of a individual's position sense [1,2]. The dynamometer moved the subject's arm passively to a reference angle: 10° internal or 10° external rotation, relative to a chosen start position. Each subject was allowed to sense the reference angle for 10 seconds before the arm was returned passively to the start position. Subsequently, the arm was moved passively towards the reference position and the subject had to indicate verbally when he/she felt that it had been reached. At that point the dynamometer was stopped by the experimenter. The absolute error in degrees (i.e. offset) between the indicated and reference position was measured

Shoulder kinematics

We used an electromagnetic tracking device to quantify shoulder kinematics. This setup consists of a transmitter creating a weak magnetic field in which the position and orientation of several receivers can be followed. Measurements were performed on both arms separately in sitting position according to standards of the International Shoulder Group (ISG). Poses (position (i.e. translation in x, y and z direction) and orientation) of the scapula relative to the thorax during rest (with arms along side the body) were used for analysis.

3. Results

It was found that: 1) both shoulders of patients with PSSP show more lateral rotation than patients without PSSP and controls; 2) both shoulders of patients with PSSP show deteriorated proprioception (both on TDPM and PRJP tests) when compared to patients without PSSP and controls; 3) the contralateral shoulder of patients with deteriorated proprioception shows more scapular lateral rotation than controls; and 4) the ipsilateral shoulder of patients with deteriorated proprioception shows more scapular lateral rotation than patients with normal proprioception and controls.

4. Conclusion

The clinical implications of the observed relationships between PSSP, shoulder proprioception and kinematics remain speculative since the design of this study does not allow for a causal relation to be established. However, we can conclude in general that patients with PSSP show more scapular lateral rotation and have deteriorated proprioception. Also patients with affected proprioception have a more laterally rotated scapula. So in determining the risk of developing PSSP, attention should be paid to a patients shoulder proprioception and kinematics. If both are altered after stroke, this could worsen the initial pathology or cause secondary pathologies and thus initiate a vicious circle of repetitive soft tissue damage leading to chronic PSSP. Another interesting implication is that measurements on the ipsilateral (non-paretic) side could be used as an indicator for the development of PSSP on the contralateral side. For stroke patients, measurements on the ipsilateral shoulder are easier, faster and more comfortable than measurements on the contralateral shoulder. If shoulder kinematics and proprioception are both affected on the ipsilateral side, this could reflect the vulnerability of the contralateral shoulder for developing PSSP during the early stages of rehabilitation.

Future studies investigating the causal relation between proprioception, shoulder kinematics and the development of PSSP should incorporate a longitudinal design and/or interventions aimed at improving shoulder proprioception and shoulder kinematics. This could also shed more light on the mechanisms leading to chronic PSSP. Additionally, more research should be done on possibility of using measurements of the ipsilateral shoulder as an indicator for the development of PSSP on the contralateral side.

References

[1]　S.M. Lephart, J.J.. Warner, P.A. Borsa and F.H. FU, Proprioception of the shoulder joint in healthy, unstable and surgically repaired shoulders. *J Shoulder Elbow Surg* **3** (1994), 371–380.

[2]　M.H. Niessen, D.H. Veeger, P.A. Koppe, M.H. Konijnenbelt, J. van Dieen and T. Janssen. Proprioception of the shoulder after stroke, *Arch Phys Med Rehabil* **89** (2008), 333–338.

[3]　M.H. Niessen, T.W. Janssen, C.G. Meskers, P.A. Koppe, M.H. Konijnenbelt, and D.H. Veeger. Kinematics of the contralateral and ipsilateral shoulder: a possible relationship with Post Stroke Shoulder Pain, *J Rehabil Med* **40** (2008), 482–486.

4.3

Poster Presentations

Rehabilitation: Mobility, Exercise and Sports
L.H.V. van der Woude et al. (Eds.)
IOS Press, 2010

doi:10.3233/978-1-60750-080-3-149

Stride time fluctuations during the six minute walk test in COPD patients

J. ANNEGARN[a], M.A. SPRUIT[b], H.H.C.M. SAVELBERG[a], P.J.B. WILLEMS[a],
E.F.M. WOUTERS[b,c], A.M.W.J. SCHOLS[c], K. MEIJER[a]

[a] *Human Movement Science, NUTRIM School for Nutrition, Toxicology and Metabolism Maastricht University Medical Centre, Maastricht, Netherlands*
[b] *Research, Development & Education, Centre for Integrated Rehabilitation of Organ failure (CIRO), Horn, Netherlands*
[c] *Respiratory Medicine, NUTRIM School for Nutrition, Toxicology and Metabolism Maastricht University Medical Centre, Maastricht, Netherlands*

Abstract. Introduction. Detrended fluctuation analyses (DFA) method provides insight in long-range correlations in gait by the scaling exponent α. Changes in α have been associated with central neurological diseases and gait unsteadiness in the elderly. It is not conclusively known if α can also reflect dysfunction of other physiological systems. We evaluated the fractal dynamics of gait in chronic obstructive pulmonary disease (COPD) patients; a population suffering from reduced muscle function and pulmonary dysfunction. Methods Healthy subjects (n=12) and COPD patients (n=15) walked continuously for six minutes as fast as possible. Stride intervals, derived with a tri-axial accelerometer, were processed with the DFA method to derive α. Results The COPD patients differed significantly (p<0.01) from healthy subjects in age (COPD 63.7 yrs±3.9; healthy 33.3 yrs±2.3), distance walked (COPD 499m±23; healthy 662m±27) stride intervals (COPD=1.08 sec.±0.08; healthy=0.95 sec.±0.08) and α (COPD 0.89±0.12; healthy 0.72±0.14). Conclusion In contrary to central neurological diseases, COPD patients show higher α compared to healthy subjects. This indicates that also muscle dysfunction or pulmonary dysfunction can influence α.

Keywords. gait, chronic disease.

1. Introduction

Analyzing walking patterns of patients can be useful in characterizing different pathological states and functional status. Recently Hausdorff (2007) suggested detrended fluctuation analyses (DFA) as method to evaluate mobility of patients and elderly with fall risk [2]. DFA provides insight in long-range correlations in gait by a single scaling exponent α [1]. An α towards 1.0 indicates healthy long-range, fractal correlations. On the other hand, an α closer to 0.5, indicating randomness, can be related to age-related and pathologic alterations in the locomotor control system. Besides physiological factors α can also be influenced by environmental factors. When healthy subjects are restricted to walk with a certain step frequency, time series fluctuations become more uncorrelated and α drops towards 0.5 [2]. Yet when subjects walk fast, α increases toward 1.0. Decrease in α have been associated with central neurological diseases, such as Parkinson and Huntington's disease and gait unsteadiness in the elderly. Although α does not alter in patients with peripheral limitations [3], it is not conclusively known if α can also reflect control processes of other physiological systems. Therefore we had a closer look at the fractal dynamics of gait in chronic obstructive pulmonary disease (COPD) patients. COPD is a highly prevalent chronic lung disease, characterized by reduced muscle function and pulmonary dysfunction.

2. Subjects and methods

Subjects

COPD patients (N=15) and healthy subjects (N=12) walked continuously as far as possible within six minutes without walking aids. All subjects were encouraged each minute during the test.

Methods

Stride interval fluctuations were derived from left and right heel strikes measured with a tri-axial accelerometer (Minimod 100Hz $\pm$ 5g) attached to the trunk [4]. Subsequently time series of stride times were processed with the DFA method to derive α, which is the slope of the line relating the average fluctuation F(n) and the box size n on an log-log plot.

3. Results

COPD patients were classified from mild to severe COPD (FEV1: 48.9 ± 15.6 % predicted). They were on average older and walked significantly ($p<0.01$) slower compared to healthy subjects. As a consequence the stride time intervals were longer in COPD patients. The distances walked by our healthy subjects were comparable to the distances measured by Troosters et al. (1999), (distance: 631m $\pm$ 93) [5]. Compared to our healthy subjects, the COPD patients had higher α (table 1).

Table 1. Subjects characteristics: *significant difference compared with the healthy subjects ($p<0.01$)

	Age [yrs]	Distance walked [m]	Stride intervals [sec.]	α
Healthy (N=12)	33.3 ± 2.3	662 ± 27	1.08 ± 0.08	0.73 ± 0.14
COPD (N=15)	$63.7 \pm 3.9^*$	$499 \pm 23^*$	$0.95 \pm 0.08^*$	$0.90 \pm 0.11^*$

4. Discussion

Surprisingly in this study α was higher in COPD patients compared to healthy subjects. The higher α could not be explained by the higher age or slower speed of the COPD patients, because in other studies α is shown to be higher in younger and faster walking subjects [2]. It should be mentioned that our fast walking healthy subjects had lower α (0.73) compared to Hausdorff (2007), (α =0.97) [2]. In our study the COPD patients and healthy subject walked in identical experimental environments. Therefore we suggest that the physiological impairments of COPD patients, like pulmonary limitations or muscle weakness, were the main determinant of the observed differences in α.

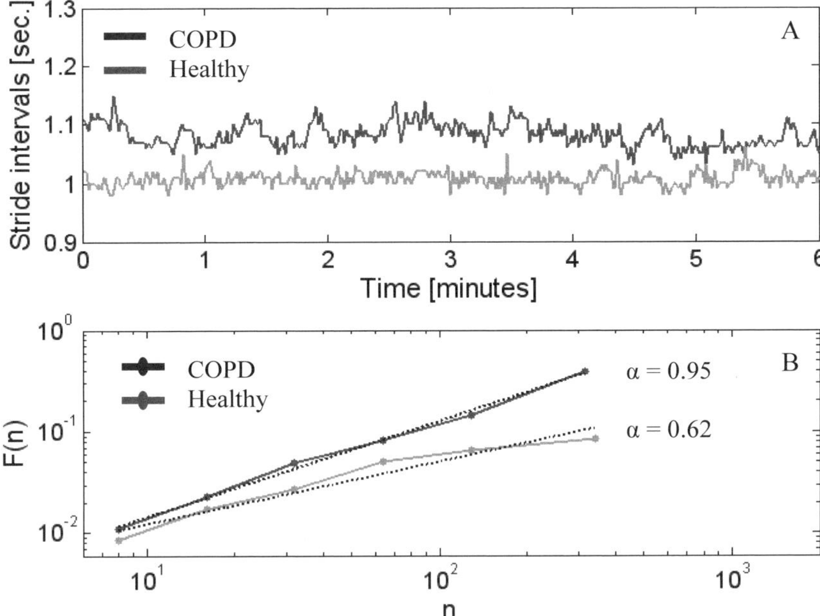

Figure 1. Example of stride interval dynamics of a healthy subject and COPD patient. Six minute stride interval time series (A) and fluctuations (B).

5. Conclusion

This study shows that different long-range correlations can exist between healthy subjects and patients who do not suffer from central neurological diseases, which indicates that also reduced muscle function and pulmonary dysfunction can influence α. Further investigation is needed to explore the underlying mechanism of the fluctuations in the time series of the stride times.

References

[1]   www.physionet.org
[2]   J.N. Hausdorff, Gait dynamics, fractals and falls: Finding meaning in the stride-to-stride fluctuations of human walking. **26** (2007), 555–589.
[3]   D.H. Gates and J.B. Dingwell, Peripheral neuropathy does not alter the fractal dynamics of stride intervals of gait. **102** (2007), 965–971.
[4]   W. Zijstra and A.L. Hof, Assessment of spatio-temporal gait parameters from trunk accelerations during human walking. **18** (2003), 1-10.
[5]   T. Troosters et al., Six minute walking distance in healthy elderly subjects. **14** (1999), 270-274

Rehabilitation: Mobility, Exercise and Sports
L.H.V. van der Woude et al. (Eds.)
IOS Press, 2010

doi:10.3233/978-1-60750-080-3-152

Muscle properties and functional recovery until one year after stroke

A.M.H. HORSTMAN[a], H.L. GERRITS[a,b], T.W.J. JANSSEN[a,b], A. DE HAAN[a,c]
*[a] Research Institute MOVE, Faculty of Human Movement Sciences, VU University
Amsterdam, the Netherlands*
[b] DNO, Rehabilitation Centre Amsterdam, Amsterdam, the Netherlands
*[c] Institute for Biomedical Research into Human Movement and Health, Manchester
Metropolitan University, Manchester, UK*

Abstract. Purpose: to investigate functional performance in relation to muscle function during first year after stroke. Methods: Maximal voluntary isometric torques of knee extensors (MVTe) and flexors (MVTf) were obtained in 14 patients with subacute stroke (bilaterally) 3.5±2 months after stroke and 3 (n=8), 6 (n=5) and 12 months (n=3) thereafter and in 12 age-matched able-bodied subjects. Maximal triplet response (intrinsic muscle strength), maximal rate of torque development (MRTD) and degree of voluntary activation of knee extensors were estimated. Patients performed 7 tests of functional performance. Results: In the paretic lower limb (PL), all parameters significantly (0.494<|r|<0.909) improved during all follow-ups. In the non-paretic lower limb (NL) most improvement occurred within the first 3 months. For NL and PL, MVTe improved 5 and 16%, respectively MVTf 3 and 20%, triplet 0 and 13%, activation 8 and 9%, MRTD 16 and 61%. Significant correlations (0.460<|r|<0.906) were found between all tests of functional performance and all muscle parameters of PL and all parameters (0.454<|r|<0.873) but triplet and MRTD of NL. Conclusion: All strength parameters correlated significantly with functional performance. Therefore, it is recommended to investigate the role of strength training of both legs during at least the first year of stroke.

Keywords: stroke, functional performance, maximal voluntary contraction, muscle properties, longitudinal study.

1. Introduction

Information about *longitudinal* changes in intrinsic muscle weakness, activation failure and fast torque development during the first year after stroke is vital for rehabilitation. This would allow proper rehabilitation strategies after stroke with the ultimate goal to achieve a level of functional independence that enables the patient to return home and integrate into community life as fully as possible. Therefore, the aim was to investigate longitudinal changes in motor control and muscle function during the first year after stroke and determine the relationship of these changes with functional impairments.

2. Methods

Subjects

Fourteen patients after their first-ever stroke and a hemi paresis of the lower extremity participated. They entered the study on average 3.5 months after stroke and 2 months after admission in the rehabilitation centre (Figure 1: t = 0) and were measured again 3 (n=8), 6 (n=5) and 12 (n=3) months after their first measurement (Figure 1: follow-up (F)1, F2 and F3 respectively). Both the paretic (PL) and non-paretic lower limb (NL) were measured. Twelve able-bodied control subjects volunteered in this study. They were matched as much as possible for age and height and were measured once with only their right leg.

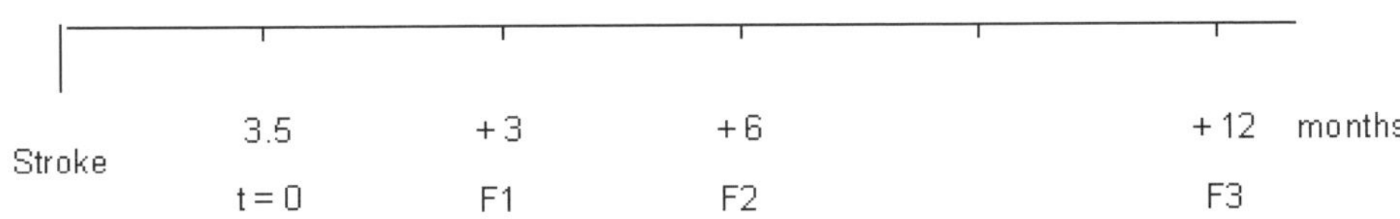

Figure 1. Time frame with measurement points. First measurement point (t=0) is 3.5 month after stroke and the three follow-up measurements (F1, F2, F3) were executed 3, 6 and 12 months after t=0, respectively.

Experimental set-up and procedures

Maximal voluntary and electrically evoked forces of the knee extensor and knee flexor muscles were measured using a custom built Lower EXtremity System (LEXS) [1]. Subjects were asked to maximally generate isometric knee extensions for 3-4 seconds to determine maximal voluntary knee extension torque (MVCe). Alternately, MVC's with the knee flexors (MVCf) were performed. Thereafter, subjects were asked to perform knee extensions as fast as possible with the command: 3, 2, 1 GO!
A modified super-imposed stimulation technique was used in which electrically evoked triplets (pulse train of three rectangular 200µs pulses applied at 300 Hz) were used to establish the subjects' capacity to voluntarily activate their knee extensor muscles [2]. First, stimulation current was increased until torque measured in response to a triplet levelled off. The current (in mA) was then increased by a further 20mA to ensure supramaximal stimulation (maximal resting triplet torque). Subsequently, subjects underwent measurements consisting of a triplet superimposed on the plateau of the force signal of the MVC.

Variables

The following muscle parameters were measured at the measurement points (Figure 1):
- **MVC torque**: peak force from the force plateau multiplied by external moment arm, during both knee extension (MVCe) and during knee flexion (MVCf).
- **Maximal rate of torque development** (MRTD): the steepest slope of torque development during fast voluntary contractions.

- (Supra maximal) **triplet torque** at resting muscle: measure for maximal (intrinsic) torque capacity of the knee extensors, independent of voluntary activation.
- **Voluntary activation** (VA): the completeness of skeletal muscle activity during voluntary contractions and was calculated by means of a modified interpolated twitch technique.

Seven **tests of functional performance**: Timed get-Up-and-Go (TUG), 10meter walk test (10m), Rivermead Mobility Index (RMI), Functional Ambulation Categories (FAC), Berg Balance Scale (BBS), Fugl Meyer (FM) and Motricity Index (MI).

3. Results

Overall, the data of the functional performance tests show improvement, especially between t=0 and F1. In PL, all muscle parameters significantly improved during all follow-ups, whereas in NL most improvement occurred within the first half year. For NL and PL MVCe improved 5 and 16%, resp., MVCf 3 and 20%, triplet 0 and 13%, activation 8 and 9%, MRTD 16 and 61% between t=0 and F1.

Significant correlations ($0.460 < |r| < 0.906$) were found between all tests of functional performance and all muscle parameters of PL and all parameters ($0.454 < |r| < 0.873$) except triplet and MRTD of NL.

4. Conclusion

As would be expected after hemi paretic stroke, we found that PL scored consistently lower than NL on all muscle parameters, and both lower limbs were significantly affected compared to controls. A new interesting finding is the considerable recovery in fast torque development. All strength parameters improved during recovery and correlated well with scores on tests of functional performance. Although we could not prove a cause-and-effect relationship, the results clearly indicate that (intrinsic) muscle strength, voluntary activation and the coherent ability to generate torque as fast ad possible are important variables which can potentially be prolific targets to improve during rehabilitation. Therefore, it is recommended to investigate the role of strength and speed training of both legs during at least the first half year after stroke.

References

[1]   A.M. Horstman, M.J. Beltman, K.H. Gerrits, P. Koppe, T.W.J. Janssen, P. Elich, A. de Haan, Intrinsic muscle strength and voluntary activation of both lower limbs and functional performance after stroke. *Clin Physiol Funct Imaging* **28**(4) (2008), 251-261.

[2]   R.D. Kooistra, C.J. de Ruiter, A. de Haan, Muscle activation and blood flow do not explain the muscle length-dependent variation in quadriceps isometric endurance. *J Appl Physiol* **98**(3) (2005), 810-816.

Rehabilitation: Mobility, Exercise and Sports
L.H.V. van der Woude et al. (Eds.)
IOS Press, 2010
© 2010 The authors and IOS Press. All rights reserved.
doi:10.3233/978-1-60750-080-3-155

How neurological disability influences the quality of life in people with Multiple Sclerosis

L. PEDRO[a] , J.L.P. RIBEIRO[b]
[a] Escola Superior de Tecnologia da Saúde de Lisboa – Politécnico de Lisboa
[b] Faculdade Psicologia Ciências Educação – U. Porto (Portugal)

Abstract. Multiple sclerosis (MS) it is a chronic neurological disease, characterized by demyelisation. The impact of multiple sclerosis on QoL is usually quite dramatic. A reported that the somatic symptoms of MS affect the functioning life, family life, economic condition, social interaction and autonomy. The aim of the present study is to examine the Influences of neurological disability in quality of life in patients with multiple sclerosis. The study is cross-sectional and correlational and utilised the Expanded Disability Status Scale (EDSS) and MSQoL- 54 Quantifying neurological disability in multiple sclerosis and MSQoL (SF-54): The results in correlations between EDSS and the domains of MSQOL-54, demonstrate de strong relation in every body dimensions of quality of life with neurological disability. These results are more important in dimensions: Physical Health and Physical Role Limitations Conclusion neurological Disability can play an important role in the quality of life of patients with multiple sclerosis.

Keywords. multiple sclerosis, quality of life, neurological disability.

1. Introduction

Multiple sclerosis (MS) it is a chronic neurological disease, characterized by demyelisation, linked with a broad spectrum of physical, emotional and social impairment. Is a chronic neurological disorder affecting young adults [1,2]. Characteristically, MS strikes between the ages of 20 and 40 and affects approximately million adults, mostly women, worldwide [3]. The cause is unknown, although it is considered to be an autoimmune disease [1]. MS is outstanding in its wide range of symptoms and unpredictable disease course, including a benign course, a relapsing-remitting course (exacerbations and remissions), which invariably turns into a secondary progressive course, and a type that is progressive from its onset [4]. The combination of a progressive and unpredictable disease process is a strong stressor, which powerfully impacts upon the quality of life of patients with MS [5].

The concept of QoL has received much attention; traditionally used measures of medical outcome such as morbidity and mortality do not simple scientific capture the full impact of medical interventions, especially in the case for chronic diseases like MS. To capture the multidimensional impact of diseases such as MS it is necessary consider physical functioning, social functioning, and emotional well being, [6,7] traditionally included in QoL assessment. Rudick et al. [8] reported that the somatic symptoms of MS affect family life, economic condition and social interaction

The aim of the present study is to examine the Influences of neurological disability in quality of life in patients with multiple sclerosis

2.   Methods

The study is cross-sectional and correlational.

Participants

Participants are 280 patients with MS were recruited via their physician at a neurology department of a central hospital in Lisbon. They were eligible for inclusion in the study if they met the following criteria: diagnosis according to relevant medical criteria, between 18 and 65 years, being diagnosed at least 1 year ago, EDSS score under 7. The mean age was 40 years (range 18- 65), 71.3% were women, 61.1% were married, 63% active workers, mean school level of 12 years, and the mean score of EDSS is 2.8.

Material

The Expanded Disability Status Scale (EDSS) [9] is a method of quantifying neurological disability in MS, and   The Multiple Sclerosis Quality of Life with 54 items (MSQoL -54) [10] is a specific traditional method to access QoL in MS. Scores on all subscales range from 0 (poor QoL) to 100 (best possible QoL). Scores on physical function, role limitations (physical and emotional), energy, health perceptions and change in health on the SF-54 are equivalent to SF-36 scores.
     Scores on the SF-54 emotional well-being are equivalent to the mental health SF-36. The SF-54 social function and pain scores include additional items to the SF-36 and these scores are therefore reported for both scales. 54 scores for cognitive function, health distress, sexual function, satisfaction with sexual function, overall quality of life, mental health composite and physical health composite.

Procedures

Ethical procedures where used accordingly with Helsinki declaration, Portuguese law and Hospital rules. Participants fill the questionnaire and if necessary the first author helps the patients with the task.

3.   Results

The correlations between EDSS and the domains of MSQOL-54: Physical Health (r=0.62, p<0.01), Physical Role Limitations (r=0.51, p<0.01), Emotional Role Limitations (r=0.29, p<0.05), Pain (r=0.29, p<0.05), Well-being (r=0.23, p<0.05), Energy (r=0.34, p<0.05), Health in General (r=0.30, p<0.05), Social function (r=0.40, p<0.01), Cognitive Function (r=0.18, p<0.05), Health Distress (r=0.32, p<0.05), Overall Qol (r=0.36, p<0.05), Sexual function , (r=0.28, p<0.05), Change Health (r=0.22, p<0.05),   and Satisfaction with sexual function (r=0.25, p<0.05),.are all statistic signification, but moderate.

4. Conclusion

There is a statistically significant correlation between the variables, suggesting that neurological Disability can play an important role in the quality of life of patients with multiple sclerosis.

This study demonstrates that there is an early, significant, evidence of disability measured by the EDSS and Quality of life with people of multiple sclerosis. Our study reinforces the prevailing view that there is a complex relationship between disability and quality of life in multiple sclerosis [25].

References

[1]   Rudick, R, A., Cohen, J. A., Weinstock-Guttman, B, Kinkel, R, P, & Ransohoff, M. Managementof multiple sclerosis, *N Engl J Med* **27**, (1997) 1604-1611.

[2]   SchiafEno, K. M., Shawaryn, M.A., & Blum, D. Assessing the psychosocial impact of multiple sclerosis: Learning from research on rheumatoid, *J Neurol Rehabil* **10**, (1996) 81-89.

[3]   Kremenchutzky, M., Rice, G., Baskerville, J., Wingerchuk, D. & Ebers, G. The natural history of multiple sclerosis: a geographically based study. 9. Observations on the progressive phase of the disease, *Brain* **129**, (2006), 584-594.

[4]   Kesselring, J. (2003). Blue Books of Pratical Neurology Multiple Sclerosis-2. W. McDonald and J.Noseworthy (Ed.),*Complications of Multiple Sclerosis:fatigue; spasticity; ataxia; pain; and bowel, bladder, and sexual dysfunction* (pp.217-302). Butterworth-Heinemann (USA).

[5]   Kobelt, G., Berg, J., Lindgren, P., Fredrikson, S .& Jonsson, B. Coast and quality of life in multiple esclerosis in Europe, *Journal Neurologic Neurosurgie Psychiatry* **77**, (2006), 918-926.

[6]   León, J., Morales, J., Navarro,J. & Mitchell, A. A review about the impact of multiple sclerosis on health-related quality of life, *Disabil Rehabil* **25**, (2003) 1291-1303.

[7]   Somerset, M., Peters, T., Sharp, D. & Campbell, R. Factors that contribute to quality of life outcomes prioritised by people with multiple sclerosis, *Qual Life Res* **12**, (2003), 21-29.

[8]   Rudick RA, Miller D, Clough JD, Gragg LA, Farmer RG. Quality of life in multiple sclerosis. Comparison with in⁻ amatory bowel disease and rheumatoid arthritis, *Arch Neurol* **49** (1992), 1237-1242.

[9]   Kurtzke, J. F. Rating neurological impairment in multiple sclerosis: An Expanded Disability Status Scale (EDSS), *Neurology* **33**, (1983), 1444-1452.

[10] Vickrey BG, Hays RD, Harooni R, Myers LW, Ellison GW. A health-related quality of life measure for multiple sclerosis, *Qual Life Res* **4** (1995), 187-206.

Rehabilitation: Mobility, Exercise and Sports
L.H.V. van der Woude et al. (Eds.)
IOS Press, 2010

doi:10.3233/978-1-60750-080-3-158

A breakthrough in Complex Regional Pain Syndrome treatment or not? A case report

M. SPIJKER, H.P.L.M. VOSSEN, R.C.J. ZONDERVAN
Heliomare Rehabilitation Centre, Wijk aan Zee, The Netherlands

Abstract. Little consensus exists, concerning cause, diagnose and treatment about Complex Regional Pain Syndrome type 1 (CRPS-1), which is also known as post traumatic dystrophy or reflex sympathetic dystrophy syndrome, a chronic pain condition. In an attempt to go out of the current concept of "with pain no gain" in which the pain limits are not overloaded, a new treatment approach was applied on a patient at Heliomare Rehabilitation Centre (Wijk aan Zee- The Netherlands). One of the manual therapist tackled movement restricted joints with mobilizations and manipulations to restore the Range of Motion (ROM). Once that was achieved active exercise took place focusing on gait patterns. After three months of treatment the patient no longer presented complaints and reached full recovery. Even though this new approach has reached good results, this was just a case study. High quality Randomized Controlled trials involving larger sample sizes and a more scientific methodology are essential before definitive conclusions can be drawn about the benefit of this therapy technique over traditional approaches or no treatment.

Keywords. complex regional pain syndrome type 1, dystrophy, manual therapy.

Published. Nederlands Tijdschrift voor Pijn en Pijnbestrijding, 25 (27), 2006

1. Introduction

Complex regional pain syndrome type 1 (CRPS-1) is a poorly understood chronic pain condition with regard to diagnosis, pathophysiology and treatment.

Our Purpose is to evaluate a treatment aiming at functional restoration, without paying respect to pain in patients complaining from Complex Regional Pain Syndrome type-1.

2. Case description

The patient was a 55-year-old female. She was suffering from CRPS-1 of the left foot, caused by a sprained ankle, since one year. Pain limited her ability to walk, climb stairs and drive a car. Conventional treatment with vitamin C, acetylcysteine and DMSO crème was unsuccessful.

Physical examination

The patient has poor motor control of foot and toes. Passive movement of several foot joints is restricted.

Treatment

Treatment was aimed at retrieving motor control and restoring range-of-motion without paying attention to the pain. In a home exercise program, the patient was encouraged to gain control over the active movements of the foot and perform strengthening and range-of-motion exercises of the left leg and foot. In addition, a proper walking technique was taught and walking distance was increased according to a graded activity approach.

Treatment frequency

The patient was treated six times, once a week.

Primary outcome measures

Treatment outcome was based on walking speed (ten meter walking test), pain (100 mm Visual Analogue Scale) and the PSK (patient specific functional scale). It scores the difficulties in executing five very important daily activities. Tests were done just before start of the treatment (T0), just after the last treatment (T1) and three months later (T2).

3. Results

After treatment, the patient no longer experienced complaints and reached full functional recovery. The PSK score diminished from an average of 90 (score 0-100) just before treatment, to 0 three months after treatment.

4. Conclusion

A physical therapy treatment aiming at functional restoration, without paying respect to an increase of pain, appears to be a promising new approach in the treatment of CRPS-1. Further research is needed to found this conclusion.

5. Discussion

This case illustrates that the method can be very successful. Yet it is not common practice in the Netherlands. Is the treatment save enough to treat all (chronic) CRPS-1 patients?

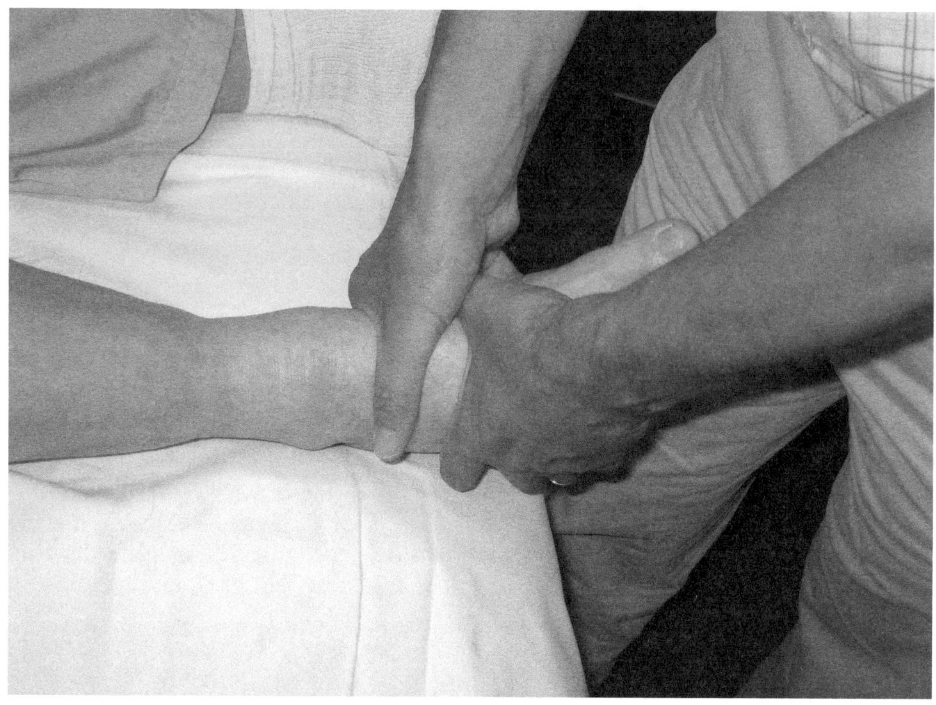

Figure 1. manual therapy

Table 1. Results

Moment of measurement	T0 (before)	T1 (after treatment)	T2 (3 months later)
Walking speed (comfort, km/h)	3	4,8	5
Walking speed (max, km/h)	3,8	11	missing
Pain score (VAS, mm)	75	50	0

References

[1]   Behandelingsprotocol complex regionaal pijnsyndroom type 1, dystrofie vereniging; RSGM Perez., site http:/pdver.atcomputing.nl/protocol.html en Ziektebeeld.
[2]   Conceptrichtlijn complex regional pijnsyndroom type 1, CBO 2005
[3]   Bepalen belastbaarheid bij complex regionaal pijnsyndroom type 1 / posttraumatische dystrofie; Margreet Oerlemans, Stimulus, 24(2005), p. 92-106
[4]   Een wonderbaarlijke genezing, J.W. Ek en J.C. van Gijn, Nr. 11 - 12 maart 2004 Medisch Contact.

Rehabilitation: Mobility, Exercise and Sports
L.H.V. van der Woude et al. (Eds.)
IOS Press, 2010
© 2010 The authors and IOS Press. All rights reserved.
doi:10.3233/978-1-60750-080-3-161

The development of an innovative rehabilitation measurement system

M. OOSTERWAAL, A.E. STATHAM[1], M. WIJNEN, M.B. HOPPENBROUWERS,
P.M.J. KOK

Monitoring Systems, TNO Science and Industry, Eindhoven, the Netherlands

Abstract. Purpose: The aim of the work was to develop a rehabilitation analysis solution that was robust, simple to use, wireless and inexpensive that could facilitate research and application in areas that were previously impractical. Methods: The embodiment of this vision was a pressure measurement insole and optical knee angle sensor system capable of wirelessly logging data. A participant was equipped with an experimental version of the system and performed various gaits along a motion-lab runway. A Vicon system tracked the participant's motion along the runway and an embedded force plate measured contact forces. The motion-lab reference data was used to validate the system and identify correlations that could aid with data interpretation and possible applications of the system. Results: Validation of the insole device showed good correlation with reference data (r>0.9) for centre of pressure location and an accuracy of +/-0.2 ms for all timing parameters. The joint angle sensor demonstrated an accuracy of within +/-3 degrees. Further correlations in the data were identified enabling classification of gait patterns. Conclusion: The system proved to be reliable, robust and accurate enough to be used in a variety of "in the field" research and rehabilitation quantification product scenarios previously rendered impractical by existing technology products.

Keywords. ambulant monitoring.

1. Introduction

Numerous methods of gait analysis have been pioneered through various veins of research. The majority of these methods is based upon motion, mechanical or magnetic measurement parameters and is restricted to use within the laboratory environment. The aim of the work presented in this publication was to develop a practical gait analysis solution that was robust, simple to use, remote/wireless and inexpensive that could facilitate research and application in "real life".

The gait analysis solution tested in this study comprised an angle sensing knee brace and 8 sensor pressure sensing insole. The knee brace was capable of measuring flexion and extension angles from 10 to 160° in one plane of motion. The pressure sensing insole was able to measure relative changes in pressure on a time base from which it was possible to determine centre of pressure location and contact times. The system was primarily designed to monitor rehabilitating knee replacement patients but also has many other potential applications in not only health but also sports settings.

---

[1] andy.statham@tno.nl , +31(0)402650647

2. Methods

8 capacitive sensors embedded into an insole were used to measure foot pressure. The signal from these sensors was read by an ankle mounted processing unit as described by Wijnen et al.[1]. An optical fibre was integrated into a knee brace to form a separate knee angle measurement system.

Validation

The pressure sensing insole was used to calculate centre of pressure (COP) location. The accuracy of the COP was compared with the higher sensor density TekScan system. The sensors were placed one upon the other on a flat concrete floor. For the first test a participant walked over the sensors and data was captured for 10 repetitions. In the second test the participant placed one foot on the sensors whilst moving through the extremes of range so as to move the centre of pressure from heel to toe, and from left to right and vice versa.

The insoles timing parameters were tested on a separate jig with the insole secured to a metal cylinder. The metal cylinder was rolled over a treadmill band and the timing of the activation of each sensor compared to that from the known speed of the rolling cylinder.

The knee brace angle measurement was validated against joint angles measured by the Vicon motion analysis system. The brace was worn by a participant who performed a number of different gaits and movements the knee angles of which were measured simultaneously with Vicon.

Complete system tests

One of the pressure sensing insoles was inserted into the right shoe of the test participant. The knee brace was also worn on the dominant (right) leg. Both the insole and the knee fed synchronised data to a wireless data logger.

The participant performed 25 different gaits varying in speed, range of motion and loading along the motion-lab runway. A Vicon system tracked the participant's motion along the runway.

3. Results

Validation of the insole device showed good correlation for centre of pressure location with reference data from the TekScan system (r>0.9) (figure. 1)

A comparison of the pressure sensor timing and the contact time from the metal cylinder tests showed an error range of +/-0.2 ms for all timing parameters.

The joint angle sensor demonstrated an accuracy of within +/-3 degrees for maximal flexion when compared to the Vicon data (figure 2).

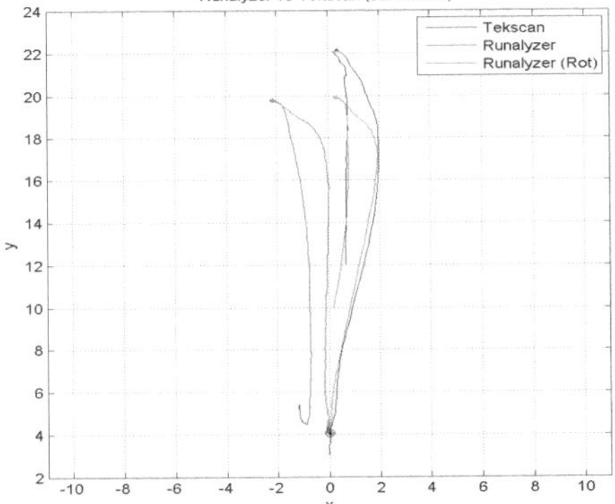

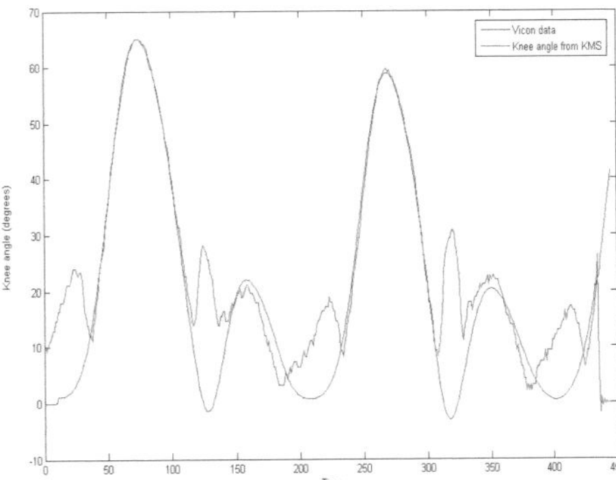

Figure 1. Comparison of x-y centre of pressure position between insole measurement system (incl. rotation to correct for sensor mis-alignment) and TekScan

Figure 2. Comparison of knee angle measurement between the knee brace system and the Vicon motion capturing system

4. Discussions & conclusions

Despite the lower sensor density the pressure sensing insole showed comparable accuracy to that achieved by the higher sensor density TekScan system (r>0.9). In the forefoot region the centre of pressure measurement was least accurate due to the low local sensor density (i.e. one sensor in the toe). The timing base of the system was shown to have an acceptable error range (+/-2ms).

The results from the angle measurement testing displayed some singularities in angle measurement for shallow angles (<10°). Despite the presence of these singularities at shallow angles and the limited accuracy of centre of pressure measurement in the locality of the forefoot the system proved to be reliable, robust and accurate enough to be used in a variety of "in the field" research and rehabilitation quantification product scenarios previously rendered impractical by existing technology products.

Future steps

In future work the system will first attempt to overcome the issue of singularities in the knee angle measurement. This should be possible with further development of the sensor.

The functionality of the rehabilitation system can also be enhanced by making the knee angle measurement capable of measuring all angles, e.g. not only in the plane of flexion and extension. A further useful feature planned for future developments is absolute pressure measurement.

References

[1] M. Wijnen, M.B. Hoppenbrouwers, J.W.M. Willems, Runalyser, ISEA *7th International conference*, 2008.

Rehabilitation: Mobility, Exercise and Sports
L.H.V. van der Woude et al. (Eds.)
IOS Press, 2010

doi:10.3233/978-1-60750-080-3-164

Ambulatory measurement of the scapulohumeral rhythm: intra- and inter-rater reliability of a protocol based on inertial and magnetic sensors

P. GAROFALO[a,b], A.G. CUTTI[b,1], I. PAREL[a,b], G. FIUMANA[c], G. PORCELLINI[d],
A. CAPPELLO[b]
[a] *INAIL Prostheses Centre, Vigorso di Budrio, Italy*
[b] *DEIS - University of Bologna, Bologna, Italy*
[c] *Shoulder Tech, Forlì, Italy*
[d] *Centre of Excellence in Shoulder Surgery, Cervesi Hospital, Cattolica, Italy*

Abstract. A new protocol has been recently proposed to measure the coordinated movement of humerus and scapula, through an inertial & magnetic measurement system, in ambulatory settings. Since the protocol requires the intervention of a rater, the aim of this study was to assess its intra- and inter-rater reliability. Results for the coefficient of multiple correlation showed a reliability of the protocol ranging from 0.84 to 1, thus supporting its use for clinical assessment.

Keywords. shoulder, ambulatory measurement, reliability, inertial sensors, magnetic sensors.

1. Introduction

A clinical parameter which is heavily affected in most of shoulder musculoskeletal disorders is the scapulohumeral rhythm (SHR). The SHR is the coordinated movement between scapula and humerus, when this latter is elevated. From the clinical view-point, the SHR is primarily analyzed by looking at two angle-angle plots: in the first, the X axis reports the humerothoracic elevation and Y the scapulothoracic medio-lateral rotation (MELA); in the second, Y reports the scapulothoracic protraction-retraction (PRRE). Despite of its importance, the measure of the SHR has been limited so far, also because of the lack of low-cost, easily-usable, ambulatory measurement systems. Recently, a protocol has been developed based on the Xsens inertial & magnetic measurement system (Xsens Technologies, NL), to overcome these limitations [1].

The Xsens system consists of lightweight boxes, called MTx, which comprise a 3D accelerometer, gyroscope and magnetometer. Through sensor-fusion algorithms, the 3D real-time orientation of each MTx is known relative to an ubiquitous global coordinate system, based on the magnetic north and the gravity.

To measure the SHR, the protocol requires to complete the following two preliminary steps:

---

[1] Corresponding Author.

- position an MTx sensor on thorax, scapula, and humerus (Fig. 1a): for the thorax the sensor is place on the sternum; for the humerus is positioned just to minimize the soft tissue artifact; for the scapula, the long side of the MTx is aligned with the cranial edge of the spine, over its central third;
- execute a static calibration with the subject standing in a pre-defined posture: upright position, elbow flexed 90°, humerus perpendicular to the ground and in neutral internal-external rotation.

These steps are required to execute the so-called "sensor-to-segment calibration", i.e. to define the anatomical coordinate systems of thorax, scapula and humerus and relate them to the technical coordinate systems of the corresponding MTx sensors.

Both steps require the intervention of a rater. In particular, to position the scapula sensor the rule has to be followed with care. The rater is also responsible to position the subject is the calibration posture, checking in particular the orientation of the humerus.

The aim of this work was therefore to assess the inter- and inter-rater reliability of the protocol in measuring the SHR.

2. Material and Methods

A group of 20 subjects (25-70 years-old, mean 45) were involved in the experiment, together with two raters (A and B) familiar with the protocol. Subjects were recovering from different shoulder pathologies, and were included in the study (after giving their informed consent) if they were able to actively and repeatedly elevate the humerus at a minimum of 70° in the sagittal plane and 45° in the frontal plane. Three measurement sessions were completed for each subject with the protocol: two by one rater and one by the other. Between acquisitions, the scapula-sensor was removed and reapplied, and the static calibration was repeated. Acquisitions were 15 minutes apart, to minimize the within-subject biological variability.

In each acquisition, a total of 10 humerus flexion-extensions (FE) and ab-adductions (AA) were measured, but 8+8 were kept for subsequent computations. For each movement the SHR waveform was computed and split in its upward (flexion, abduction) and downward (extension, adduction) phase [2].

Before computing the intra- and inter-rater reliability, for each subject we checked the intra-subject repeatability of the SHR waveforms, by computing the adjusted coefficient of multiple correlation, in the within-session form (CMC_1) [2]. Only for those subjects with a very-good repeatability ($CMC_1 > 0.85$) we computed the intra- and inter-rater reliability of the protocol.

The intra- and inter-rater reliability was quantified for each of the remaining subjects by assessing the similarity of his/her SHR waveforms with-in and between-rater, through the CMC in the between-session form (CMC_2) [2], after removing the offset between the waveforms of the different raters.

The distribution of CMC_2 values over subjects was evaluated with box-and-whisker plots, as this was not normal; median and whiskers were extracted; values were interpreted as in [2]: 0.75-0.85: good; 0.85-0.95: very-good; 0.95-1: excellent.

Finally, statistically significant differences in the MELA and PRRE ROM measured by the raters were searched for through an ANOVA with repeated measures.

3. Results and Discussion

Among the 20 subjects, 11 presented a CMC_1 greater than 0.85 in all sessions and for all the components of the SHR, and were then considered for the intra- and inter-rater assessment. As discussed in [2], the selection of subjects based on CMC_1 was required, since the CMC_2 can be lowered by a low intra-subject repeatability, altering therefore the estimation of the intra-rater and inter-rater reliability of the *protocol*.

As shown in Figure 1b, higher repeatability was found for the MELA both intra- and inter-rater and both for FE and AA, with values within-whiskers generally in the excellent range. For the PRRE, values within-whiskers were in the very-good to excellent range (1 value out of 22 in the good range). The intra- and inter-rater reliabilities were comparable for all movements, MELA and PRRE.
No statistically significant differences ($p > 0.05$) were found between the ROMs measured by the raters.

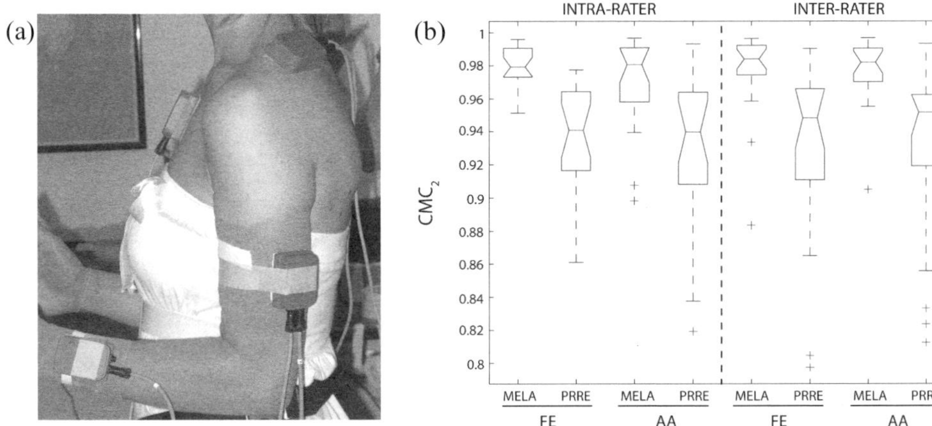

Figure 1a,b: (a) Xsens sensors set-up. The MTx on the forearm was not used in the present study. (b) Distributions of CMC_2, intra- and inter-rater, for the FE and the AA task, for MELA and PRRE. The CMC_2 values for the upward and downward phase were merged for brevity (22 values are reported in each box-plot).

4. Conclusion

The results support the robustness of the protocol for longitudinal studies and to changes in rater. As a side results, it seems that CMC_1 could be a useful parameter to monitor the level of mobility restoration of subjects, as those presenting a lower CMC_1 were actually the subjects clinically evaluated as in need for continuing the physical therapy. Further studies are however required to draw conclusions.

References

[1]   Cutti AG, et al., Ambulatory measurement of shoulder and elbow kinematics through inertial and magnetic sensors, *Med Bio Eng Comput* **46** (2008), 169-178.
[2]   Garofalo P, et al., Inter-operator reliability and prediction bands of a novel protocol to measure the coordinated movements of shoulder-girdle and humerus in clinical settings, *Med Bio Eng Comput*, DOI 10.1007/s11517-009-0454-z

Rehabilitation: Mobility, Exercise and Sports
L.H.V. van der Woude et al. (Eds.)
IOS Press, 2010

doi:10.3233/978-1-60750-080-3-167

Long-term functional outcome and quality of life after Steindler flexorplasty in patients with a traumatic brachial plexus injury

B.J. DUIJNISVELD, S. HOGENDOORN, T. VERHAAF, R.G.H.H. NELISSEN
Department of Orthopedics, Leiden University Medical Center, Leiden, The Netherlands

1. Introduction

Traumatic brachial plexus injuries (TBPI) often lead to long-term functional disabilities. The Steindler flexorplasty could restore active flexion of the paralyzed elbow by transposition of the flexor-pronator origin to a more proximal location on the humerus. The purpose of this study was to assess the functional outcome and quality of life after Steindler flexorplasty.

2. Methods

From 1991 to 2008, a prospective follow-up study was performed including 41 adult TBPI patients who received Steindler flexorplasty. Pre- and post-operatively, the range of motion (ROM) and strength (MRC score from 0 to 5) were assessed together with the quality of life questionnaires DASH and SF-36 on a scale from 0 (dissatisfied) to 100 (satisfied). The median follow-up was 3.2 years (IQR 1.5 to 8.5 years). One patient was lost to follow-up.

3. Results

Pre-operatively, the median active elbow flexion was 0° (Interquartile range (IQR) 0° to 0°) with a median MRC biceps strength of 1 (IQR 0 to 2). At final follow-up, the median active elbow flexion was increased to 110° (IQR 85° to 120°) with a median MRC strength of 4 (IQR 4 to 4), the median flexion contracture was 10° (IQR 0° to 20°), the median active pronation 90° (IQR 90° to 90°) and the median active supination 25° (IQR 0° to 40°). The median DASH score was 70 (IQR 45 to 85) and the median SF-36 score was 75 (IQR 55 to 85). The correlation of active elbow flexion with DASH was 0.35 (Pearson's rho, $P = 0.058$) and with SF36 was 0.15 (Pearson's rho, $P = 0.48$). Seven patients had temporarily ulnar hypesthesia. Patients were reoperated: 1 for refixation and 1 because of infection.

4. Conclusions

The Steindler flexorplasty improves elbow flexion ROM and strength. Because the correlation of active elbow flexion with the quality of life questionnaires was poor, we suggest developing a new questionnaire specifically for TBPI. To improve functional outcome and quality of life, TBPI patients with residual functional impairment should be considered for operative treatment in their rehabilitation program.

Rehabilitation: Mobility, Exercise and Sports
L.H.V. van der Woude et al. (Eds.)
IOS Press, 2010
doi:10.3233/978-1-60750-080-3-169

169

Do arm motions help to recover from a trip?

I. KINGMA, M. PIJNAPPELS, J.H.VAN DIEËN
Research Institute MOVE, Faculty of Human Movement Sciences,
VU University Amsterdam

Abstract. When someone is tripped during gait, an angular momentum is induced in all planes of motion. We measured full-body 3D kinematics in subjects who were tripped during mid-swing. We analyzed the effect of the arm swing on body rotations in all planes of motion during recovery from the trip.

Keywords. tripping, balance recovery, arm motion.

1. Introduction

When someone is tripped during gait, the body obtains a large forward angular momentum in the sagittal plane. This momentum needs to be counteracted for successful recovery from the trip [1,2]. Most likely, a main goal of recovery responses is to prolong the step of the tripped leg, so that this leg can be placed forward far enough in order to break the forward angular momentum of the body [3]. Elderly fallers have been shown to have a reduced capability to break the forward angular momentum, which may in part be due to lower peak ankle moments. [4]. Another candidate variable that may limit reduction of the angular momentum in elderly is limited ability to generate vigorous arm movements in the recovery phase [5]. However, as of yet, the actual contribution of the arms to balance recovery after tripping, which could occur through sagittal plane motions as well as through motion in other planes, has not yet been investigated. Therefore, the goal of the present study was to analyze body rotations in all planes of motion during tripping and subsequent recovery. Furthermore, we aimed to uncover the role of the arms in trip recovery by comparing the actual body rotations after tripping to the body rotations that would have occurred if the arms would not have contributed.

2. Methods

Ten healthy young adults (6 males and 4 females) walked 70 times over a 12 x 2.5 m. platform at a self-selected velocity. In about 10 trials subjects were tripped over an obstacle that suddenly appeared from the floor. On-line kinematic data were used to select which of 14 hidden obstacles should pop up 100 ms prior to collision in order to catch the left leg at mid swing [2,3]. Subjects wore a safety harness connected to a ceiling-mounted rail in order to prevent injury in case of a fall. Full body 3D kinematics were recorded at a sample rate of 100 Hz (Optotrak, Northern Digital), and smoothed with a second order 6 Hz low-pass butterworth filter. Only the first trip was analyzed for the present study. The body angular momentum was calculated in all 3 planes of motion according to:

$$\mathbf{L}_{body} = \sum (I_j \cdot \mathbf{\omega}_j + (m_j \cdot \mathbf{r}_j \times \dot{\mathbf{r}}_j)) \qquad (1)$$

where I_j is the instantaneous inertia tensor of the jth segment relative to its centre of mass (COM), $\mathbf{\omega}_j$ is the angular velocity vector of the segment, m_j is the segment mass, $\mathbf{r}_j$ is the position vector from the segment COM to the body COM and $\dot{\mathbf{r}}_j$ is the velocity vector of the segment COM relative to the body COM. To analyze the role of the arms, we focused on the rotation of the trunk plus legs ($\mathbf{L}_{trunk+legs}$) both in presence and absence of the arms. First, we applied equation (1) to all body segments except the arms in order to calculate the angular momentum that actually occurred in the trunk+legs during and after tripping. The next step was to calculate how the trunk+legs would have rotated in the absence of the arms, or, more precisely, when the arms would be removed from the instant of collision with the obstacle onwards. First, we assumed that the trunk+legs would need to 'take up' the angular momentum of the arms at the instant of tripping as well as the angular momentum of the arms that actually occurred after tripping. Second, we calculated how the trunk+legs would have rotated if the arms would be removed without transferring their angular momentum at the instant of tripping. In both cases, we subsequently determined the angular velocity of the trunk+legs from:

$$L_{trunk+legs} = I_{trunk+legs} \cdot \omega_{trunk+legs} \qquad (2)$$

Finally, by numerically integrating $\omega_{trunk+legs}$, we determined how much the trunk+legs rotated between the instant of tripping and the instant of recovery foot placement. This was done for the actual rotation, for the simulated condition without arms with transfer (transfer&cut), and for the simulated condition without arms without transfer (cut).

3. Results

Calculation of the actual trunk+legs rotation showed that, at landing of the recovery foot relative to trip initiation, the trunk+legs had rotated 20.4° (SD 6.3) forward in the sagittal plane (Figure 1). For the 'cut' simulation, the increase in forward body rotation did not reach significance. For the 'transfer&cut' simulation, the trunk+legs rotated, on average, 5.7° more forward between tripping and recovery foot landing. In the frontal plane, the trunk+legs actually rotated 10.4° (SD 3.5) to the tripped side. If the trunk+legs would have had to take up the angular momentum of the arms at the instant of tripping, and would not have profited from arm movements after trip initiation, the trunk would have rotated 19.5° (SD 12.6) towards the tripped side. This indicates that in the frontal plane the arm motions were beneficial as well. In the transverse plane, the actual rotation of the trunk+legs appeared to be slightly to the non-tripped (right) side (-3.0°, SD 8.1), despite induction of a leftward rotation by the trip. However, when virtually cutting the arms and transferring the angular momentum at the instant of tripping to the trunk+legs, a large 18.8° (SD 20.9) rotation to the tripped (left) side was calculated. Importantly, this would strongly reduce the length of the recovery step. Surprisingly, the disadvantage of cutting away the arms was completely canceled out if the arms would keep their angular momentum at cutting.

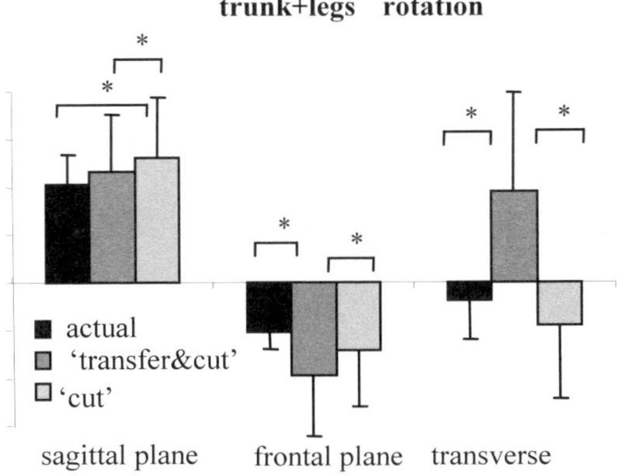

Figure 1. Average (and SD) rotation of the trunk+legs for the actual tripping condition and the 'transfer&cut' and 'cut' simulations in 3 planes from impact with the obstacle until landing of the recovery foot. Positive directions are forward rotation in the sagittal plane; towards the non-tripped side in the frontal plane, and towards the tripped side in the transverse plane. Statistical significant differences ($p < 0.05$) between analytical and actual tripping conditions are indicated with a *.

4. Conclusion

The effects of virtually removing the arms in the transverse plane highly depended on whether or not the angular momentum of the arms at the instant of tripping was transferred at the instant of tripping. This can be understood when considering the arm swing during normal gait. Because of equal signs of the left and right arm contributions, the transverse plane body rotation is strongly affected by the arm swing during normal gait [6]. We tripped our subjects at the instant of about maximum arm swing velocity. During normal gait, the angular momentum of the arms is transferred to the trunk+legs after this point in time.

When tripped during mid-swing, subjects essentially prolong their arm swing, thereby delaying the transfer of angular momentum to the trunk+legs. While the 'transfer&cut' simulation may have somewhat overestimated what would happen if the arms would do nothing more than during normal gait, it does indicate that arm movements can substantially contribute to recovery, especially by enlarging the recovery step through transverse plane rotation. It remains to be investigated to what extent reduced arm motion can explain limitations in recovery responses in elderly.

Acknowledgements
The authors would like to thank Daphne Wezenberg and Guus Reurink for data collection and initial analysis and the Netherlands Organisation for Scientific Research (NWO) for their financial support (grant # 916.76.077).

References

[1] Pavol, M. J., Owings, T. M., Foley, K. T. et al., 2001, Mechanisms leading to a fall from an induced trip in healthy older adults, J Gerontol A Biol Sci Med Sci, 56, M428-37.

[2] Pijnappels, M., Bobbert, M. F. and van Dieën, J. H., 2004, Contribution of the support limb in control of angular momentum after tripping, Journal of Biomechanics, 37, 1811-8.

[3] Pijnappels, M., Bobbert, M. F. and van Dieën, J. H., 2005, How early reactions in the support limb contribute to balance recovery after tripping, Journal of Biomechanics, 38, 627-34.

[4] Pijnappels, M., Bobbert, M. F. and van Dieën, J. H., 2005, Push-off reactions in recovery after tripping discriminate young subjects, older non-fallers and older fallers. Gait Posture ,21(4): 388-94.

[5] Roos, P. E., McGuigan, M. P., Kerwin, D. G. et al., 2008, The role of arm movement in early trip recovery in younger and older adults, Gait Posture, 27, 352-6.

[6] Bruijn, S. M., Meijer, O. G., van Dieën, J. H. et al., 2008, Coordination of leg swing, thorax rotations, and pelvis rotations during gait: the organisation of total body angular momentum, Gait Posture, 27, 455-62.

Rehabilitation: Mobility, Exercise and Sports
L.H.V. van der Woude et al. (Eds.)
IOS Press, 2010
© 2010 The authors and IOS Press. All rights reserved.
doi:10.3233/978-1-60750-080-3-172

The effects of proprioceptive reinforcement on the dynamic balance performance and Cobb angle of patients with mild adolescent idiopathic scoliosis

S. NAMDAR TAJARI [a,1], N. FARAHPOUR [b]
[a] *Islamic Azad University of Iran, branch saveh*
[b] *Bu Ali Sina University of Iran*

Abstract. It is reported that idiopathic scoliosis is associated with the deficits on the proprioceptive performance. The main purpose of this study was evaluate the effects of balance proprioceptive reinforcement on the scoliotic deformity in mild adolescent idiopathic scoliosis. In conclusion, this study showed that the balance training has a significant effect on the treatment of the scoliotic deformity and proprioceptive performance.

Keywords. Adolescent Idiopathic Scoliosis, balance performance, proprioceptive reinforcement.

1. Introduction

Adolescent Idiopathic Scoliosis (AIS) has been described as a three-dimensional deformity of the rib cage and the spine. Despite of many studies on the etiology of Adolescent Idiopathic Scoliosis (AIS), its cause still remains unknown. Some studies implying the Scoliosis is associated with motor control deficit (balance performance) and another one are reported that idiopathic scoliosis is associated with the deficits on the proprioceptive performance. Exercise has been recommended during conservative treatment of the AIS. However, there is some weak evidence on the effectiveness of the exercise. In some research is used strength, aerobic and stretch exercise in therapeutic program.

It is interesting to know if balance training may eliminate curve progression and/or reduce the curve amplitude. The purpose of this study was to evaluate the effects of balance training with reference to the proprioceptive training on the dynamic balance performance and Cobb angle of patients with mild adolescent idiopathic scoliosis.

2. Methods

In this study, we use the one group pretest – post test design. Twenty girls with adolescent mild idiopathic scoliosis with mean height and weight of 157.1 (± 5.22) cm and 42.8 (± 5.9) kg respectively were screened from all of 7000 student in guidance

---

[1] somayehnamdar@yahoo.com

school. Their minimum and maximum Cobb angle was measured using AP radiography and was 10 and 16 degrees. Used a dynamic stability platform (BIODEX) to record the deviation of postural orientation (balance performance), so called postural deviation (PD) from vertical line. PD was in 3 orientation, anteroposterior (AP), mediolateral (ML), and total. PD was measured in different upright standing conditions.

The first test condition was performed with open eyes and on quasi-stable platform (Ankle strategy) and the second condition was on unstable platform (Hip strategy). Patients underwent four months balance training with special reference to the proprioceptive training. The measurements were repeated after the exercise therapy. ANOVA was used for statistical analysis.

3. Results

Table1 illustrate postural deviation pre and post exercise trophy in ankle strategy(quasi-stable stable position) and   hip strategy (unstable position) when they are upright standing whit open eyes. Results showed that the postural deviation (PD) of the patients was reduced significantly (p=0.01). The greatest improvement in balance performance was obtained when hip strategy was involved. In ankle strategy, deference between total postural deviation in after treatment and before treatment was 0.23° but in hip strategy it was 0.57 °.

Figure 1 summarizes the Cobb angles variations in scoliotic patients after the exercise therapy. Before the treatment, the range of the Cobb angles was between 10 to 16 degrees. The average Cobb angles were significantly reduced by 2° (p < 0.01). Exercise training was resulted in the reduction 1 to 11 degrees of the Cobb angle in twelve subjects. In three patients the Cobb angle was not changed and in four patients, there was only one degree increase on their Cobb angle.

Table 1. PD in before and after the treatment

		AP	ML	TOTAL
Ankle strategy	Before	1.78±.40	1.41±.41	1.14±.48
	After	1.21±.40	1.09±.41	.87±.25
Hip strategy	Before	2.95±1.93	2.47±1.63	1.72±1.10
	After	1.76±.52	1.48±.48	1.15±.32

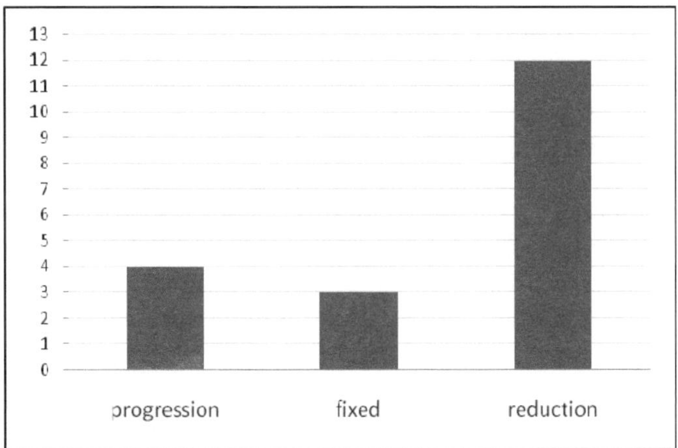

Figure 1. Cobb angle variations.

4. Conclusion

This study showed that the balance training based on the proprioceptive training has a significant effect on the treatment of the scoliotic deformity. In 60% of the patients Cobb was reduced between 1 to 11 degrees. Balance training with special focus on proprioceptives reinforcement is recommended for mild scoliosis for further researches. In additional this study showed that the balance training has a significant effect on the proprioceptive performance and improved control posture or balance performance.

References

[1]   Byl N.N, Gray J.M, Complex balance reaction in different sensory conditions: Adolescents with and without idiopathic scoliosis, *Orthopedic Research journal* **11**, (1993), 215-217.

[2]   Obeirne J, Goldberg C, Dowling FE, Fogarty EE, Equilibrium dysfunction in scoliosis: Cause or effect, *Spinal Disorder journal* **2** (1989), 184-9.

[3]   Younes M. Robitaille A. Scoliosis Correction Objectives in Adolescent Idiopathic Scoliosis. *Journal of Pediatric Orthopaedics* **27** (2007), 775-781.

[4]   Gerome C, Gauchard P, Influence of different types of progressive idiopathic scoliosis on static and dynamic postural control, *Spine journal* **26**, (2001), 1052-1058.

Rehabilitation: Mobility, Exercise and Sports
L.H.V. van der Woude et al. (Eds.)
IOS Press, 2010

doi:10.3233/978-1-60750-080-3-175

Circumvention of suddenly appearing obstacles in young and older adults

M. PIJNAPPELS[a,1], I. KINGMA[a], J.H. VAN DIEËN[a]
[a] *Research Institute MOVE, Faculty of Human Movement Sciences,
VU University, Amsterdam, the Netherlands*

Abstract. Reduced ability to circumvent an obstacle, which is noticed only shortly before collision, could be a cause of falls and injury, especially in older adults. In this study, we investigated differences in strategies and their characteristics between young and older adults when circumventing a suddenly appearing obstacle. We measured young and older adults while walking over a platform, while in some trials an obstacle suddenly appeared halfway, blocking their passage. Obstacle appearance was timed to provide available response times (ART) of 850, 1000 or 1150 ms. Circumvention strategies could be classified as either side stepping or cross-over stepping, which were observed in both age groups. Strategy choice was affected by ART and age; older adults preferred the side step strategy, especially when ART was shorter. Peak ground reaction forces were higher for the side step strategy. Older adults performed similar circumvention strategies as young adults, with a stronger preference for side stepping. This strategy appears to be more stable, although it is more demanding in terms of force generation.

Keywords. falls, elderly, obstacle avoidance, lateral balance.

1. Introduction

Reduced ability to circumvent an obstacle, which is noticed only shortly before collision, could be a cause of falls and injury, especially in older adults. Previous studies on obstacle circumvention [1,2] have shown age-related velocity reduction when circumventing an obstacle that was visible well in advance. When externally perturbed in the medio-lateral direction during stance, cross-over stepping and side stepping strategies have been observed in both young and older adults [3,4]. When perturbed in the medio-lateral direction during walking in place, both young and older adults prefer side stepping, although older adults showed more steps and interlimb collisions [5]. In studies on stepping over an unexpected obstacle on a treadmill, success rates were shown to decrease when the available response time (ART) decreased, especially in older adults, and strategy choice was found to change [6,7].
The aim of this study was to test for differences in strategies and their characteristics between young and older adults in circumventing a suddenly appearing obstacle during gait under critical time conditions.

---

[1] Corresponding Author.

2. Methods

Twenty-one young (24±3 years, 10 females) and ten older (69±4 years, 4 females) adults walked down a 12-m platform at 1.2 m/s, while in 16 out of 96 trials an obstacle (horizontal poles at ankle and shoulder height) appeared halfway, blocking their passage. Obstacle appearance was timed based on on-line kinematic data, around right heel strike in front of the obstacle, to provide Available Response Times (ARTs) of 850, 1000 or 1150 ms. Subjects were asked to circumvent the obstacle to the right and to continue walking. Gait kinematics, ground reaction forces and muscle activity were measured. Strategy, foot position, peak forces and velocity changes were analyzed.

3. Results

In both age groups, circumvention strategies could be classified as either side stepping or cross-over stepping (Figure 1). Side stepping was characterized by a shortened left foot step, followed by a step to the right by the right leg. Cross-over stepping was characterized by crossing the left foot in front of the right foot to circumvent the obstacle.

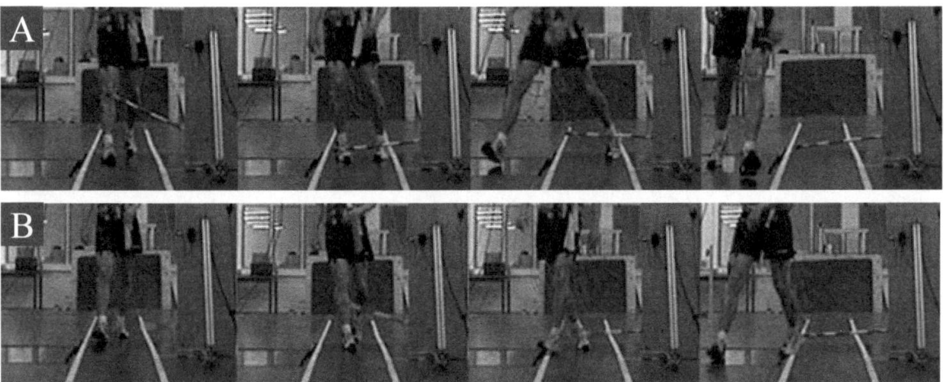

Figure 1. Strategies observed during obstacle circumvention: (A) side stepping or (B) cross-over stepping.

Strategy choice was significantly affected by ART and age; older adults preferred the side step strategy, especially when ART was shorter (Figure 2). Backward and sideward peak ground reaction forces, resulting in forward velocity reduction and sideward velocity increase, were more pronounced for side stepping than for cross-over stepping. Young adults reduced their forward velocity by 0.55 (SD 0.22) m/s during side stepping and by 0.36 (SD 0.13) m/s during cross-over stepping, whereas older adults reduced their velocity by 0.73 (SD 0.18) m/s and 0.56 (SD 0.39) m/s during side stepping and cross-over stepping, respectively. Relatively more velocity reduction in the older adults at similar walking velocity indicates that they generated larger braking forces when circumventing the obstacle.

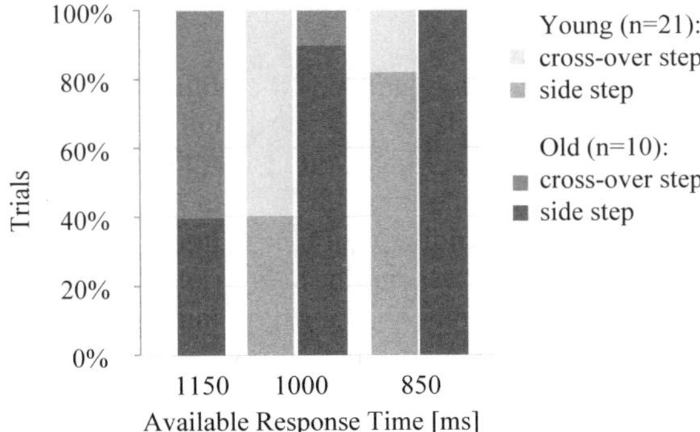

Figure 2. Strategy distribution for young and older adults over ARTs

4. Discussion

Two strategies are observed for obstacle circumvention. Cross-over stepping requires less force generation but is probably also more dangerous in terms of collision with the obstacle [4,5] and stability. Side stepping might therefore be preferred by older adults, because it is safer, especially when the available time to respond is shorter, even though it requires higher forces to perform this strategy. Future research is required to investigate the dynamic stability of both strategies for young and older adults and to evaluate if stability impairments in older adults might be related to falls or collisions.

In conclusion, older adults perform similar strategies as young adults to circumvent a suddenly appearing obstacle during gait, with a stronger preference for side stepping for shorter ART. This strategy appears a more stable strategy although it is more demanding in terms of force generation.

Acknowledgements

The authors would like to thank the Netherlands Organisation for Scientific Research (NWO) for their financial support (grant # 916.76.077).

References

[1]   Gérin-Lajoie M, Richards CL, McFadyen BJ. The circumvention of obstacles during walking in different environmental contexts: A comparison between older and younger adults. *Gait Posture* 2006;24(3):364-369.

[2]   Lowrey CR, Reed RJ, Vallis LA. Control strategies used by older adults during multiple obstacle avoidance. *Gait Posture* 2007;25(4):502-508.

[3]   Rogers MW, Mille ML. Lateral stability and falls in older people. *Exerc Sport Sci Rev* 2003;31:182-187.

[4]   Mille ML, Johnson ME, Martinez KM, Rogers MW. Age-dependent differences in lateral balance recovery through protective stepping. *Clin Biomech* 2005;20(6):607-616.

[5]   Maki BE, Edmondstone MA, McIlroy WE. Age-related differences in laterally directed compensatory stepping behavior. *J Gerontol A Biol Sci Med Sci* 2000;55(5):M270-277.

[6]   Chen HC, Ashton-Miller JA, Alexander NB, Schultz AB. Effects of age and available response time on ability to step over an obstacle. *J Gerontol A Biol Sci Med Sci* 1994;49(5):M227-233.

[7]   Weerdesteyn V, Nienhuis B, Duysens J. Advancing age progressively affects obstacle avoidance skills in the elderly. *Human Mov Sci* 2005;24(5-6):865-880.

Rehabilitation: Mobility, Exercise and Sports
L.H.V. van der Woude et al. (Eds.)
IOS Press, 2010

doi:10.3233/978-1-60750-080-3-178

Energy expenditure of stroke patients during upright standing

N. TER HOEVE[a], C.F.J. NOOIJEN[a], C.J.C. LAMOTH[b], D. RIJNTJES[c], M. TOLSMA[c], J.H.P. HOUDIJK[a,c]

[a] *Research Institute MOVE, Faculty of Human Movement Sciences, VU University Amsterdam, The Netherlands*
[b] *Center for Human Movement Science, University Medical Center Groningen, University of Groningen, The Netherlands*
[c] *Heliomare Rehabilitation Research and Development, Wijk aan Zee, The Netherlands*

Abstract. Purpose: To study the energy expenditure needed for balance control of stroke patients during upright standing, and to determine the relationship between energy expenditure and measures of balance control and muscle activity. Methods: Ten stroke patients and twelve healthy controls performed four upright standing tasks; one without and three with balance perturbations. Energy expenditure was assessed using a pulmonary gas measurement system. Conventional and dynamic balance measures were calculated from center of pressure time series, obtained with a force plate. Muscle activity of the ankle plantar flexors and dorsal flexors was measured using electromyography. Results: On average, energy expenditure during standing was 125% higher in stroke patients. Challenging balance caused a significant increase in energy expenditure (21-52%) for both groups, but no significant interaction (group x condition) was found. Balance control was impaired and muscle activity was higher in stroke patients in all standing conditions. Significant, though moderate to low, correlations were found between energy expenditure and measures of balance control and muscle activity. Conclusion: This study shows that the increased effort for maintaining balance can have a clinically relevant effect on energy expenditure of stroke patients. Besides balance control, other factors responsible for the increased energy expenditure during upright standing in stroke patients should be explored.

Keywords. energy expenditure, stroke, balance control.

1. Introduction

Stroke patients frequently complain of excessive fatigue [1]. This fatigue could be caused by a general reduction in physical capacity of the patients, but may also be associated with a higher energetic load these patients experience during activities of daily live. Although the exact cause of the higher energetic load is unclear, a possible explanation is an increased energy requirement for the impaired balance control seen in stroke patients [2,3]. However, limited data on the relation between balance control and energy expenditure is available. Information about this relation could be used to improve rehabilitation programs. The focus on balance training can be expanded and walking aids can be prescribed more adequately in order to reduce energy expenditure.

The aims of the present study were (1) to compare the energy expenditure of stroke patients and healthy controls during quiet standing, (2) to investigate the influence of challenging balance on the energy expenditure and on balance control of stroke patients and healthy controls, and (3) to determine the relation between energy expenditure and different measures of balance control and muscle activity.

2. Methods

The patient group consisted of 10 stroke patients which were included from the stroke unit at the rehabilitation centre Heliomare (Wijk aan Zee). All patients were able to stand without aids or assistance for at least two minutes and had a maximal score of 45 on the Berg Balance scale. The control group consisted of 12 able-bodied age- and weight- matched subjects.

Subjects had to perform a quiet standing task in four different conditions:
- Standing upright on firm surface (SU)
- Standing upright on firm surface while blindfolded (SUB)
- Standing upright on foam surface (SUF)
- Standing upright on a firm surface with feet placed parallel against each other (SUP)

Energy expenditure (J/min/kg) was measured using respirometry (Oxycon Delta Jaeger, Germany). From center of pressure (CoP) data obtained with a force plate (AMTI, USA), the amount of sway and of twisting and turning, regularity, and local stability were quantified by respectively the mean CoP distance, the root mean square of CoP time series, the normalized sway path, the sample entropy and the maximum Lyapunov exponent [4]. Surface EMG data (TMSi, Enschede, the Netherlands) of the m. gastrocnemius and m. tibialis was collected, and the root mean square and co-contraction index (%) were calculated as measures for muscle activity.

A repeated measures ANOVA (group x condition, p<0.05) was performed, and Pearson correlation coefficients were calculated to determine the relations between energy expenditure and the measures of balance control and muscle activity.

3. Results

On average, energy expenditure was 125% higher in stroke patients compared to able-bodied subjects. Challenging balance significantly increased energy expenditure (21-52%) in both groups, with a larger effect in the patient group. However, no significant group x condition interaction was found (Figure 1).

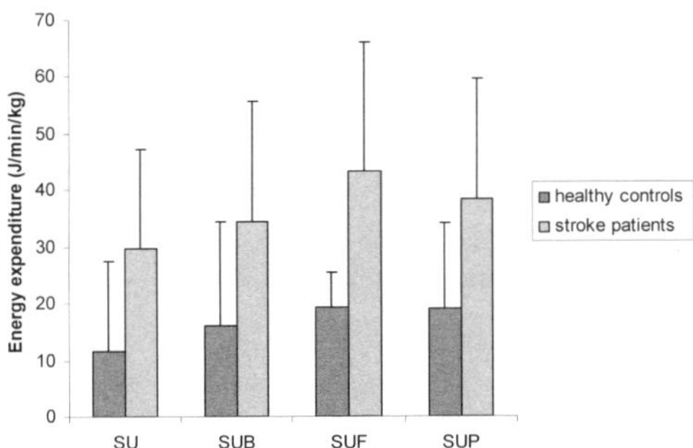

Figure 1. Average energy expenditure during the four upright standing conditions for the control subjects and stroke patients. Error bars represent standard deviations.

Balance control, in terms of CoP sway magnitude, twisting and turning, regularity and local stability, was impaired in stroke patients. When balance was challenged, balance control deteriorated in both groups with a more pronounced effect in stroke patients. Furthermore, muscle activity was higher in stroke patients. Challenging balance in the SUF and SUP condition resulted in a higher amount of co-contraction in both groups. No interaction effect (group x condition) was found.

Moderate to low though significant correlations were found between energy expenditure and measures of balance control and muscle activity (Table 1).

Table 1. Correlations between energy expenditure and measures of balance control and muscle activity

	r	p
Amount of sway (mean CoP distance)	0.19	0.08
Amount of sway (sway path length)	0.61	<0.01*
Twisting and turning	0.62	<0.01*
Regularity	-0.41	<0.01*
Local stability	0.49	<0.01*
Muscle activity (m. gastrocnemius)	0.22	0.04*
Muscle activity (m. tibialis ant.)	0.41	<0.01*

4. Conclusion

This study shows that the energy expenditure during upright standing is considerable higher in stroke patients compared to able-bodied controls. This higher energy expenditure is partly related to poor balance control and increased muscle activity. However, correlations between energy expenditure and measures of balance control and muscle activity were low to moderate. Therefore additional factors (e.g. muscle tone or increased muscle activity of hip and trunk muscles due to abnormal posture) which contribute to the higher energy expenditure should be considered.

In view of the fact that the energetic demand for balance control was already considerably elevated during quiet upright standing, the effects during more complex and dynamic tasks of daily life are probably even larger. More research is necessary to further investigate the energetic load for balance control during these tasks. This could provide guidelines for improved rehabilitation programs and a more adequate prescription of aids for stroke patients.

References

[1]   M. Stulemeijer, L. Fasotti & G. Bleijenberg, *Fatigue as a window to the brain*. MIT Press, Cambridge, 2005.
[2]   M. de Haart, A.C. Geurts , S.C. Huidekoper, L. Fasotti & J. van Limbeek, Recovery of standing balance in postacute stroke patients: a rehabilitation cohort study, *Archives of Physical Medicine and Rehabilitation* **85** (2004), 886-895.
[3]   I.C. Chen, P.T. Cheng, A.L. Hu, M.Y. Liaw, L.R. Chen, W.H. Hong & M.K. Wong, Balance evaluation in hemiplegic stroke patients, *Chang Gung Medical Journal* **23 (6)** (2000), 339-347.
[4]   C.J.C.Lamoth, R.C. van Lummel & P.J. Beek, Athletic skill level is reflected in body sway: a test case for accelerometry in combination with stochastic dynamics, *Gait Posture*, **29** (2009), 546-551.

Rehabilitation: Mobility, Exercise and Sports
L.H.V. van der Woude et al. (Eds.)
IOS Press, 2010
© 2010 The authors and IOS Press. All rights reserved.
doi:10.3233/978-1-60750-080-3-181

Cancer rehabilitation exercise-mediated improvements over a twelve-year period in cancer survivors

S.D. CARTER[a,b], C.P. REPKA[a], L.K. SPROD[a], R. HAYWARD[a], C. M. SCHNEIDER[a]

[a]*Rocky Mountain Cancer Rehabilitation Institute, University of Northern Colorado, Greeley, CO*
[b]*Regional Breast Center of Northern Colorado, Greeley, CO*

Abstract. Cancer detection and treatment have improved in recent years, resulting in millions of cancer survivors living with the negative side effects of cancer therapies. The increase in the number of cancer survivors necessitates the development of strategies that can counteract these side-effects. One such strategy could be the implementation of prescriptive exercise interventions. Purpose: To summarize the exercise response in cancer survivors following exercise training over a 12-year period. Methods: Five hundred-nineteen cancer patients participated in fitness assessments which examined cardiorespiratory fitness, pulmonary function and muscular endurance. In addition, patients completed inventories that assessed fatigue, depression and quality of life. Patients were divided according to treatment status: following treatment (n=446) and during treatment (n=73). Following the exercise assessments, patients participated in an individualized exercise intervention 2-3 days per week for 3 months. Results: Significant improvements were found across time (p< .05) in blood pressure (-3.6%), resting heart rate (-7%), treadmill time (+28%), pVO$_2$max (+15%), FEV1 (+2.3%), upper body endurance (+46.8%), lower body endurance (+58%), and core endurance (+22.3%) with concomitant improvements in fatigue (-33.9%), depression (-27.3%), and quality of life (+5.6%) in the following cancer group. The patients during treatment showed improvements in blood pressure (-3.2%), treadmill time (+16.5%), upper body endurance (+39.3%), lower body endurance (+10.3%), and core endurance (+36.8%) with concomitant improvements in fatigue (-21%), depression (-11%), and quality of life (+6.3%). No differences were found between cancer type, treatment type, or cancer stage. Conclusion: Cancer survivors have physiological and psychological improvements with the implementation of individually prescribed exercise. Additionally, the response to exercise appears to be patient specific not cancer, treatment or stage specific. Our animal studies suggest that there are likely several mechanisms involved with the beneficial effects of exercise. Such mechanisms may include adaptations in antioxidant defenses, expression of heat shock proteins, regulation of apoptosis, as well as the expression and function of nitric oxide synthase.

Keywords. cancer, rehabilitation, exercise, survivors.

1. Introduction

Mortality rates from cancer have decreased 18.4% and 10.5%, respectively, in males and females [1]. While this is an encouraging trend, there is an ever-growing population of cancer survivors living with the negative side effects of cancer treatments which result in a reduction of physical function due to damage of healthy tissue [2,3]. The detriments to physical function and psychological well-being are variable due to differing etiologies, symptoms, target tissues, patient populations, and treatment strategies.

While exercise has been shown to improve various physiological functions and psychological well-being in a healthy population [4], less is known about the benefits of exercise in cancer survivors during and after cancer treatment.

2. Methods

Five hundred-nineteen cancer patients participated in fitness assessments over a 12-year period which examined cardiorespiratory fitness, pulmonary function, muscular endurance, fatigue, depression, and quality of life. Patients were divided according to treatment status: following treatment (n=446) and during treatment (n=73). Following the exercise assessments, patients participated in an individualized exercise intervention 2-3 days per week for 3 months with cancer exercise specialists. Exercise sessions typically included a 10-minute warm-up, 40 minutes of aerobic exercise, resistance training, and flexibility and balance training, and concluded with a 10-minute cool-down.

Statistical Analysis: The main effect of supervised exercise training was determined pre to post-exercise intervention using repeated-measures (ANOVA). Tukey HSD post hoc tests were used to determine where significance occurred.

3. Results

Characteristics of the study participants did not differ in age, height, or weight. Significant improvements were found across time ($p < .05$) in blood pressure (-3.6%), resting heart rate (-7%), treadmill time (+28%), pVO_2max (+15%), FEV1 (+2.3%), upper body endurance (+46.8%), lower body endurance (+58%), and core endurance (+22.3%) with concomitant improvements in fatigue (-33.9%), depression (-27.3%), and quality of life (+5.6%) in the following cancer group. The patients during treatment showed improvements in blood pressure (-3.2%), treadmill time (+16.5%), upper body endurance (+39.3%), lower body endurance (+10.3%), and core endurance (+36.8%) with concomitant improvements in fatigue (-21%), depression (-11%), and quality of life (+6.3%). No differences were found between cancer type, treatment type, or cancer stage [5-8].

4. Conclusions

Cancer treatments negatively affect physiological and psychological health, leading to a reduction in physical function and quality of life. Cancer survivors have physiological and psychological improvements with the implementation of individually prescribed exercise. Additionally, the response to exercise appears to be patient specific not cancer, treatment or stage specific.

Potential mechanisms for the protection afforded by exercise have been found in our animal studies. We have demonstrated that regular exercise attenuates the cardiovascular dysfunction associated with 5-fluorouracil, goserelin acetate, HER2 inhibitors, and anthracyclines. In these studies, cardioprotection was associated with an up regulation of cardiac heat shock proteins, a preservation of α-myosin heavy chain expression, less anthracycline accumulation in the hearts of exercised animals, and a preservation of cardiomyocytes cross-sectional area [9-11].

In conclusion, moderate exercise during and following cancer treatment is an effective and advisable method of improving cardiorespiratory function and muscular endurance while reducing fatigue and depression and improving quality of life in cancer survivors.

References

[1]   American Cancer Society, *Cancer Facts and Figures*, Atlanta, 2007.

[2]   DeVita, V. T., Lawrence, T.S., & Rosenberg, S.A., *Cancer, principles and practice of oncology,* (8th ed.). Lippincott, Williams & Wilkins, Philadelphia, 2008.

[3]   Schneider, C. M., Dennehy, C. A., & Carter, S. D., *Exercise and Cancer Recovery*. Human Kinetics Publishing, Champaign, IL, 2003.

[4]   American College of Sports Medicine, *ACSM's Resource Manual for Guidelines for Exercise Testing and Prescription*, (6th ed.). Lippincott, Williams & Wilkins, Philadelphia, 2010.

[5]   Hsieh, C.C., Sprod , L.K., Hydock, D.S., Carter, S.D., Hayward, R, & Schneider, C.M., Effects of a Supervised Exercise Intervention on Recovery from Treatment Regimens in Breast Cancer Survivors. *Oncology Nursing Forum* **35** (2008), 909-915.

[6]   Schneider, C.M., Hsieh, C.C., Sprod, L.K., Carter, S.D. & Hayward, R., Cancer Treatment-induced Alterations in Muscular Fitness and Quality of Life: the Role of Exercise Training, *Annals of Oncology* **18**(12) (2007), 1957-1962.

[7]   Schneider, C.M., Hsieh, C.C., Sprod, L.K., Carter, S.D. & Hayward, R., Effects of Supervised Exercise Training on Cardiopulmonary Function and Fatigue in Breast Cancer Survivors During and After Treatment, *Cancer* **110** (2007), 918-925.

[8]   Schneider, C.M., Hsieh, C.C., Sprod, L.K., Carter, S.D. & Hayward, R., Exercise Training Manages Cardiopulmonary Function and Fatigue During and Following Cancer Treatment in Male Cancer Survivors, *Integrative Cancer Therapies* **6**(3) (2007), 235-241.

[9]   Wonders,K.Y., Hydock, D.S., Schneider, C.M., & Hayward, R., Endurance Exercise Training Preserves Cardiac Function in Rats Receiving Doxorubicin and the HER-2 Inhibitor GW2974, *Cancer Chemotherapy and Pharmacology* (in review).

[10] Hydock, D.S., Lien, C-Y., Schneider, C.M.& Hayward, R., Exercise Preconditioning Protects Against Doxorubicin-Induced Cardiac Dysfunction, *Medicine and Science in Sports and Exercise* **40** (2008), 808-817.

[11] Hydock, D.S., Lien, C-Y., Schneider, C.M., & Hayward, R., Effects of Voluntary Wheel Running on Cardiac Function and Myosin Heavy Chain in Chemically Gonadectomized Rats, *American Journal of Physiology: Heart and Circulatory Physiology* **293** (2007), H3254-H3264.

Chapter 5

Exercise Capacity

5.1

Keynote

Rehabilitation: Mobility, Exercise and Sports
L.H.V. van der Woude et al. (Eds.)
IOS Press, 2010
© 2010 The authors and IOS Press. All rights reserved.
doi:10.3233/978-1-60750-080-3-187

Cardiovascular disease, SCI, and exercise: risks and focused countermeasures

M.S. NASH[1]
Departments of Neurological Surgery and Rehabilitation Medicine; The Miami Project to Cure Paralysis, University of Miami Miller School of Medicine, Miami, Florida USA

Abstract. Heightened risks for all-cause cardiovascular diseases (CVD) are widely reported in persons with spinal cord injuries (SCI). These risks occur earlier in life, develop silently, and are defined by fasting and non-fasting dyslipidemias, vascular inflammation, and other archetypical CVD hazards. Fasting studies typically show depressed levels of cardioprotective high-density lipoprotein cholesterol (HDL), and less often elevated total cholesterol and low-density lipoprotein cholesterol. Low HDL is especially revealing, as it typically foretells low fitness levels. Post-prandial risks for hypertriglyceridemia have also been reported after SCI, and may also be associated with sedentary lifestyle. Reduction of this risk is important for decreasing feeding-induced vascular inflammation. Both cross-sectional and prospective studies support exercise conditioning in effective treatment of SCI-associated dyslipidemia. Acute exercise, not longitudinal conditioning, however, better treats post-prandial CVD risks. The latter evidence may require a change in the exercise conditioning paradigms for those with SCI. Risks of CVD must be better understood and effective exercise interventions adopted, if best health, life quality and longevity are to be preserved.

Keywords. cardiovascular disease, lipids, inflammation, diet, exercise, risks.

1. Introduction

Heightened risks for all-cause cardiovascular disease (CVD) are widely-reported in persons with spinal cord injuries (SCI).[1-3] These hazards appear relatively early in life, progress silently, and manifest as fasting dyslipidemias, obesity, and other archetypical CVD risks[1-4]. They also tend to cluster,[1,3] which significantly amplifies patient risk. These hazards must be understood, and targeted interventions adopted, if persons with SCI are to lead healthy, productive, and independent lives.

2. Risks of Fasting and Non-Fasting Dyslipidemias

The most pervasive CVD risk accompanying SCI is physical deconditioning,[2] and thereafter dyslipidemia[1,3] and obesity.[4] Most studies have reported low levels of high-density lipoprotein cholesterol (HDL-C), and less often elevation of total

[1] Corresponding Author: Mark S. Nash, Ph.D., The Miami Project to Cure Paralysis, Lois Pope LIFE Center, 1095 NW 14th Terrace, R-48, Miami, Florida USA; E-mail msnash@miami.edu.

cholesterol (TC), low-density lipoprotein cholesterol (LDL-C) and triglycerides (TG). While fasting dyslipidemias are a *sine qua non* of atherogenesis, humans spend most of their lives in the postprandial, not fasted state, making postprandial TG appearance and removal critical to atherogenesis. An exaggerated postprandial lipemia (PPL) is an important stimulus for this process, as delayed removal of blood-borne TG-rich lipoproteins fosters arterial deposition and atheroma formation.[5] Exaggerated PPL in persons with paraplegia follows ingestion of a high fat test meal[6] and has been noted in persons having unremarkable fasting TGs, thus making the threat covert.

3. Risks of Inflammatory Vascular Stress

Recent models of atherosclerosis have gone "beyond cholesterol" to describe CVD as a process involving inflammation. Elevated fasting and post-prandial TG are both pro-inflammatory, and instigate endothelial dysfunction and oxidative stress (VOS). Blood-borne concentrations of inflammatory cytokines, including C-reactive protein (CRP), are commonly increased after SCI, and accompany infection, bacteriuria, skin breakdown, activity-induced musculoskeletal injury, and heterotypic ossification.[5]

Several studies have reported elevated serological inflammatory products in persons with SCI. These levels exceed criterion scores for elevated vascular risk, even without evidence of frank CVD or inflammatory disorder. Other studies of persons with SCI have observed significant associations among inflammatory cytokines and common CVD risks, including insulin resistance, elevated TG, elevated Framingham risk scores, increased abdominal sagittal diameter, fasting glycemia, elevated fasting and post-load insulin, low HDL-C, and elevated body mass index.[5]

4. Diet as a CVD Risk

A pattern of suboptimal dietary intake is a CVD risk in persons with SCI.[7] The diet is typically excessive in calories and mismatched for daily caloric expenditure. The mismatch is most profound in those sustaining adrenergic dysfunction from injuries above the T1 spinal level, which lowers resting metabolism, attenuates thermic effects of food intake, and blunts metabolism both during and following exercise. Caloric excess creating an 'obesogenic' environment has recently been described.[7]

Several studies have examined changes in diet composition after SCI. However, significant caloric restriction may worsen the lipid profile by lowering HDL-C. A six month program of nutrition education, exercise, and behavior modification appears to best favor weight loss, although dietary effects on other CVD risks still require study.

5. Exercise as a CVD Risk Countermeasure

Persons with SCI are ranked at the lowest end of the fitness continuum, and many experience deconditioning so severe that it challenges independent daily living. Fortunately, exercise is an effective and widely-adopted countermeasure for deconditioning, as well as dyslipidemia and other CVD risks. It is also most effective of non-pharmacological treatments for PPL when performed within 16-18 hours of TG intake. Both endurance and resistance exercises improve fitness in persons with SCI.[8,9] Endurance exercise, interval training, resistance exercise, and recreational sports also lessen CVD risks of fasting dyslipidemia.[2,8,9] In a cross-sectional comparison of active and sedentary males with tetraplegia Dallmeijer (1997) reported that regular sport activities (1.5 – 6 hours/week) increase the HDL-C and ApoA1:ApoB ratio while reducing the TC:HDL ratio. El-Sayed (2005) reported increased HDL-C in paraplegics undergoing 30 minutes of arm exercise for 12 weeks at 60-65% of peak oxygen consumption. Hooker et al. (1989) observed a similar increase in HDL-C with lowered TG, LDL-C, and TC:HDL ratio following eight weeks of wheelchair ergometry at 70-80% of heart rate reserve (HRR). Interval training by de Groot (2003) favored a dose-dependent reduction of the TC:HDL-C and TG at 70-80% HRR. In two studies using circuit resistance training for young and middle-aged persons with paraplegia, Nash et al. reported significant improvements in fitness (i.e., endurance, strength, and anaerobic power) with increases in HDL-C and reduction of LDL, LDL:HDL ratio, and the TC:HDL ratio. In one study the lowering of the TC:HDL ratio reflected a CVD risk reduction of almost 25%.

6. Conclusions

Antecedents to CVD are incompletely understood after SCI, although deconditioning is clearly among them. Imposition or adoption of a sedentary lifestyle poses significant CVD risks, and forecasts complications such as dyslipidemia, obesity, and cardio-metabolic syndrome. Physical activity is an effective countermeasure to these risks. Resistance exercise may be the best at enhancing all fitness attributes and reducing CVD risks of dyslipidemia, although recreational and endurance activities are also successful in achieving these goals. Persons with SCI should adopt engaging and fulfilling exercise to achieve sustained compliance and durable lifestyle modification.

The health scenario for those with SCI continues to improve. Still, a better understanding of CVD hazards is needed so that targeted therapies can be improved. Dietary intervention looks promising when coupled with exercise and education, but less promising as a monotherapy. Exercise needs to be more widely adopted as a healthy lifestyle and recreational alternative. Guideline-driven primary intervention must become a widely-adopted clinical standard,[1] as secondary prevention will likely be less effective in treating disease that has already developed, cardiovascular damage that is already manifested, or lifestyle habits that are too entrenched to change.

References

[1]   Nash M.S. (Ed.) Cardiovascular Disease After SCI. *Top Spinal Cord Inj Rehabil* 2009;14(3):1-104.
[2]   Nash M.S. Central Nervous System: Spinal Cord Injury. *In*: Exercise in Rehabilitation Medicine, pp. 191-205, W.R. Frontera, et al. (Eds). Human Kinetic Publishers, Champaign, IL, 2006.
[3]   Bauman W.A. and A.M. Spungen AM. Coronary heart disease in individuals with spinal cord injury: assessment of risk factors. *Spinal Cord* 2008;46(7):466-76.
[4]   Nash M.S. and D.R. Gater, Jr. Exercise To Reduce Obesity in SCI. *Top Spinal Cord Inj Rehabil* 2007;12(4):76-93.
[5]   Nash M.S. and A.J. Mendez. Non-Fasting Lipemia and Inflammation as Cardiovascular Disease Risks after SCI. *Top Spinal Cord Inj Rehabil* 2009;14(3):32-45.
[6]   Nash M.S., J.deGroot, A. Martinez-Arizala, and A.M. Mendez. Evidence for an Exaggerated Post-Prandial Lipemia in Chronic Paraplegia. *J Spinal Cord Med*. 2005;28:320-5.
[7]   Feasel S. and S.L. Groah. The Impact of Diet on Cardiovascular Disease Risk in Individuals with Spinal Cord Injury. *Top Spinal Cord Inj Rehabil* 2009;14(3)58-68.
[8]   Valent L., A. Dallmeijer, H. Houdijk, E. Talsma, and L. van der Woude. The effects of upper body exercise on the physical capacity of people with a spinal cord injury: a systematic review. *Clin Rehabil* 2007;21(4):315-330.
[9]   Cowan R.E., L. Malone, and M.S. Nash. EXERCISE is Medicine©: Exercise Prescription after SCI to Manage   CVD   Risk   Factors.   *Top   Spinal   Cord   Inj   Rehabil*   2009;14(3):69-83

Rehabilitation: Mobility, Exercise and Sports
L.H.V. van der Woude et al. (Eds.)
IOS Press, 2010

doi:10.3233/978-1-60750-080-3-190

Genetics and exercise

M.T. E. HOPMAN

Radboud University Nijmegen Medical Centre, Nijmegen, The Netherlands

Spinal cord injured individuals are prone to inactivity and related health problems. Physical activity plays an important role in health related risk management. Exercise training in healthy individuals and in those with cardiovascular disease or risk factors improves cardiovascular function, thereby lowering the cardiovascular risk. However, current knowledge about the underlying mechanisms is limited, especially regarding the role of genes. Last decade, research possibilities in the field of physiological genomics have expanded intensively, and translational research has become highly appreciated. This presentation summarizes the current knowledge on genes that potentially play a role in vascular adaptation to exercise in healthy and spinal cord injured individuals. Specifically, I will focus on animal and human in vivo measures of exercise, inactivity and vascular function, combined with gene expression of the nitric oxide pathway, growth factors and their receptors, antioxidative enzymes and several alternative vasoactive factors. Accordingly, I aim to link activity and inactivity with gene expression to gain better insight into the mechanisms of exercise-induced adaptations. While the limited available translational research suggests a relationship between expression of certain (groups of) genes and functional adaptations of the cardiovascular and muscular system, a large gap remain to be closed between fundamental and applied functional research.

5.2

Oral Presentations

Rehabilitation: Mobility, Exercise and Sports
L.H.V. van der Woude et al. (Eds.)
IOS Press, 2010

doi:10.3233/978-1-60750-080-3-193

Physical capacity after 7 weeks of low-intensity wheelchair training

R. VAN DEN BERG[a], S. DE GROOT[b,c], C.M.A. SWART[a],
L.H.V. VAN DER WOUDE[c,1]

[a] *Research Institute MOVE, Faculty of Human Movement Sciences, Vrije Universiteit, Amsterdam*
[b] *Rehabilitation Centre Amsterdam*
[c] *Centre for Human Movement Sciences, University Medical Centre Groningen, University of Groningen, Groningen, The Netherlands*

Abstract. The aim of this study was to evaluate the effect of a 7-week low-intensity hand rim wheelchair training program on the physical capacity in able-bodied individuals. In total 25 able-bodied participants participated; 10 participants exercised three times a week at 30% heart rate reserve for 30 minutes (training group), and 15 participants participated in a control group. Physical capacity (maximal isometric strength, sprint power, peak power output and peak oxygen uptake) and submaximal performance were assessed before and after training. Levels of upper body discomfort were determined with the use of the LEO-questionnaire (Dutch version Local Perceived Discomfort). The experimental group improved significantly on sprint power and peak power output compared to the control group. The participants did not experience high levels of discomfort during the program, as indicated by the LEO-questionnaire. A low-intensity training program can improve physical capacity in able-bodied individuals. Its effectiveness must be tested in a wheelchair-dependent population.

Keywords. wheelchair training, spinal cord injury, able-bodied, low-intensity.

1. Introduction

People with a spinal cord injury (SCI) have a reduced physical capacity compared to able-bodied individuals, which is the result of a loss of active muscle mass, and a relative inactive lifestyle. This inactive lifestyle will lead to a further decrement of physical capacity and as a consequence a vicious downward circle may occur.[1] Furthermore, overuse complaints are common in people with SCI, because activities of daily life (ADL) are very straining for the upper extremities.

To achieve training effects in physical capacity, the general accepted guidelines of the American College of Sports Medicine (ACSM) recommend an aerobic exercise intensity of 50-85% Heart Rate Reserve (HRR), with a duration of 20-30 minutes, and a frequency of 3-5 days a week.[2] Haskell[3] did put these ACSM guidelines into a somewhat different perspective in terms of intensity, duration and frequency, especially in de-conditioned people such as those with a chronic disease or disability. It is argued that exercising at a lower intensity is accompanied with greater safety, would be

---

[1] Corresponding Author: Lucas H.V. van der Woude; l.h.v.van.der.woude@med.umcg.nl

perceived as achievable, reduces the risk of overuse complaints and can improve motivation to remain active, while still becoming more fit.[3]

The aim of the present study was to investigate if a 7-weeks low-intensity (30% HRR) and norm-duration (30min/session) wheelchair training program can induce favourable effects in physical capacity. We hypothesized that a low-intensity norm-duration wheelchair training program improves physical capacity in able-bodied individuals, inexperienced in wheelchair propulsion.

2. Methods

Participants

25 Able-bodied participants were assigned to an experimental and control group after signing an informed consent. The experimental group (N=10) received a 7-week hand rim wheelchair exercise training program on a motor-driven treadmill, 3 sessions/week at 30% HRR, 30 min/session. The control group (N=15) did not participate in any exercise program. All participants were instructed not to change their usual physical activities during the study period. The study was approved by the local ethic committee.

Tests

In the standardized pre- and posttest the maximal isometric strength (Fiso), anaerobic sprint power (P30), submaximal performance (VO_2, HR, mechanical efficiency (ME)), the peak aerobic power output (PO_{peak}), and the peak oxygen uptake (VO_{2peak}), were measured in a wheelchair ergometer.[4] During the first and last training session on a treadmill the oxygen uptake (VO_2), the energy expenditure (EE) and heart rate (HR) were measured. The Local Perceived Discomfort (LPD) (in Dutch) was used to measure local upper-body discomfort after each training session.

Statistics

An independent t-test was performed to determine potential differences in participant characteristics and physical capacity (F_{iso}, P30, $VO_2$20, $VO_2$40, HR20, HR40, PO_{peak}, and VO_{2peak}) at baseline between the experimental and the control group.

With repeated measures ANOVA the effect of the training program on physical capacity was determined. The outcomes of the pre-test were added as a covariate if necessary to adjust for differences between the groups at baseline. Differences in physical capacity between the groups (experimental group and control group) and within tests (pre- vs. post-test) and their interaction were determined. A paired sample t-test was used to compare outcomes of the first and last training session (VO_2, EE and HR). The significance level was set at $P < 0.05$ in all analyses.

3. Results

The groups were comparable with regard to personal characteristics. Physical capacity variables, measured at baseline, revealed differences between groups on F_{iso} and VO_{2peak}. The increases in the experimental group over the training period for P30 and PO_{peak} were significantly higher than in the control group. The experimental group showed a significant drop in submaximal VO_2 (p=0.009) and submaximal HR (p= 0.030) compared to the control group. ME improved significantly in the experimental group compared to the control group (p=0.009).

The results of the analysis of the first (training 1) versus the last (training 21) training showed that at the same power output HR, VO2, and EE decreased significantly over the training program in the experimental group compared to the control group.

Table 1. Mean (SD) of the outcome measures maximal isometric strength (F_{iso}), anaerobic sprint power (P30), peak aerobic power output (PO_{peak}), and peak oxygen uptake (VO_{2peak}) on pre- and posttest per group, and the results of the interaction of the repeated measures ANOVA.

		Control	**Experimental**	**T-test**	**Rep. measures ANOVA**
F_{iso} (N)	Pre	294.3 (94.8)	471.6 (80.6)	0.000	
	Post	309.8 (123.8)	494.8 (109.0)		
P30 (W)	Pre	112.1 (19.6)	113.5 (31.6)		
	Post	120.9 (21.5)	148.7 (29.2)		0.001
PO_{peak} (W)	Pre	54.9 (16.3)	56.4 (10.0)		
	Post	55.0 (16.8)	75.6 (12.6)		0.000
VO_{2peak} ($l \cdot min^{1}$)	Pre	1.54 (0.28)	2.13 (0.30)	0.001	
	Post	1.64 (0.37)	2.09 (0.28)		

4. Discussion

The experimental group significantly improved compared to the control group with respect to P30, PO_{peak}, submaximal VO_2, HR, RER and ME, while no significant improvements were found for F_{iso}, and VO_{2peak}. These results may seem surprising in the light of the ASCM exercise intensity guidelines.[2] Yet, one needs to consider that the ASCM guidelines essentially are prescriptions for large muscle (i.e. lower-limb) exercise, not for upper-limb exercise. Besides, the current training program was given to individuals, fully inexperienced in upper-limb exercise and the specific task.

In conclusion, a 7-week low-intensity norm-duration wheelchair training can improve the physical capacity in able-bodied individuals. This low-intensity training might be suitable during rehabilitation, because it might increase the physical capacity while the risk to develop overuse complaints is assumed to be low. Future studies should test the effectiveness of the training in a wheelchair-dependent population.

References

[1]   J.A. Haisma, L.H.V. Van der Woude, H.J. Stam, M.P. Bergen, T.A. Sluis, J.B. Bussmann, Physical capacity in wheelchair-dependent persons with a spinal cord injury: A critical review of the literature, *Spinal Cord* **44** (2006), 642-652.

[2]   American College of Sports Medicine: The recommended quality and quantity of exercise for developing and maintaining cardiorespiratory and muscular fitness, and flexibility in healthy adults, *Med Sci Sports Exerc.* **30** (1998), 975-991.

[3]   W.L. Haskell, Health consequences of physical activity: Understanding and challenges regarding dose-response, *Med Sci Sports Exerc* **26** (1994), 649-660.

[4]   L.H.V. Van der Woude, J.J. Van Croonenborg, I. Wolf, A.J. Dallmeijer, A.P. Hollander, Physical work capacity after 7 wk of wheelchair training: Effect of intensity in able-bodied subjects, *Med Sci Sports Exerc* **31** (1999), 331-341.

Rehabilitation: Mobility, Exercise and Sports
L.H.V. van der Woude et al. (Eds.)
IOS Press, 2010
© 2010 The authors and IOS Press. All rights reserved.
doi:10.3233/978-1-60750-080-3-196

Eucapnic voluntary hyperpnea testing in spinal cord injured athletes

J.M. LABRECHE[ab,1], D.C. MCKENZIE[a]
[a]*University of British Columbia*
[b]*Canadian Sport Centre Pacific*

Abstract. Purpose: Eucapnic voluntary hyperpnea (EVH) is a sensitive test for airway hyperresponsiveness (AHR). It is accepted by the IOC Medical Commission and used extensively in able bodied (AB) athletes to confirm the diagnosis of asthma. AHR has been shown in spinal cord injury (SCI), however EVH testing has not been reported. The purpose of this study was to compare airway responsiveness in two athletic populations; SCI rugby players and elite AB swimmers. Methods: Sixteen swimmers (AB) and twelve rugby players (SCI - tetraplegia) performed the standard EVH test. A drop of >10% in FEV_1 was considered a positive test. Results: Positive test incidence was 81% and 69% for the AB and SCI groups respectively. Although FEV_1/FVC was normal in the SCI group (84%), predicted FVC and FEV_1 were significantly lower (80%, 81%) when compared to AB (122%, 109%). Mean ventilations during hyperpnea were also significantly lower (SCI=95.9L/min, AB=154.5L/min). Conclusion: EVH testing in SCI produces prevalence levels similar to previous tests for airway hyperresponsiveness in this population. However, due to smaller ventilatory capacities, the EVH test may not be as sensitive a tool for the SCI population (compared to an AB population). Additional testing may be required.

Keywords. exercise induced asthma, hyperresponsiveness, spinal cord injury.

1. Introduction

Exercise induced bronchoconstriction (EIB) is a term used to describe a transient airway narrowing during or following exercise. It is generally expressed as a percent reduction in forced expiratory volume in 1 second (FEV_1) pre to post exercise as per the American Thoracic Society (ATS) and the European Respiratory Society (ERS) standards [1,2]. The main stimulus is water loss by evaporation causing drying and cooling of the airway surface. This leads to release of inflammatory mediators, vasoconstriction of the pulmonary vessels and eventual obstruction of the airway.

The eucapnic voluntary hyperpnea (EVH) test is the current gold standard to test for EIB in Olympic athletes. Both the International Olympic Committee (IOC) and the International Paralympic Committee (IPC) accept this test in application for therapeutic use exemption of β_2 agonist. However, most data reported in the literature is on able-bodied athletes. Various studies have reported a high incidence of airway hyperreactivity in spinal cord injured athletes (C4-8 lesion level) using chemical challenge protocols such as methacholine and histamine [3-6]. No studies to date have

---

[1] Corresponding Author: JM Labreche, University of British Columbia, Vancouver, BC, Canada.
E-mail: labreche@interchange.ubc.ca

reported EVH test results in this population. The purpose of this study was to evaluate the EVH test response in this population compared to an able-bodied population with a similarly high incidence of positive tests.

2. Methods

Athletes from two Canadian National teams were recruited. The spinal cord injured group (SCI) consisted of twelve male wheelchair rugby players with lesion level C4-C8. The able bodied group (AB) consisted of sixteen male swimmers.

All subjects performed the eucapnic voluntary hyperpnea test according to the protocol of Anderson et al 2001 [7]. Baseline spirometry was performed (2 x FEV_1 maneuvers within 5%) followed by a 6 minute hyperpnea challenge set at 30 x FEV_1. Subjects inhaled dry gas containing 5% CO_2, 21% O_2 and balance N_2 at room temperature for the challenge portion. Follow up spirometry occurred at 5, 10, 15, and 20 minutes post challenge. A drop in FEV_1 of >10% was considered a positive test.

3. Results

Descriptive data are presented in Table 1 along with baseline pulmonary function results and ventilations for hyperpnea. Predicted FVC, FEV_1 and mean ventilation were significantly lower in the SCI group (p <0.01). Nine of 13 in the SCI group and 13 out of 16 in the AB group had a drop in FEV_1 of >10%. The incidence of positive tests was 81% and 69% for the AB and SCI groups respectively. The average drop in FEV_1 (of those who tested positive) was 17% in the AB group and 16% in the SCI group.

Table 1. Descriptive and baseline pulmonary data for the two the AB and SCI groups. Both baseline and predicted values are included where appropriate. Values are expressed as means and (standard deviations) except for the ratios. All means are significantly different between groups (p > 0.01).

Variable	Able-Bodied	Spinal Cord Injured
Height (cm)	191.3(4.3)	181.3(9.4)
Weight (kg)	85.9(4.3)	68.9(13.0)
FVC_{base} (L)	7.7(0.9)	4.4(0.7)
FEV_{1base} (L)	5.6(0.7)	3.7(0.5)
FVC_{pred}(%)	122.0(12.4)	80.1(11.8)
FEV_{1pred}(%)	108.5(12.9)	81.1(9.9)
FEV_1/FVC_{base}(Ratio)	0.74	0.84
Target Ventilation (L/min)	169.4(19.7)	109.8(14.5)
Actual Ventilation (L/min)	154.5(17.6)	95.9(18.3)

4. Conclusion

Respiratory complications are common in tetraplegia. Disruption to the respiratory muscle innervation results in reduction of active respiratory muscle mass available to expire forcibly. The consequence is a decrease in functional lung volumes and flow rates [8]. In addition, sympathetic outflow is compromised resulting in a lack of vasodilatation and a decrease in circulating epinephrine levels [9]. These factors influence airway response to exercise but may also influence ability to complete the EVH protocol appropriately. In this study, the SCI group was only able to attain ~80% of predicted values of FVC and FEV_1 at baseline. They may also be susceptible to fatigue during the hyperpnea challenge. Due to this unique set of circumstances, researchers should be aware of airway challenge protocols and their mechanism of stressing the system to produce the desired outcome.

Swimmers have been shown to have a bronchoconstrictive response to exercise due to repeated exposure to chlorine and chlorine derivatives [10]. While this hyperreactivity in swimmers is induced by chemical irritants, in a wheelchair population hyperreactivity may appear to be present due to a lack of muscle innervation and abnormal function of the autonomic nervous system. These two populations have both displayed a high incidence of EIB via the EVH test. As the mechanisms responsible may be entirely different, the question needs to be asked: Is this test appropriate in diagnosing EIB in a population with a compromised respiratory system? Further research should be conducted comparing EIB test protocols in an SCI population (particularly tetraplegics).

References

[1]   R. Crapo, A. Morris, R. Gardner, Spirometric Values Using Techniques and Equipment That Meet ATS Recommendations *American Review of Respiratory Disease* **123** (1981), 659-664.

[2]   P. Sterk, L. Fabbri, P. Quanjer, D. Cockcroft, P. O'Byrne, Anderson SD, et.al., Airway Responsiveness. Standardized Challenge Testing With Pharmacological, Physical and Sensitizing Stimuli in Adults. Report Working Party Standardization of Lung Function Tests, European Community for Steel and Coal. Official Statement of the European Respiratory Society, *European Respiratory Journal - Supplement* **16** (1993), 53-83.

[3]   R.V. DeLuca, D.R. Grimm, M. Lesser, W.A. Bauman, P.L. Almenoff, Effects of a β_2-Agonist on Airway Hyperreactivity in Subjects With Cervical Spinal Cord Injury, *Chest* **115** (1999), 1533-1538.

[4]   D.R. Grimm, D. Chandy, P.L. Almenoff, G. Schilero, M. Lesser, Airway Hyperreactivity in Subjects With Tetraplegia Is Associated With Reduced Baseline Airway Caliber, *Chest* **118** (2000), 1397-1404.

[5]   P.V. Dicpinigaitis, A.M. Spungen, W.A. Bauman, A. Absgarten, P.L. Almenoff, Bronchial Hyperresponsiveness After Cervical Spinal Cord Injury, *Chest* **105** (1994), 1073-1076.

[6]   E. Singas, M. Lesser, A.M. Spungen, W.A. Bauman, P.L. Almenoff, Airway Hyperresponsiveness to Methacholine in Subjects With Spinal Cord Injury, *Chest* **110** (1996), 911-915.

[7]   S. Anderson, G.J. Argyros, H. Magnussen, K. Holzer, Provocation by Eucapnic Voluntary Hyperpnoea to Identify Exercise Induced Bronchoconstriction, *British Journal of Sports Medicine* **35** (2001), 344-347.

[8]   J. Ledsome, J. Sharp, Pulmonary Function in Acute Cervical Cord Injury, *American Review of Respiratory Disease* **124** (1981), 41-44.

[9]   Schmid, M. Huonker, J.M. Barturen, F. Stahl, A. Schmidt-Trucksass, D. Konig, D. Grathwohl, M. Lehmann, J. Keul, Catecholamines, Heart Rate, and Oxygen Uptake During Exercise in Persons With Spinal Cord Injury, *Journal of Applied Physiology* **85** (1998), 635-641.

[10] J. Potts, Factors Associated With Respiratory Problems in Swimmers, *Sports Medicine* **21** (1996), 256-261.

Rehabilitation: Mobility, Exercise and Sports
L.H.V. van der Woude et al. (Eds.)
IOS Press, 2010
© 2010 The authors and IOS Press. All rights reserved.
doi:10.3233/978-1-60750-080-3-199

Lung volumes in spinal cord injury - a distinct restrictive pattern

G. MUELLER[a,b,1], C. PERRET[b], F. MICHEL[b]
[a] *Swiss Paraplegic Research, Nottwil, Switzerland*
[b] *Swiss Paraplegic Centre, Nottwil, Switzerland*

Abstract. Purpose: Functioning of the respiratory pump is an important determinant of physical exercise in spinal cord injury (SCI). The higher respiratory limitations are the more exercise capacity and general health may be affected. The purpose of this study was to analyze lesion specific lung volumes in order to better understand individual difficulties of breathing in SCI. Methods: Routine lung volume measurements by bodyplethysmography. Individuals aged between 18 and 70 years with chronic (> 1 year), traumatic, motor complete (ASIA A+B) SCI. Results: 146 SCI individuals with lesion levels between C4 and L4 met the inclusion criteria. Their mean age was 46±12y, height 1.75±0.08m, weight 72±13kg and they were 15.4±11.7y post injury. Compared to the able-bodied population, all lesion levels showed increased residual volumes (RV) and reduced expiratory reserve volumes (ERV). As a consequence, functional residual capacity (FRC) was around normal values. Nevertheless, relative to total lung capacity, FRC increased with higher lesion levels. Conclusion: Due to the loss of innervated inspiratory muscle mass, most lung volume parameters of individuals with SCI show a distinct restrictive breathing pattern. The additional loss of innervated expiratory muscle mass leads to lesion dependent increases in RV and decreases in ERV. This fact seems to cause the rapid shallow breathing pattern during exercise tasks in SCI.

Keywords. bodyplethysmography, lung function testing, spinal cord injury, breathing pattern.

1. Introduction

SCI can result in diminished pulmonary function, due to lesion dependent paralysis of respiratory muscles. Coughing and forced breathing, which requires activity of expiratory muscles, is often impaired especially in tetraplegic individuals. Depending on the level and completeness of the lesion, respiratory function of subjects with SCI is affected to different extents, decreasing with increasing lesion level [1,2]. Due to a lower physical activity in persons with SCI, less respiratory muscle mass is stimulated in daily life. This fact may also explain the weakened respiratory system, particularly for persons with tetraplegia [3]. During exercise, inefficient rapid shallow breathing patterns, which are characterized by high breathing frequencies and low breathing volumes, are often seen in individuals with SCI. Nevertheless, very few is known on the relation of lesion specific impairments in exercise capacity and decreased lung

---

[1] Corresponding Author: Gabi Mueller, Coordinator Clinical Research, Swiss Paraplegic Centre, CH-6207 Nottwil, Switzerland; E-mail: gabi.mueller@paranet.ch

volumes. Thus, the aim of our study was to evaluate lesion specific differences in lung volumes of individuals with SCI, measured by bodyplethysmography. The advantage of measurements by bodyplethysmography is that not only forced vital capacity (FVC), forced expiratory volume in 1s (FEV_1) and peak expiratory flow (PEF), but also total lung capacity (TLC), expiratory reserve volume (ERV), residual volume (RV) and functional residual capacity (FRC) can be measured. To our knowledge, these additional parameters are very rarely documented in the SCI literature, but values seem to differ substantially to those of able-bodied individuals [4].

2. Methods

This study is based on routine lung volume measurements by bodyplethysmography, including FVC, FEV_1, PEF, TLC, RV, FRC and ERV. Relative lung volumes (% of able-bodied predicted) [5] of all individuals that met the inclusion criteria and who were measured between May 2004 and December 2007 were entered in a database. Inclusion criteria were: men and women, 18-70 years of age with traumatic SCI for > 1 year, ASIA A or B and lesion level C4-L4. Exclusion criteria were: progressive neuromuscular diseases, patient does not fit into the bodyplethysmography cabin, bad cooperation of the patient, agoraphobia, tracheotomy, acute or chronic respiratory diseases. Subjects were grouped into the following 7 functional lesion level groups: C4, C5, C6, C7-C8, T1-T6, T7-T12, L1-L4. For each of the 7 lesion groups and all measured parameters, mean ± SD were calculated. Data are presented descriptively.

3. Results

146 SCI individuals met the inclusion criteria. Their mean age was 46±12y, height 1.75±0.08m, weight 72±13kg and they were 15.4±11.7y post injury. FVC, FEV_1, PEF and TLC decreased gradually with increasing lesion level (Figure 1). Compared to able-bodied predicted values, all lesion groups showed increased RV and reduced ERV. As a consequence, FRC was around normal values (Figure 1). Nevertheless, FRC increased with higher lesion levels, relative to TLC (Figure 2).

4. Conclusion

Due to the loss of innervated inspiratory muscle mass and possibly also stiffening of the chest wall, most lung volume data of SCI individuals showed a distinct restrictive breathing pattern. The additional loss of innervated expiratory muscle mass leads to lesion dependent increases in RV and decreases in ERV. This fact seems to cause a rapid shallow breathing pattern during exercise tasks in SCI.

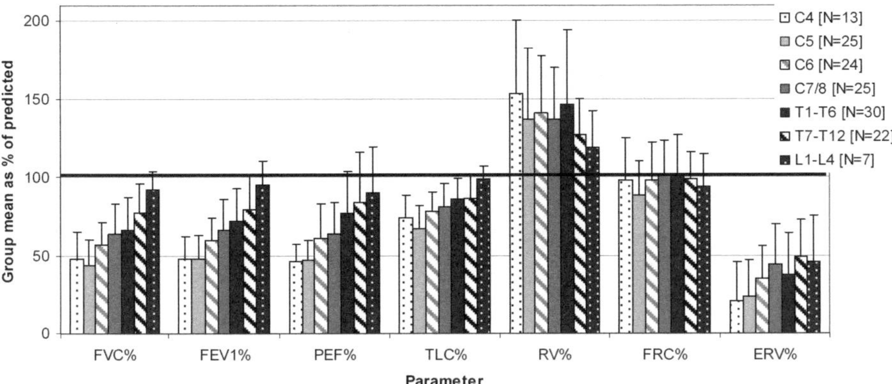

Figure 1. Lung volumes as % predicted of able-bodied individuals for the 7 different lesion level groups.

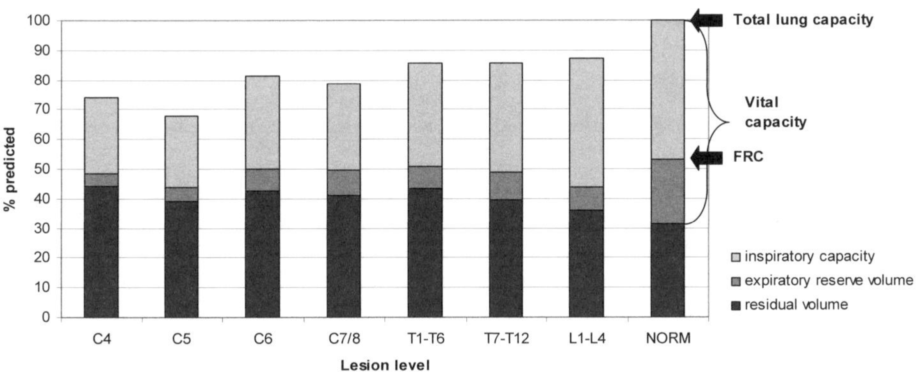

Figure 2. Total lung capacity as % predicted of able-bodied individuals and relative compartments of residual volume, expiratory reserve volume and inspiratory capacity.

References

[1] Almenoff PL, Spungen AM, Lesser M, et al. Pulmonary function survey in spinal cord injury: influences of smoking and level and completeness of injury. *Lung* **173** (1995), 297-306.

[2] Linn WS, Adkins RH, Gong H, Jr., et al. Pulmonary function in chronic spinal cord injury: a cross-sectional survey of 222 southern California adult outpatients. *Arch Phys Med Rehabil* **81** (2000), 757-763.

[3] Noreau L, Shephard RJ. Spinal cord injury, exercise and quality of life. *Sports Med* **20** (1995), 226-250.

[4] Stepp EL, Brown R, Tun CG, et al. Determinants of lung volumes in chronic spinal cord injury. *Arch Phys Med Rehabil* **89** (2008), 1499-1506.

[5] Quanjer PH, Tammeling GJ, Cotes JE, et al. Lung volumes and forced ventilatory flows. Report Working Party Standardization of Lung Function Tests, European Community for Steel and Coal. Official Statement of the European Respiratory Society. *Eur Respir J Suppl* **16** (1993), 5-40.

Rehabilitation: Mobility, Exercise and Sports
L.H.V. van der Woude et al. (Eds.)
IOS Press, 2010
© *2010 The authors and IOS Press. All rights reserved.*
doi:10.3233/978-1-60750-080-3-202

Examining community organizations' capacity to disseminate evidence-based physical activity promotion initiatives for people with spinal cord injury

A.E. LATIMER[a,b,1], L.R. BRAWLEY[a,c], C. CONLIN[a,d], K.A. MARTIN GINIS[a,d]

[a] *SCI Action Canada, Hamilton, Ontario, Canada*
[b] *School of Kinesiology & Health Studies, Queen's University, Canada*
[c] *College of Kinesiology, University of Saskatchewan*
[d] *Department of Kinesiology, McMaster University*

Abstract. To estimate the potential for systematically promoting physical activity (PA) in the spinal cord injury (SCI) population, we examined the capacity of community organizations in a large Canadian province to implement PA promotion initiatives. Representatives from 23 community PA (n=7), sports (n=8) and advocacy (n=8) organizations for people with disabilities completed a community capacity questionnaire and a follow-up telephone interview. Organizations' strategic priorities and available resources for promoting PA were obtained. Descriptive statistics for questionnaire data and recurring themes from participants' interview responses were analyzed. While 96% of organizations valued PA, only 65% had a strategic priority to promote PA. The majority (>73%) were willing to integrate PA promotion into current services (e.g., peer support programs) or link with other organizations already promoting PA (e.g., post a website ad). However, their capacity was limited; 40% indicated needing resources to foster PA promotion. Capacity building at multiple levels is needed for successful dissemination of evidence-based PA promotion initiatives for people with SCI.

Keywords. physical activity promotion, community capacity, dissemination.

1. Introduction

Participation in physical activity (PA) can reduce the personal and social burdens associated with inactivity in the SCI population[1]. Yet there have been no systematic efforts to increase PA in the SCI community. In fact, PA programs and information on how PA can promote health are two of the services most desired but least available to people with SCI[1]. Thus, to meet the needs of the SCI population, evidence-based interventions should be disseminated widely in collaboration with existing community organizations. The purpose of the current study was to examine the capacity of community organizations from a large Canadian province to implement PA promotion initiatives. Specifically, we examined whether organizations had the knowledge, skills,

---

[1] Corresponding Author. Amy E. Latimer, School of Kinesiology & Health Studies, Queen's University, 69 Union St., Kingston, Ontario, Canada K7L 3N6; E-mail: amy.latimer@queensu.ca

commitment and resources at the individual and organizational level to effectively promote PA participation.

2. Method

Participants

Participants were 23 representatives from community organizations for sport (n=8) PA (n=7) and advocacy (n=8) organizations for people with disabilities. Recruitment letters and information were initially sent to 61 organizations that served residents from Ontario, Canada.

Measures and procedure

A questionnaire plus follow-up interview protocol was used for the study. Organizations were contacted by telephone to inform them that they would be receiving a copy of a community capacity questionnaire. Questionnaires were mailed or e-mailed according to participant preference.

The 8-item questionnaire[2] assessed the following domains of community capacity in which participants indicated, on behalf of their organizations : 1) general commitment to PA promotion: participants indicated whether their organizations valued PA and had strategic priorities for PA, 2) capacity to deliver PA promotion interventions for individuals with SCI: participants indicated whether they could integrate PA promotion into existing policies, programs, or facilities and/or link with other organizations already engaged in PA promotion in the SCI population, and 3) resources needed to deliver PA promotion for individuals with SCI: participants identified whether they had adequate administrative support, qualified staff, physical resources (e.g., informational materials, infrastructure), and resources to sustain a PA promotion. Each question had three response options: "Yes," "Currently no, but can be" or "No, does not fit." In the questionnaires for the PA and advocacy organizations, PA promotion was defined as initiatives to increase PA awareness, improve behaviour management skills and make the environment more accessible for PA. In the sport organization questionnaire, PA promotion was defined as athlete-development initiatives.

Two weeks after the initial mailing, organizations that did not respond received reminder postcards, as well as follow-up e-mails and telephone calls over a five week period. Organizations that returned the questionnaire were scheduled for a follow-up interview within two weeks of returning their survey. During the interview, participants were asked to explain their rationale for each of their responses.

Descriptive statistics for questionnaire data and recurring themes from participants' interview responses were analyzed.

3. Results

Overall, 96% of organizations valued PA; yet, only 65% had a strategic priority to promote PA. The majority (>73%) were willing to integrate PA promotion into current services or link with other organizations already promoting PA. However, their capacity was limited to these forms of dissemination. Many organizations indicated needing resources and sustainable funding to foster PA promotion. Advocacy groups, in particular, indicated a very limited capacity and inadequate resources to integrate PA promotion into their existing services.

Table 1. Percentage of organizations who indicated having capacity in each domain

Organization type	Commitment		Delivery		Needs			
	Value	Strategic priority	Integrate	Link	Admin Support	Staff Support	Physical resources	Sustain funding
Sport	100.0%	75.0%	71.4%	75.0%	62.5%	57.1%	62.5%	28.6%
Exercise	85.7%	85.7%	85.7%	100.0%	85.7%	85.7%	57.1%	57.1%
Advocacy	100.0%	37.5%	62.5%	87.5%	25.0%	25.0%	62.5%	0.0%
Overall (*M*)	95.7%	65.2%	72.7%	87.0%	56.5%	54.5%	60.9%	28.6%

In the follow-up interview, ideas for integrating PA promotion into existing services included increasing emphasis on athlete development, information provision, and opportunity for social recreation. Websites, newsletters, and bulletin boards were suggested as potential strategies for sharing information and linking organizations. Advocacy organizations considered these linking options as a feasible strategy for PA promotion. Organizations identified a variety of resources needed to promote PA including additional informational and promotional materials, staff training, facilities, and financial support.

4. Discussion

Community organizations serving the SCI population are a potential channel through which PA can be promoted. To successfully disseminate evidence-based PA promotion initiatives, community organizations require additional capacity.

In the current study, gaps in capacity were particularly apparent in advocacy groups. While most of these groups valued PA, PA promotion was not a strategic priority and resources for promoting PA were lacking. Advocacy groups, however, are an important channel for dissemination; these organizations typically serve more people with SCI than other organizations. Thus, building capacity in advocacy groups and strengthening links between advocacy groups and PA and sport organizations is essential.

The success of partnerships between advocacy groups and PA and sport organizations will hinge on the ability of PA and sport organizations to deliver programs that meet the needs of the SCI population. To fulfill this mandate, PA and sport organizations require trained staff, physical resources, and sustainable funding.

Taken together, the findings from this study highlight the importance of systematically building the capacity of advocacy, PA, and sport organizations for effective dissemination of evidence-based PA promotion initiatives.

References

[1] D. L. Wolfe, K. A. Martin Ginis, A. E. Latimer, B. L. Foulon, J. J. Eng, J. T. C. Hsieh, Physical activity following spinal cord injury. *Spinal Cord Injury Rehabilitation Evidence (SCIRE)* [Internet]. 2008 [cited 2009 April 02]; Available from: www.icord.org/scire/

[2] G. Bell Woodard, *Health Promotion Capacity Checklists: A Workbook for Individual, Organizational and Environmental Assessment* [Internet]. 2005 [cited 2009 April 02]; Available from: http://www.prhprc.usask.ca/publications/finalworkbook.pdf

5.3

Poster Presentations

Rehabilitation: Mobility, Exercise and Sports
L.H.V. van der Woude et al. (Eds.)
IOS Press, 2010
© 2010 The authors and IOS Press. All rights reserved.
doi:10.3233/978-1-60750-080-3-207

Seated double-poling ergometer – a new training device for persons with spinal cord injury

A. BJERKEFORS[a,b], F. TINMARK[a,b], L. NOLAN[a,b], A. ARNDT[c], S. UCHIYAMA[a,d], J. NILSSON[a,b], A. THORSTENSSON[a,b]

[a]Department of Neuroscience, Karolinska Institutet, Sweden
[b]The Swedish School of Sport and Health Sciences (GIH), Sweden
[c]Department of Clinical Science, Intervention and Technology, Karolinska Institutet, Sweden
[d]School of Physical Education, Tokai University, Japan

Abstract. Purpose: To introduce a new training device and its applicability for persons with spinal cord injury. Method: A person with a T4 spinal cord injury (SCI) and an able-bodied person (AB) performed double poling exercise at incremental intensities, submaximal to maximal, on a new ergometer. Forces in the right pole and movements were measured in 3D with a piezoelectric force sensor (Kistler) and an optoelectronic system (ProReflex), respectively. Results: Stroke rates showed similar ranges for the two subjects, 27-38 strokes/min in SCI and 24-35 strokes/min in AB. Mean power per stroke, calculated over 5 strokes, ranged 29-124 W for SCI and 30-255 W for AB. The highest single pole forces attained were 153 N (SCI) and 307 N (AB). Sagittal upper trunk movement increased with intensity in both subjects, 29-37 deg (SCI) and 8-20 deg (AB), the larger amplitude in SCI being due to additional backward lean. Conclusion: The results hitherto obtained in this study in progress have indicated that the new ergometer for seated double poling is a suitable tool for training of the upper body in persons with spinal cord injury. It provides a large range of controllable intensities making possible both endurance and strength/sprint type of training.

Keywords. double poling, ergometer, kinematics, paraplegia, reaction force, training.

1. Introduction

Spinal cord injury (SCI) results in a complete or partial loss of motor and/or sensory function below the injury level. An SCI causes extensive functional impairment compelling many persons to wheelchair usage. Maintaining an adequate strength and control of trunk and shoulder muscles becomes essential, as the majority of every day tasks will be performed in sitting position. Moreover, physical exercise is crucial to avoid risks connected with a sedentary life-style (1). Therefore, it becomes important to find suitable, effective and attractive physical activities to retrain and improve motor functions achieved during rehabilitation. Ideally, such a training activity should be versatile and have the potential to improve several capacities beneficial to everyday life and thereby increase the independence of persons with SCI.

Sit-skate (Fig.1) is a leisure activity that is accessible for individuals with SCI and appears to have a potential to develop various desirable physical capacities, such as endurance, balance and strength. Training indoors on a double-poling ergometer is an alternative to outdoor skating, having the advantage of not being weather-dependent. Double-poling standing ergometers are commercially available for able-bodied persons, and are widely used among competitive cross-county skiers (2), but to our knowledge not adjusted or tested for persons with SCI.

The purpose of this study was therefore to introduce a new training device (Fig. 2) and its applicability for persons with SCI.

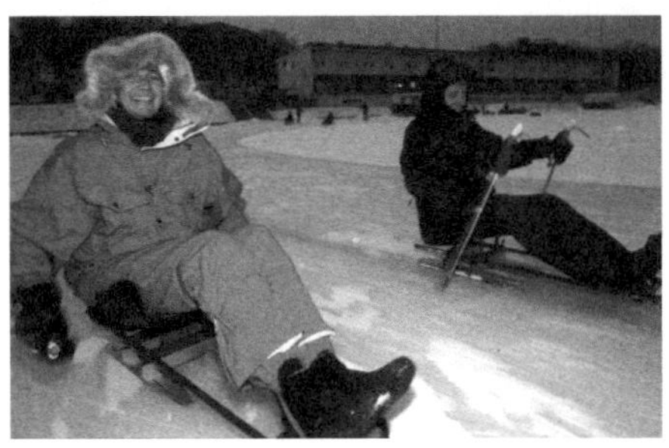

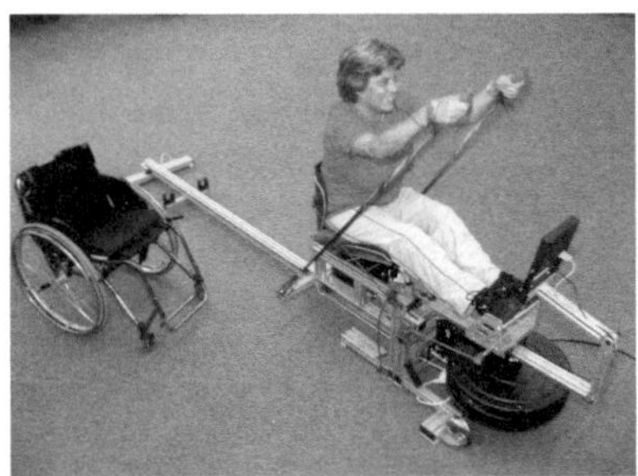

Figure 1. Double-poling outdoors on the sit-skate   **Figure 2.** Double-poling indoors on the ergometer

2. Methods

Pilot data were collected from two healthy habitually active men, one with a thoracic SCI, clinically classified as complete at T4 level, and one matched able-bodied (AB) person. Subjects performed double poling exercise on the new ergometer at four submaximal incremental intensities and in one maximal test.

Movement data measured in 3D were recorded using an optoelectronic system (ProReflex, Qualisys Medical AB, Sweden) at a sampling frequency of 120 Hz. The camera set-up included 7 cameras that were placed in a circle approximately 3 m around the subjects. Reflective markers were attached on the head, trunk, seat, left and right arm and pole, respectively (Fig. 3). The data were used to calculate 3D angular displacement of the poles and body segments, using the software package Visual3D (C-motion Inc., Maryland USA).

A piezoelectric force sensor (Kistler Instrument AG, Switzerland), was used to continuously record the forces below the handgrip in the right pole at a sampling frequency of 1200 Hz. The transducer was connected to an amplifier (Kistler Instrument AG, Switzerland) and signals were A/D converted.

The kinetic and kinematic data were used to calculate stroke frequency, stroke length, mean power during the stroke cycle, peak pole force and upper trunk angle in the sagittal plane during the stroke cycle.

Subjects were given both oral and written information about all aspects of the study and gave their written consent to participate. Approval was granted from the Regional Ethics Review Board in Stockholm.

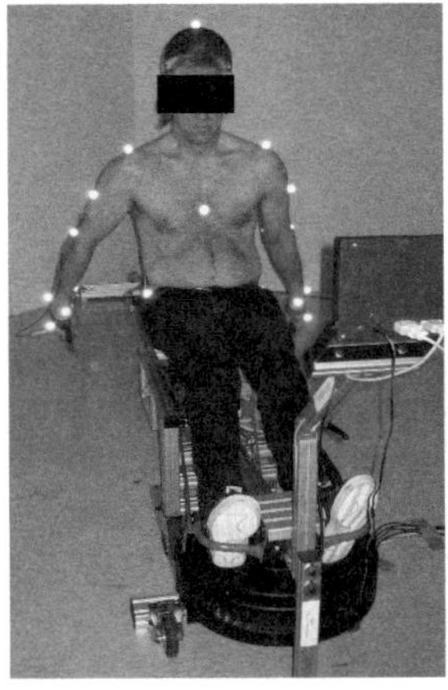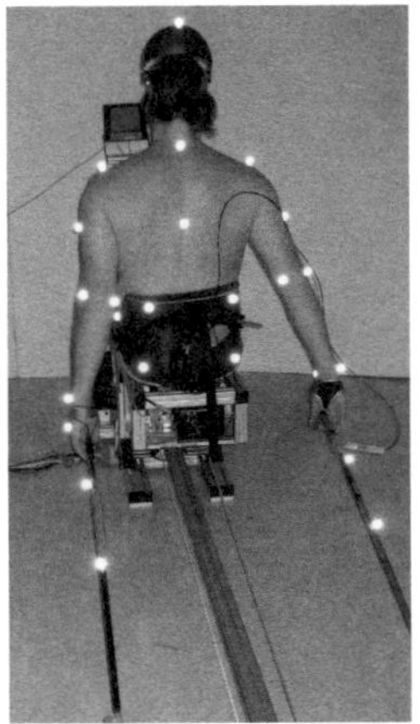

Figure 3. Markers attached on the subject with SCI. The force transducer was mounted 7 cm below the right ski-pole handgrip.

3. Results

The double poling exercis did not lead to any shoulder problems or other overload symptoms. Stroke rates and stroke lengths showed similar ranges for the two subjects, 27-38 strokes/min and 1.32-1.65 m in SCI, and 24-35 strokes/min and 1.29-1.78 m in AB. Mean power per stroke, calculated over 5 strokes, ranged 29-124 W for SCI and 30-255 W for AB. The highest single pole forces attained were 153 N (SCI) and 307 N (AB). Sagittal upper trunk movement increased with intensity in both subjects, 29-37 deg (SCI) and 8-20 deg (AB), the larger amplitude in SCI being due to additional backward lean.

4. Discussion

The main finding of this study in progress is that the new ergometer for seated double poling is a suitable tool for training of the upper body in persons with SCI. The smooth character of the movement during double poling also promotes this training device, since shoulder pain associated with more jerky movements can be a major problem for persons with SCI (e.g. 3). A great advantage with the ergometer is also that it provides a large range of controllable intensities making possible both endurance and strength/sprint type of training. Information provided from the display on intensity, speed and stroke rate can also motivate the trainees during exercises. Further studies are needed to evaluate if, and to what extent, a period of training on the double poling ergometer could influence functional performance as well as specific qualities, such as, muscle strength, balance control and oxygen uptake in persons with SCI.

References

[1] Davies DS and McColl MA. Lifestyle risks for three disease outcomes in spinal cord injury. Clin Rehabil. 2002 Feb;16 (1):96-108.

[2] Nilsson JE, Holmberg HC, Tveit P, Hallén J. Effects of 20-s and 180-s double poling interval training in cross-country skiers. Eur J Appl Physiol. 2004 Jun;92 (1-2):121-7.

[3] van Drongelen et al. Upper extremity musculoskeletal pain during and after rehabilitation in wheelchair-using persons with a spinal cord injury. Spinal Cord. 2006 Mar;44 (3):152-9.

Rehabilitation: Mobility, Exercise and Sports
L.H.V. van der Woude et al. (Eds.)
IOS Press, 2010
© *2010 The authors and IOS Press. All rights reserved.*
doi:10.3233/978-1-60750-080-3-210

The effects of Osteopathic treatment on common femoral artery blood flow in SCI individuals and able-bodied controls

G.A.W. DENISSEN[a], D. MURRAY[b], M.M.T. HOPMAN[a], M.J. MACDONALD[b]
[a] *Department of Physiology, Radboud University, Nijmegen, The Netherlands*
[b] *Department of Kinesiology, McMaster University, Hamilton, Ontario, Canada*

Abstract: Introduction: Pressure sores have been shown to be the major secondary health complication in spinal cord injured (SCI) individuals, and are associated with decreased blood flow and reduced healing potential. The goal of this study was to determine the effect of 3 different sessions of osteopathic treatment on mean leg blood flow (MLBF) in the left common femoral artery (CFA) of SCI individuals compared to able-bodied (AB) individuals. Methods: Six individuals (five male, one female; age 44 ± 17.5 years) with chronic SCI (C6-T12; ASIA A-B; 3.7 ± 4.6 years post-injury) and six AB individuals (five male, one female, 38.3 ± 9.7 years) participated in our study. The protocol consisted of 1 control 'familiarization' session of 40 minutes and 3 osteopathic treatment days, where our participants received manual therapy treatment focusing on the cranium (session 1), abdomen (session 2) and the lower extremities (session 3). Doppler ultrasound was used to determine the diameter and mean blood velocity (MBV) in the CFA before, during and after each session. Results: Two-way ANOVA statistical analysis revealed no difference in the maximal change in MLBF and leg vascular resistance (LVR) between groups or between the different treatment days. However, the maximal change in (MBV) was higher and maximal change of mean diameter was lower in SCI individuals (1.9 ± 2.0 cm/s; 0.03 ± 0.03 cm) compared to AB individuals (0.4 ± 1.3 cm/s; 0.06 ± 0.06 cm) across all treatments. There were no differences in absolute MLBF or LVR between treatments. Conclusion: Osteopathic treatment did not have an effect on CFA MLBF in either SCI or AB individuals. There was, however, a difference in the maximal change in MBV and diameter from rest to during treatment between groups. These, were however, so small that absolute flow was not observed to be different from baseline.

Keywords: osteopathic therapy, spinal cord injuries, blood flow, ultrasound.

1. Introduction

A decreased blood flow in the paralyzed legs of SCI individuals has been associated with many secondary complications (1-3). Pressure sore development is one of the most common complications associated with a decreased blood flow (1;2). It is hypothesized that in SCI, there is a reduced healing potential due to the decreased blood flow, which contributes to pressure sore development. These secondary complications of decreased leg blood flow can lead to an extreme decrease in the quality of life for an individual. Therefore reductions in these complications can result in decreased pain and discomfort.

In our study, we examined the effects of osteopathic therapy on blood flow in the lower extremities of individuals with SCI and age-matched able-bodied (AB) individuals. The goal of this osteopathic therapy is to create a balance between and within many of the regulatory systems of the body, including the musculoskeletal, cardiovascular, nervous and digestive systems. Most of the manual forces used are very light and should not create any discomfort or pain.

There has been no research to date examining the effect of osteopathic treatment on lower limb blood flow in individuals with SCI. Therefore, the objectives of this study were I) to determine the effects of 3 sessions of osteopathic treatment on blood flow in the left CFA of individuals with chronic, ASIA A-D SCI and able-bodied individuals and II) to determine which of the different osteopathic techniques/treatments may be most effective. We hypothesized that the different osteopathic treatments would result in an increase in femoral diameter and mean leg blood flow in SCI individuals compared to AB individuals cause their flow was more impaired at the outset of treatment.

2. Methods

Six spinal cord Injured individuals (44 ± 17.5 years) with complete and incomplete injuries (C6-T12; ASIA A-B; 3.7 ± 4.6 years post-injury) and six AB individuals (38.3 ± 9.7 years) participated in our study. Because the groups were age and sex-matched, there were no significant differences between ages in both groups and both groups composed of 5 males and 1 female. The protocol consisted of one control 'familiarization' session of 40 minutes and three osteopathic treatment days, each lasting for approximately 50 minutes.

The three osteopathic treatment days involved manual therapy consisting of different types of osteopathic treatments. Of these sessions; first session focused more on the dura, cranium, spinal cord, occiput, sacrum and diaphragm, second session focused on the abdomen and pelvis and the structures in the lower extremities (femoral artery) and the third session focused on the lower extremities, with special attention to the interosseous membrane, fibula and tibia and the femoral artery. Each session took place 1 week apart.

Doppler ultrasound was used to determine the diameter and blood velocity in the CFA and blood pressure was measured in the brachial artery before, during and after the control and treatments days.

3. Results

Two-way ANOVA statistical analysis revealed no difference in maximal change in mean leg blood flow (MLBF) and leg vascular resistance between both groups and between the different treatment days. However, maximal change of mean blood velocity (MBV) was higher and maximal change of mean diameter was lower in SCI individuals (1.9 ± 2.0 cm/s; 0.03 ± 0.03 cm) compared to AB individuals (0.4 ± 1.3 cm/s; 0.06 ± 0.06 cm). One-way repeated measures ANOVA did not show any differences in MLBF or LVR during the different treatments.

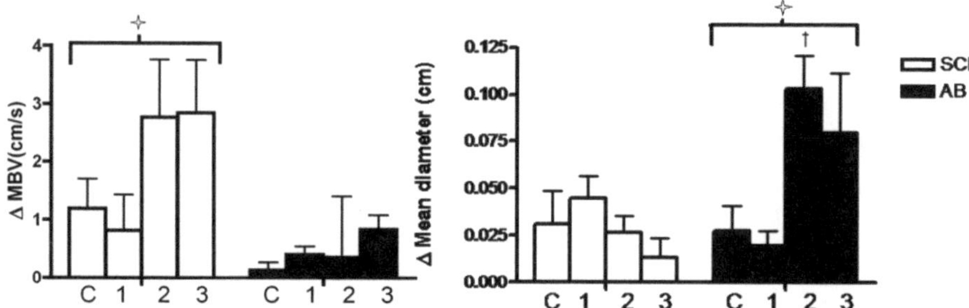

Figure 1. Maximal changes in MBV (a) and mean diameter (b) (mean ± SEM). C= control session; 1,2,3 = number of treatment days.   <0.05, † , 0.05.

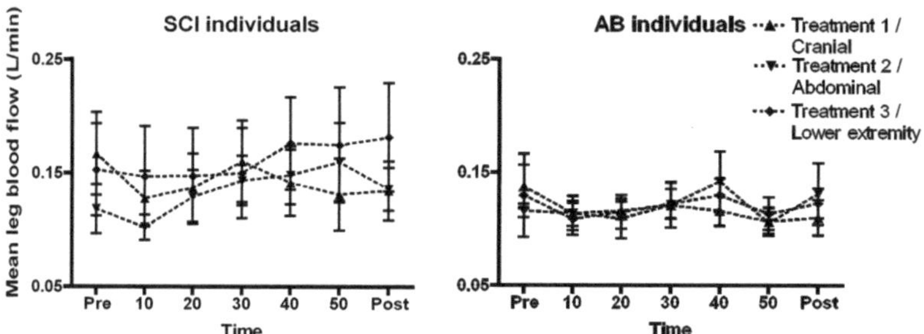

Figure 2. Changes in mean leg blood flow over time in SCI individuals (A) and AB individuals (B). Mean ± SE.

4.   Conclusion

After the application of three different treatment days of osteopathic manipulation therapy, no significant changes were observed in MLBF and LVR. The results show, however, that SCI individuals had greater changes in the CFA MBV, compare to AB individuals who had greater changes in CFA diameter. These changes were the largest after treatment of the abdomen and the leg. The findings were too small to result in detectable increases in MLBF or LVR. This is the first research to investigate the effect of osteopathic manipulation on MLBF. Individuals only received the therapy for three weeks while many other intervention studies demonstrate the effects of an intervention after extended periods of time. Therefore, it would be beneficial to examine the effects of osteopathic therapy over a longer period of time in order to determine if greater differences would result. It would also be useful to determine the skin blood flow or skin temperature to see if there is a significant change in blood flow distribution with osteopathic therapy.

References

[1]   R.L. Johnson, K.A. Gerhart, J. McCray, J.C. Menconi, G.G. Whiteneck, Secondary conditions following spinal cord injury in a population-based sample. *Spinal Cord* **36(1)** (1998 January), 45-50.
[2]   L. Noreau, P. Proulx, L. Gagnon, M. Drolet, M.T. Laramee, Secondary impairments after spinal cord injury: a population-based study. *Am J Phys Med Rehabil* **79(6)** (2000 November), 526-35.
[3]   L. Giangregorio, A. Hicks, C. Webber, S. Phillips, B. Craven, J. Bugaresti et al., Body weight supported treadmill training in acute spinal cord injury: impact on muscle and bone. *Spinal Cord* **43** (2005), 649-57.

Rehabilitation: Mobility, Exercise and Sports
L.H.V. van der Woude et al. (Eds.)
IOS Press, 2010
© 2010 The authors and IOS Press. All rights reserved.
doi:10.3233/978-1-60750-080-3-213

Relationship between physical capacity and the four dimensions of psychopathology in patients with heart conditions

E.M. NIEUWENBURG- VAN TILBORG[a,1], M.N. EVERSDIJK[a], B. ZWARTS[a],
E. ANGENOT[a], S. DE GROOT[a,b]
[a] *Rehabilitation Center Amsterdam*
[b] *Centre for Human Movement Sciences, University Medical Centre Groningen,
University of Groningen*

Abstract. The purpose of this study was to determine whether distress, depression, anxiety or somatisation result in a diminished physical capacity in patients with heart conditions. Data on the Dutch version of the four dimensional symptom questionnaire (4DKL, with the components distress, depression, anxiety and somatisation) and physical capacity, expressed in peak oxygen uptake (VO2peak) and peak power output (POpeak) were collected on all patients who followed the rehabilitation program in the Rehabilitation Centre Amsterdam between January 2004 and August 2008. A total of 445 patients completed a symptom-limited bicycle exercise test and the 4DKL. Scores on the 4DKL were classified into low, medium or high for the four different dimensions. Differences in VO2peak and POpeak between these three groups were analysed. On the dimensions distress, depression and anxiety no differences were found in VO2peak or POpeak. Patients with a high somatisation score had a significantly lower POpeak (p=0.02) than patients with a low somatisation score while no difference was found in VO2peak. Except for somatisation, psychopathology has no diminishing effect on physical capacity in patients with heart conditions. The effect of somatisation on physical capacity might be explained by actual physical complaints apart from psychological well-being.

Keywords. physical capacity, 4DKL, heart conditions.

1. Introduction

Psychopathology, such as anxiety, depression, distress and somatisation, are common in patients with heart conditions [1]. These four dimensions of psycho-pathology are associated with virtually all established cardiovascular risk factors, including diminished physical activity [2]. A diminished physical activity results in a lower physical capacity.

Therefore, the purpose of this study was to determine whether distress, depression, anxiety or somatisation result in a diminished physical capacity in patients with heart conditions.

---

[1] Corresponding Author: Liesbeth Nieuwenburg- van Tilborg; E-mail: l.v.tilborg@rcamsterdam.nl

2. Methods

Participants

445 Patients with heart conditions participated in this study. All patients followed the cardiac rehabilitation program in Rehabilitation Centre Amsterdam between January 2004 and August 2008. 71% Of the patients were male. The average age of the patients was 53.6 (SD=11.9) years, and the body mass index was on average 27.7 (SD=5.7) kg•m^{-2}.

Psychopathology

The Dutch version of the four dimensional symptom questionnaire (4DKL) was administered at the start of rehabilitation program to evaluate the baseline level of distress, depression, anxiety and somatisation. Scores on the 4DKL were categorized into low, medium, and high per dimension.

Physical capacity

All patients completed a symptom-limited bicycle exercise test. Baseline level of physical capacity was determined by the peak oxygen consumption (VO2peak, ml/min/kg) and peak power output (POpeak, Watt).

Statistics

To determine differences in physical capacity (VO2peak and POpeak) between patients with low, medium or high scores on the 4DKL a One-Way ANOVA was performed (p<0.05).

3. Results

The distribution of scores on the four dimensions of the 4DKL are shown in Figure 1.

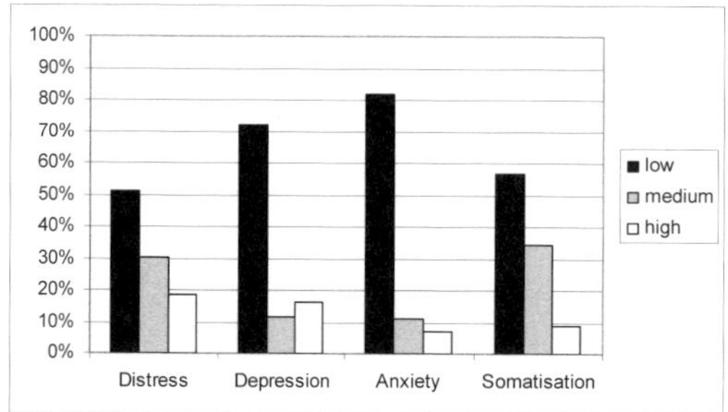

Figure 1. Distribution of the scores on the 4 dimensions of psychopathology (low, medium, high) in patients with heart disease.

Most patients had low scores on the four dimension of the 4 DKL. However, 49% of the patients had a medium (30%) or high (19%) distress score. The somatisation score was medium (34%) or high (9%) in almost half of the patients. 28% and 19% Of the patients had a medium or high score on respectively depression and anxiety.

On the dimensions distress, depression and anxiety no differences were found in VO2peak or POpeak. Patients with a high somatisation score had a significantly lower POpeak (p=0.02) than patients with a low somatisation score while no difference was found in VO2peak.

Table 1. Mean (M) and standard deviations (S) of VO2peak (ml/min/kg) and POpeak (W) of people with different psychopathology levels (low, medium, high). * = significant difference at p<0.05.

	Distress			*Depression*			*Anxiety*			*Somatisation*		
	Low	*Med*	*High*	*Low*	*Med*	*High*	*Low*	*Med*	*High*	*Low*	*Med*	*High*
VO2peak												
Mean	19.1	17.8	19.0	19.0	17.5	18.1	18.7	17.9	19.7	19.1	18.2	17.4
SD	6.1	5.9	5.8	6.0	6.6	5.8	6.2	5.5	5.4	6.3	5.9	5.0
POpeak												
Mean	108.1	99.9	106.5	107.6	96.2	101.6	105.5	101.0	109.4	109.8*	101.3	91.8*
SD	43.2	40.2	36.2	41.9	41.3	36.7	42.2	36.1	36.0	43.1	39.8	26.9

4.　Conclusions

Although most of the patients had low scores on the 4DKL dimensions, up to 49% of the patients show medium to high score on distress and somatisation.

Except for somatisation, psychopathology has no diminishing effect on physical capacity in patients with heart conditions. The effect of somatisation on physical capacity might be explained by actual physical complaints apart from psychological well-being.

References

[1] Revalidatiecommissie NHS/NVVC, Richtlijn Hartrevalidatie 2004. Den Haag: Nederlandse hartstichting 2004.
[2] Egger E. et al. Depression and anxiety symptoms affect change in exercise capacity during cardiac rehabilitation. *Eur J Cardiovasc Prev Rehabil.* 2008 Dec;15(6):704-8.

Rehabilitation: Mobility, Exercise and Sports
L.H.V. van der Woude et al. (Eds.)
IOS Press, 2010

doi:10.3233/978-1-60750-080-3-216

Repeatability and validity of the combined arm-leg (Cruiser) ergometer

E.K. SIMMELINK[a], J.B. WEMPE[a,b], J.H.B. GEERTZEN[a,c], R. DEKKER[a,c]
[a]*Center for Rehabilitation, University Medical Center Groningen, The Netherlands*
[b]*Department of Pulmonology, University Medical Center Groningen, The Netherlands*
[c]*Graduate School for Health Research (SHARE), University of Groningen, The Netherlands*

Abstract. The measurement of physical fitness of lower limb amputees is difficult as the commonly used ergometer tests have limitations. A combined arm-leg (Cruiser) ergometer might be valuable. The aim of this study was to establish the repeatability and validity of the combined arm-leg (Cruiser) ergometer. Thirty healthy volunteers performed three incremental exercise tests, once on the bicycle ergometer and twice on the Cruiser ergometer. The repeatability of the Cruiser ergometer was assessed by studying the means of the test-retest and the validity by studying the means of the bicycle and the two Cruiser ergometer tests. Intraclass Correlation Coefficient (ICC) for repeated measurements on the Cruiser ergometer was 0.84 for the maximal oxygen consumption (V_{O2} max) and 0.71 for the maximal heart rate (HR max). ICC for the measurements on the bicycle ergometer and the Cruiser ergometer was 0.86 for the V_{O2} max and 0.73 for HR max. Bland and Altman plots for V_{O2} max and HR max showed a bias close to zero and a great accuracy. The conclusion of this study is that the Cruiser ergometer provides a repeatable and valid measurement of the physical fitness in healthy volunteers. Its value in clinical practice for lower limb amputees needs further to be established.

Keywords: physical fitness, combined arm-leg (Cruiser) ergometer, exercise test, repeatability, validity.

1. Introduction

Patients with a lower limb amputation experience a decline in physical fitness. Walking with a prosthesis costs more energy than walking with two sound legs [1]. Evidence from Chin et al. suggests that when prosthetic rehabilitation only covers walking training with a prosthesis, maximal aerobic capacity of amputees does not improve to the level of able-bodied persons [2]. Therefore, training in prosthetic walking should accompany some kind of endurance exercise training with the aim of improving fitness of amputees.

Before commencing aerobic training, an appropriate maximal exercise test is necessary. Up to now, different types of ergometers are available for exercise testing and training. For a reliable measurement of aerobic capacity and safety, it is best to choose an ergometer on which the subject uses a large muscle mass during exercising thus reaching higher maximal oxygen uptake and maximal heart rate [3]. In a pilot study, Vestering et al. developed a maximal exercise testing protocol for lower limb amputees using a combined arm-leg ergometer: the Cruiser ergometer [4]. She concluded that the Cruiser ergometer can indeed be used in limb amputees for determination of maximal aerobic capacity and in fact elicited a higher oxygen uptake and heart rate than arm ergometry. At this moment, no data are present on the repeatability and validity of the combined arm-leg (Cruiser) ergometer. The aim of this study is to establish the repeatability and validity of the Cruiser ergometer.

2. Methods

30 Healthy volunteers (16 men and 14 women) age between 20 and 61 years participated in this study. The subjects performed three incremental exercise tests, once on the bicycle and twice on the Cruiser ergometer. ECG recordings were made and blood pressure was measured. The repeatability was assessed by studying the mean values of the test-retest and the validity by studying the mean values of the bicycle and the two Cruiser ergometer tests. In rest, after the warming-up period and at the point of maximal load the Borg 10-point category scale with ratio properties was used to rate the perceived exertion[5]. Dyspnoea, leg muscle fatigue (bicycle and cruiser ergometer) and arm muscle fatigue (cruiser ergometer) were measured using the Borg score.

3. Results

No significant differences were found for the maximal oxygen consumption (VO2max), maximal heart rate (HRmax), maximal ventilation (VEmax) and anaerobic treshold (ATmax) between the two tests on the Cruiser ergometer and between the test on the bicycle ergometer and Cruiser ergometer.

The maximal load (Wmax) reached on the bicycle ergometer was significant higher than on the Cruiser ergometer and the Wmax at the second test on the Cruiser ergometer was higher than at the first test. [Table 1]

The ICC for repeated measurements on the Cruiser ergometer was 0.84 for the VO2max and 0.71 for the HRmax. ICC for the measurements on the Cruiser ergometer was 0.86 for the VO2max and 0.73 for HRmax. Bland and Altman plots for VO2max and HRmax showed a bias close to zero and a great accuracy. Borg scores for muscle fatigue were significantly higher than for dyspnoea on all tests.

4. Discussion

This study shows that the Cruiser ergometer provides a repeatable and valid measurement of physical fitness in healthy volunteers.

There are some limitations of our study. Firstly, getting acquainted to the Cruiser-ergometer may be more important than to the bicycle ergometer as the movement is more complex and less familiar. This is supported by the higher load on the second Cruiser test and a lower VO_2 in the second steady state period

Secondly, our subjects were all healthy persons. Before using the Cruiser ergometer for patients with a lower limb amputation, we have to adapt our protocol because these patients will reach a lower maximal load.

Finally, ECG-recordings were not accurate in all subjects because of too much noise. Accurate ECG-recording is absolutely necessary in patient such as lower limb amputees, often with concomitant cardiovascular disease.

5. Conclusion

This study shows that the Cruiser ergometer provides a repeatable and valid measurement of the physical fitness in healthy volunteers. The bicycle ergometer is preferred above the Cruiser ergometer because it is more energy efficient and ECG recording is possible. However, for patients with a lower limb amputation the Cruiser ergometer seems to be a good alternative. Further research is needed before the Cruiser ergometer can be used in lower limb amputees.

Table 1. Comparison of the three exercise tests.

	Bicycle	Cruiser 1	Cruiser 2
mean (SD) N=30			
V_{O2} max (l/min)	2.70 (0.60)	2.62 (0.63)	2.64 (0.67)
V_{CO2} max (l/min)	3.06 (0.68)	2.84 (0.69) *	3.00 (0.90)
V_E max (l/min)	91.62 (21.14)	89.89 (22.18)	98.21 (33.11)
HR max (beats/min)	167.50 (13.94)	164.77 (14.88)	167.60 (12.19)
Load max (W)	240.00 (54.20) **	196.00 (42.31) *	208.67 (48.00) ***
AT max	1.70 (0.37)	1.81 (0.42)	1.80 (0.47)

* significant difference between test on the Biycle ergometer and first test on the Cruiser ergometer
** significant difference between test on the Biycle ergometer and second test on the
    Cruiser ergometer
*** significant difference between the tests on the Cruiser ergometer

Abbreviations	
V_{O2} max:	maximum oxygen consumption
V_{CO2} max:	maximum carbon dioxide output
V_E max :	maximum ventilation
HR max :	maximum heart rate
Load max:	maximum load
AT max:	anaerobic treshold at maximum load

References

[1]   Waters RL, Perry J, Antonelli D, Hislop H (1976). Energy cost of walking of amputees: influence of level of amputation. *J Bone Joint Surg Am* **58**, 42-46.

[2]   Chin T, Sawamura S, Fuijta H., Oijma I., Oyabu H. et al. (2002). VO2max as an indicator of prosthetic rehabilitation outcome after dysvascular amputation. *Prosthet Orthot Int* **26**, 44-49.

[3]   Bostom AG, Bates E, Mazzarella N, Block E, Adler J (1987). Ergometer modification for combined arm-leg use by lower extremity amputees in cardiovascular testing and training. *Arch Phys Med Rehabil* **68**, 244-247.

[4]   Vestering MM, Schoppen T, Dekker R, Wempe J, Geertzen JHB (2005). Development of an exercise testing protocol for patients with a lower limb amputation: results of a pilot study. Int J Rehabil Res 28, 237-244.

[5]   Borg GAV (1982). Psychophysical bases of perceived exertion. *Med Sci Sports Exerc* **14**, 377-381.

Rehabilitation: Mobility, Exercise and Sports
L.H.V. van der Woude et al. (Eds.)
IOS Press, 2010

doi:10.3233/978-1-60750-080-3-219

Arterial haemoglobin oxygen saturation and power output are maintained at peak oxygen consumption in upper compared to lower body exercise in normobaric hypoxia

C.D. THAKE[a,1], C. SIMONS[b], M.J. PRICE[a]

[a] *Faculty of Health and Life Sciences, Coventry University, Coventry, UK*
[b] *Myerscough College, Preston, Lancashire, UK*

Abstract. Purpose: To examine the effect of reduced F_IO_2 and the magnitude of reduction in $\dot{V}O_2$ peak, peak power output (PPO) and arterial haemoglobin oxygen saturation (SpO_2) in upper compared to lower body exercise. Methods: Nine healthy able-bodied male participants (age mean 22 ± 2 years) undertook three upper and three lower body discontinuous (30 sec intervals) incremental exercise tests to volitional exhaustion (UBX; LBX) whilst breathing either normoxia (N) or normobaric hypoxia (H_1 and H_2); F_IO_2s $\approx$ 0.21, 0.15 and 0.13 respectively. Data were examined using general linear model analysis of variance. Results: UBX $\dot{V}O_2$ peak was 71 $\pm$10 and 76 $\pm$8% whereas PPO was 50 $\pm$5 and 55 $\pm$3% of that in LBX at H_1 and H_2 respectively; demonstrating that $\dot{V}O_2$ peak and PPO were maintained in UBX relative to LBX in H_2. Correspondingly SpO_2 was 79 $\pm$4% in UBX versus 73 $\pm$4% in LBX at H_2 compared to 85 $\pm$5% in UBX versus 83 $\pm$4% in LBX at H_1. Conclusion: UBX $\dot{V}O_2$ peak and PPO do not decline in the same manner as LBX with reduced F_IO_2. This may be explained by the smaller reduction in SpO_2 observed during UBX compared to LBX.

Keywords. arterial oxygen saturation, upper body exercise.

1. Introduction

At sea level upper body exercise (UBX) elicits approximately 70% $\dot{V}O_2$ peak and 50% peak power output (PPO) of that attained during lower body exercise (LBX) in non specifically trained individuals.[1] Although it is well established that $\dot{V}O_2$ peak and PPO decline with increasing altitude during LBX [2] responses to UBX remain equivocal. [3, 4] For example, even though hyperoxia has been shown to increase $\dot{V}O_2$ peak during arm cranking in able-bodied participants a reduced inspired oxygen fraction $(F_IO_2) = 0.15$ did not reduce $\dot{V}O_2$ peak from that in normoxia[3]. Furthermore arterial haemoglobin oxygen saturation (SpO_2) data were not reported in this investigation. In contrast the percentage reduction in $\dot{V}O_2$ peak (c. 10%) observed in trained participants at $F_IO_2 = 0.146$ did not vary between UBX and LBX. [4] However

---

[1] Corresponding Author: C. Douglas Thake, Faculty of Health and Life Sciences, James Starley Building, Coventry University, Coventry, CV1 5FB, UK; d.thake@coventry.ac.uk.

the mode of UBX was doublepoling ergometry for cross country skiing and was unlikely to have exclusively engaged the upper body, in comparison to a more isolated exercise mode (leg cycling) used for LBX. Therefore we examined the effect of reduced F_IO_2 and the magnitude of reduction in $\dot{V}O_2$ peak and PPO in UBX (arm cranking) compared to LBX (leg cycling) in able-bodied participants.

2. Method

Using a randomized cross-over type design nine healthy male participants (age 22 ± 2 yrs; body mass 78.7 ± 12.2 kg; height 180.6 ± 8.2 cm; estimated fat mass 15.8 ± 6.4 %; estimated muscle mass 57.5 ± 6.5 %; haemoglobin 14.9 ± 0.7 g·dl^{-1}) undertook three UBX and three LBX discontinuous (30 sec intervals) incremental tests to volitional exhaustion whilst breathing either normoxia (N) or normobaric hypoxia (H_1 and H_2); F_IO_2s ≈ 0.21, 0.15 and 0.13 respectively. Exercise commenced with a resistance of 70 W for cycle ergometry and 35 W arm cranking and was increased by 30 and 15 W, respectively, every 3 min thereafter. Cadence was maintained at 70 rpm throughout. Expired gas was collected (Douglas bag technique), for subsequent analysis, during the last 60 sec of each exercise stage. Heart rate (HR) and arterial haemoglobin oxygen saturation (SpO_2) were monitored continually. Data were examined using general linear model analysis of variance.

3. Results

Physiological responses are given in Table I. UBX $\dot{V}O_2$ peak was 72 ± 3, 71 ± 10 and 76 ± 8% whereas PPO was 50 ± 6, 50 ± 5 and 55 ± 3% of that in LBX at N, H_1 and H_2

Table 1. Physiological variables at peak exercise (mean $\pm s$)

		LBX			UBX		
		N	H_1	H_2	N	H_1	H_2
Peak Power output (W)	#, †	273 ± 49	250 ± 37	223 ± 28	135 ± 27	127 ± 20	123 ± 18
$\dot{V}O_2$ peak (L·min^{-1})	#, †, Φ	3.52 ± 0.50	3.04 ± 0.46	2.68 ± 0.27	2.53 ± 0.35	2.15 ± 0.40	2.04 ± 0.34
HR (bt·min^{-1})	#, δ	189 ± 12	188 ± 12	183 ± 13	180 ± 13	180 ± 13	176 ± 14
SpO_2 (%)	#, †, Φ	96 ± 2	83 ± 4	73 ± 4	96 ± 2	85 ± 5	79 ± 4

#$P<0.001$ exercise mode; †$P<0.001$, δ$P<0.01$ F_IO_2; Φ$P<0.05$ exercise mode × F_IO_2; effect size eta^2 = 0.03 to 0.80.

respectively; demonstrating that $\dot{V}O_2$ peak and PPO were maintained in UBX relative to LBX in H_2. SpO_2 was 79 ± 4% in UBX vs. 73 ± 4 % in LBX at H_2 ($P<0.01$) compared to 85 ± 5 % in UBX versus 83 ± 4 % in LBX at H_1. There was a tendency for

HR to remain lower in UBX (183 $\pm$ 13 vs. 176 $\pm$ 14 bt·min^{-1}; P=0.07 at H$_2$). Exercise durations of 27.11 $\pm$ 5.74 *vs.* 26.58 $\pm$ 6.61, 24.06 $\pm$ 4.21 vs. 24.53 $\pm$ 4.98 and 21.22 $\pm$ 3.31 vs. 23.56 $\pm$ 4.27 min for LBX vs. UBX in N, H$_1$ and H$_2$, respectively were observed and declined with F$_I$O$_2$ (P<0.001). Peak blood lactate was >10 mmol.L^{-1} in UBX and LBX and did not vary with F$_I$O$_2$. However, during LBX RER increased from 1.19 $\pm$ 0.04 to 1.21 $\pm$ 0.06 and 1.27 $\pm$0.04, while UBX elicited an RER of 1.18 $\pm$ 0.08, 1.28 $\pm$ 0.10 and 1.34 $\pm$0.11 for N, H$_1$ and H$_2$, respectively. $\dot{V}_E/\dot{V}O_2$ and $\dot{V}_E/\dot{V}CO_2$ were highest during UBX compared to LBX at all F$_I$O$_2$s (P<0.001) e.g. $\dot{V}_E/\dot{V}O_2$ 44.03 $\pm$ 5.59 vs. 50.75 $\pm$ 9.57 L·L^{-1} and $\dot{V}_E/\dot{V}CO_2$ 34.49 $\pm$ 3.86 vs. 37.84 $\pm$ 5.68 L·L^{-1} in H$_2$ for LBX and UBX respectively.

4. Discussion

UBX $\dot{V}O_2$ peak and PPO do not decline in the same manner as during LBX with reduced F$_I$O$_2$ in participants not specifically UBX trained. This may be explained by the smaller reduction in SpO$_2$ observed during UBX compared to LBX. The 6% greater S$_P$O$_2$ in UBX in H$_2$ not only contributes to the maintenance of oxygen delivery but may also maintain the oxygen diffusion gradient across the capillary to active muscle. Arguably $\dot{V}O_2$ peak and PPO are able to be maintained between H$_1$ and H$_2$ in UBX compared to LBX as central circulatory function is not limiting in UBX and muscle oxygen extraction can be increased due to the relatively better maintenance of SpO$_2$ in UBX compared to LBX. Several factors may account for the observed difference in SpO$_2$ at $\dot{V}O_2$ peak between UBX and LBX in H$_2$ i) Smaller proportion of total venous return from UBX compared to LBX ii) Reduced red blood cell pulmonary transit time during peak UBX iii) Increased P$_A$O$_2$ due to relative hyperventilation during peak UBX. Evaluating both UBX and LBX responses to hypoxia pre and post UBX training will help elucidate factors determining the maintenance of SpO$_2$ during UBX. This is potentially relevant to understanding the preparation for and management of athletic and occupational activities predominantly involving UBX at altitude.

References

[1] M. N. Sawka, Physiology of upper body exercise, *Exercise and Sport Science Reviews* **14** (1986), 175-211.

[2] J. A. L. Calbet, R. Boushel, G. Radegran, H. Sondergaard, P. D. Wagner, B, Saltin, Determinants of maximal oxygen uptake in severe acute hypoxia, *American Journal of Physiology-Regulatory Integrative and Comparative Physiology* **284** (2003), R291-R303.

[3] M. E. T. Hopman, S. Hotman, J. T. Groothuis, H. T. M. Folgering, The effect of varied fraction inspired oxygen on arm exercise performance in spinal cord injury and able-bodied persons, *Archives of Physical Medicine and Rehabilitation,* **85** (2004) 319-323.

[4] M. Angermann, H. Hoppler, M. Wittwer, C. Dapp, H. Howald, M. Vogt, Effect of acute hypoxia on maximal oxygen uptake and maximal performance during leg and upper-body exercise in Nordic combined skiers, *International Journal of Sports Medicine,* **27** (2006), 301-306.

Rehabilitation: Mobility, Exercise and Sports
L.H.V. van der Woude et al. (Eds.)
IOS Press, 2010
© 2010 The authors and IOS Press. All rights reserved.
doi:10.3233/978-1-60750-080-3-222

Continuous versus discontinuous protocols using a graded one-legged peak exercise test for lower limb amputees

D. WEZENBERG[a,b,1], J.H.P. HOUDIJK[a,b], L.H.V. VAN DER WOUDE[c],
A. DE HAAN[a]

[a] *Research Institute MOVE , Faculty of Human Movement Sciences, VU University, Amsterdam, The Netherlands*
[b] *Heliomare R&D, Wijk aan Zee, The Netherlands*
[c] *Center for Human Movement Sciences,
University Medical Center Groningen, University of Groningen, Groningen, The Netherlands*

Abstract. Testing patients with a uni-lateral leg amputation using a graded one-legged peak exercise test (GOPET) poses difficulties. The smaller muscle mass results in increased intramuscular tension, thereby restricting blood flow to the active muscle. This ultimately leads to enhanced local fatigue in the active muscles. This is aggravated when vascular problems are present, such as often seen in persons who underwent amputation. This study investigated the influence of a discontinuous protocol when performing a GOPET in healthy participants. It is hypothesized that the resting phase following the exercise phase will restore blood flow, postponing local fatigue resulting in a higher measured aerobic capacity. Eight healthy participants performed three GOPET's: a continuous protocol (CON) and two discontinuous protocols in which an exercise phase of 60 (DIS60) or 90 s (DIS90) was followed by a 30 s rest period. No difference in aerobic capacity and peak heart rate were found among the three protocols. Peak workload and exercise duration were significantly higher in both discontinuous protocols compared to the continuous protocol. Subjectively, participants experienced the DIS protocols as more comfortable. A discontinuous protocol elicits similar aerobic capacities and peak heart rates, but higher peak workloads and lower discomfort, compared to a continuous protocol. Given the subjective preference, a discontinuous protocol may be advantageous over a continuous protocol, which may especially apply for patients with an amputation due to vascular problems.

Keywords. amputees, exercise testing, discontinuous, aerobic capacity.

1. Introduction

A graded peak exercise test is accepted as a useful method to determine exercise capacity and cardiac, respiratory or vascular limitations in a variety of patients. Due to a prolonged period of inactivity prior and post operation, people who underwent a lower limb amputation show a considerable decrease in aerobic capacity (VO_{2peak}). In

---

[1] Corresponding Author: D. Wezenberg, Faculty of Human Movement Sciences, VU University Amsterdam, Van der Boechorststraat 9, 1081 BT, Amsterdam, The Netherlands; E-mail: d.wezenberg@fbw.vu.nl ; www.progait.nl

addition, these people often suffer from atherosclerosis of the coronary arteries. A graded peak exercise test could evaluate these problems. Studies have postulated that a graded peak exercise test should be performed prior to start of rehabilitation, ensuring a safe and effective training program [1]. Additionally, it has been used as a predictor of prosthetic rehabilitation outcome [2,3].

If used, it is of great importance that the test performed provides valid results. Due to the lower limb amputation, patients are limited in the use of active muscle mass. Arm ergometry has often been used as the instrument of choice. However, using only the arms has shown to result in a lower VO_{2peak}, higher blood lactate concentration and higher intramuscular pressure compared to leg exercise [4]. Since cardiac problems are often present in this group of patients, it is questionable whether arm ergometry really is the best test of choice. Moreover, arm ergometry is not specific when evaluating leg tasks. A graded one-legged peak exercise test (GOPET) might be an adequate alternative, since a bigger muscle group is used thereby limiting intramuscular pressure. Moreover, it is more specific when evaluating walking performance. The influence of the high intramuscular pressure can be further reduced by allowing blood flow to the active muscle mass at regular intervals. This could be accomplished using a discontinuous exercise protocol. During the resting phase the intramuscular pressure is reduced and the circulatory system is given the time to exchange metabolites over the capillary membrane. The transport of metabolites over the cell membrane will also reduce the feeling of local fatigue.

The purpose of this research was to determine whether a discontinuous protocol has an advantage over a continuous protocol on measured VO_{2peak} while performing a GOPET.

2. Method

Eight healthy participants, two women and six men (age 29.8 years, range [19-47]) and mean BMI 23.5 range [21.1-29.8]) participated in this research. Participants visited the research lab three times. Exercise was performed on an electronically braked cycle ergometer (Lode Excalibur, Lode NV, Groningen, the Netherlands). Heart rate and respiratory gas exchange were measured (COSMED quark b^2, COSMED, Rome, Italy)

After familiarization, the starting workload and magnitude of increments were individually determined, this to ensure similar test durations between participants. Participants performed three randomly assigned GOPET's: a continuous protocol (CON) and two discontinuous protocols in which an exercise phase of 60 s (DIS60) or 90 s (DIS90) was followed by a 30 s rest period. VO_{2peak}, peak heart rate (HR_{peak}) and peak workload (W_{peak}) were determined as the highest value obtained during the last or the penultimate exercise phase. Perceived local fatigue was measured using a VAS score. Differences between obtained VO_{2peak} HR_{peak}, W_{peak} and test duration were evaluated using a repeated measurement ANOVA (SPSS 16.0). Significance was set at p<0.05.

3. Results

No differences were found in obtained VO_{2peak} (figure 1) and HR_{peak} between different protocols (p=0.205 and p=0.201, respectively). W_{peak} differed significantly between all protocols (p<0.001). Test duration differed between the CON and both discontinuous protocols (figure 1). No differences were found in perceived local fatigue at the end of exercise. When asked, participants experienced the discontinuous protocols as more comfortable.

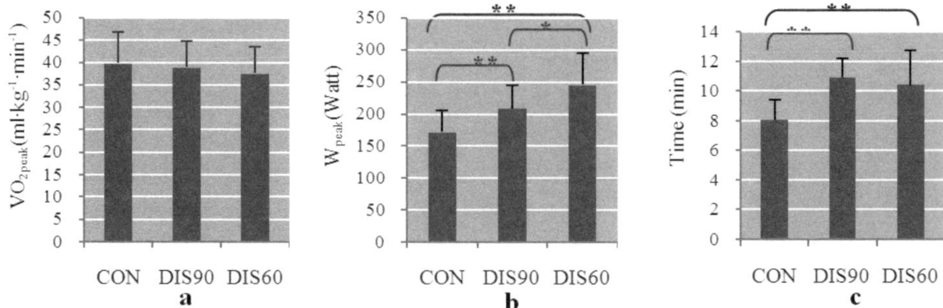

Figure 1. Mean (± standard deviation) VO_{2peak} (**a**), W_{peak} (**b**) and test duration (**c**). CON is the 2 min increment continuous protocol. DIS90 and DIS60 are the discontinuous protocols where 90 or 60 s exercise phases are followed by a 30 seconds rest, respectively. Peak values are determined as the highest value reached during the last or penultimate last exercise step. Significant differences are denoted using *($p < 0.05$) and **($p < 0.001$).

4. Conclusion

Introducing rest phases in between exercise steps elicited similar VO_{2peak} and HR_{peak} values but higher W_{peak} when performing a GOPET. Although, test duration was higher it was still within acceptable limits. Performing a GOPET using a discontinuous protocol was found to be better tolerable. This could be associated with a reduced feeling of local fatigue, owing to blood flow during the resting phases.

A discontinuous protocol may well result in higher peak values when testing patients suffering from vascular problems.

References

[1] T. Chin, Sawamura S, Fujita H, Ojima I, Oyabu H, Nagakura Y, Otsuka H, and Nakagawa A. %VO2max as an indicator of prosthetic rehabilitation outcome after dysvascular amputation. Prosthetics and Orthotics International 26 (2002), 44-49.

[2] H.E. Cruts, de Vries J, Zilvold G, Huisman K, van Alste JA, and Boom HB. Lower extremity amputees with peripheral vascular disease: graded exercise testing and results of prosthetic training. Archives of Physical Medicine and Rehabilitation 68(1987), 14-19.

[3] T. Erjavec, Presern-Strukelj M, and Burger H. The diagnostic importance of exercise testing in developing appropriate rehabilitation programmes for patients following transfemoral amputation. European Journal of Physical and Rehabilitation Medicine 44(2008), 133-139.

[4] N. Olivier, Legrand R, Rogez J, Berthoin S, Prieur F, and Weissland T. One-leg cycling versus arm cranking: which is most appropriate for physical conditioning after knee surgery? Archives of Physical Medicine and Rehabilitation 89(2008), 508-512.

Chapter 6

Everyday Physical Activity

6.1

Oral Presentations

Rehabilitation: Mobility, Exercise and Sports
L.H.V. van der Woude et al. (Eds.)
IOS Press, 2010
© 2010 The authors and IOS Press. All rights reserved.
doi:10.3233/978-1-60750-080-3-227

Activities of daily living and CHD risk factors among individuals with chronic spinal cord injury

S.P. HETZ [a,1], A.E. LATIMER[a], K.A. MARTIN GINIS[b], A.C. BUCHHOLZ[c],
SHAPE-SCI RESEARCH GROUP

[a] *School of Kinesiology and Health Studies, Queen's University, Kingston, Ontario, Canada*
[b] *Department of Kinesiology, McMaster University, Hamilton, Ontario, Canada*
[c] *Department of Family Relations and Applied Human Nutrition, University of Guelph, Guelph, Ontario, Canada*

Abstract. The purpose of the study was to evaluate the relationships between participation in activities of daily living (ADL) and coronary heart disease (CHD) risk factors in individuals with SCI. Participants completed the Physical Activity Recall Assessment for People with Spinal Cord Injury (PARA-SCI) and CHD risk factor assessment including waist circumference, total cholesterol, LDL-cholesterol (LDL), HDL-cholesterol (HDL), and triglycerides. Using generalized linear models, controlling for leisure time physical activity and covariates, increased Mobility ADL (transferring and wheeling) were associated with lower plasma total cholesterol and LDL. No other significant relationships emerged. Further investigation is needed to determine causality between Mobility ADL and CHD risk.

Keywords. activities of daily living, non-exercise physical activity, coronary heart disease risk factors, spinal cord injury, SHAPE-SCI.

1. Introduction

Although there is accumulating evidence to support the negative relationships between leisure time physical activity (LTPA) and coronary heart disease (CHD) risk, the relationships between activities of daily living (ADL; normal day-to-day fundamental tasks which are essential to every day life, such as mobility and domestic related activities) and CHD risk remain unknown. Therefore, the primary purpose of this study was to examine the relationships between ADL participation and CHD risk factors including waist circumference, total cholesterol, LDL-cholesterol (LDL), HDL-cholesterol (HDL), and triglycerides in the SCI population.

---

[1] Samuel P. Hetz, School of Kinesiology and Health Studies, Physical Education Centre, 69 Union Street, Queen's University, Kingston, ON, Canada, K7L 3N6, samuel.hetz@queensu.ca

2.   Materials and Methods

This study involved an analysis of seventy-five individuals who participated in the Study of Health and Activity in People with Spinal Cord Injury (SHAPE-SCI) [1]. A full list of measurements as well as inclusion and exclusion criteria of the SHAPE-SCI are reported elsewhere [1]. Sixty-one men and 14 women were included in the study (51% had paraplegia; M_{age} = 42.39±11.78, $M_{years\ post\ injury}$ = 14.94±10.57).

Participants completed a biometric evaluation consisting of venous blood sampling and waist circumference measurements in the individuals' home and the Physical Activity Recall Assessment for People with SCI (PARA-SCI) via the telephone. The PARA-SCI [2] is a valid and reliable self-report measure of all activities performed over a 3-day recall period. Similar to past analyses using the PARA-SCI, activities which required similar functional movements were clustered [3]. For example, wheeling and transferring were combined into the 'Mobility ADL' class. Cleaning, food preparation, laundry, and yard work were combined into the 'Domestic ADL' class. This categorization helped to increase statistical power and provide more generalizable information regarding a class of activities (e.g. mobility and domestic activities) rather than specific activities (e.g. mopping the floor).

3.   Results

Participants spent an average of 118.81±121.29 minutes per day (min/d) engaged in Total ADL (Range= 0.00min/d to 468.83min/d), 17.35±27.07 min/d engaged in Mobility ADL (Range= 0.00min/d to 160.03min/d), and 15.78±30.45 min/d engaged in Domestic ADL (Range= 0.00min/d to 150.00min/d).

The relationships between each ADL category (Total, Mobility, and Domestic) and each biometric indicator (waist circumference, total cholesterol, LDL, HDL, and triglycerides) were examined using a unique generalized linear model. An assessment of potential covariates indicated that women had higher HDL levels than men (F=12.11, df=1, p=.001), age was positively associated with waist circumferences (r=.34, p<.01), and triglycerides were positively associated with alcohol consumption (r=.40, p<.01). These associations, in addition to LTPA were controlled for in subsequent analyses. Due to three relationships being examined for each CHD risk factor, a Bonferroni correction was employed such that the p-value was set at .016. Individuals who spent more time participating in Mobility ADL had lower total cholesterol and LDL levels (B=-.005, Wald Chi-Square≥7.79, p≤.005). No other significant relationships emerged.

4.   Discussion

It has been well established that individuals with SCI spend a great deal of time participating in ADL [4]. However, there is limited evidence supporting the potential beneficial effects of ADL in decreasing the risk of CHD. The current study examined the relationships between ADL and CHD risk factors in individuals with chronic SCI.

Mobility ADL were associated with lower total cholesterol and LDL. The specific physiological mechanisms underlying the study findings are complex and poorly understood. The aerobic characteristics of Mobility ADL may have contributed to these findings. It has been suggested that aerobic activities may be more effective than resistance training at decreasing LDL and total cholesterol [5].

Although Mobility ADL were associated with lower LDL and total cholesterol, we were not able to demonstrate similar findings with the other biometric indicators. The inconsistencies between our study and previous research [6] examining the relationship between short bouts of non-exercise physical activity and CHD risk factors may be due to measurement differences (self-report vs. objective measures of physical activity) or indicative of the variation between sample populations (able bodied individuals vs. individuals with SCI). Moreover, it is quite possible that the SCI specific ADL performed by the current sample were not of adequate intensity or duration to affect certain biomarkers.

Total and Domestic ADL were unrelated to CHD risk factors. Total ADL encompasses very sedentary activity such as desk and office work. These sedentary activities likely weakened the relationships between ADL and CHD risk factors. Furthermore, it is possible that Domestic ADL are not performed for the same duration as the majority of Mobility ADL and that Mobility and Domestic ADL differ in the amount of physical exertion required to accomplish these tasks [7].

5. Conclusion

By classifying and examining SCI specific ADL, our preliminary findings suggest that increased Mobility ADL participation may be a strategy worth investigating as a means of decreasing CHD risk factors, particularly LDL and total cholesterol in individuals with SCI. The practical implications of the findings are that Mobility ADL participation should be promoted by practitioners in addition to LTPA in the SCI population. Notably, practitioners encouraging Mobility ADL participation should also remind clients of safe ADL practices in order to prevent injury.

References

[1] K.A. Martin Ginis, A.E. Latimer, A.C. Buchholz, S.R. Bray, B.C. Craven, K.C. Hayes, A.L. Hicks, M.A. McColl, K. Smith, D.L. Wolfe, Establishing evidence-based physical activity guidelines: Methods for the study of health and activity in people with spinal cord injury (SHAPE SCI), *Spinal Cord* **46** (2008), 216-221.

[2] K.A. Martin Ginis, A.E. Latimer, A.L. Hicks, B.C. Craven. Development and evaluation of an activity measure for people with spinal cord injury. *Med Sci Sports Exerc* **37** (2005), 1099–1111.

[3] S.P. Hetz, A.E. Latimer, K.A. Martin Ginis. Relationships between physical fitness and leisure time physical activity and activities of daily living in individuals with spinal cord injury. *Spinal Cord* In press (2008)

[4] A.E. Latimer, K.A. Martin Ginis, B.C. Craven, A.L. Hicks. The physical activity recall assessment for people with spinal cord injury: validity. *Med Sci Sports Exerc* **38** (2006), 208-216.

[5] J.L. Durstine, P.W. Grandjean, P.G. Davis, M.A. Ferguson, N.L. Alderson, K.D. DuBose. Blood lipid and lipoprotein adaptations to exercise: a quantitative analysis. *Sports Med* **31** (2001), 1033-1062.

[6] G.N. Healy, D.W. Dunstan, J. Salmon, E. Cerin, J.E. Shaw, P.Z. Zimmet, N. Owen. Breaks in Sedentary Time beneficial associations with metabolic risk. *Diabetes Care* **31** (2008), 661-666.

[7] T.W. Janssen, C.A. van Oers, H.E. Veeger, A.P. Hollander, L.H. van der Woude, R.H. Rozendal. Relationship between physical strain during standardized ADL tasks and physical capacity in men with spinal cord injuries. *Paraplegia* **32** (1994), 844-859.

Rehabilitation: Mobility, Exercise and Sports
L.H.V. van der Woude et al. (Eds.)
IOS Press, 2010

doi:10.3233/978-1-60750-080-3-230

Estimation of energy expenditure derived from a body-worn sensor versus indirect calorimetry in wheelchair users

R.A. TANHOFFER[a,1], A.I.P. TANHOFFER[a], K.R. PITHON[c], E.H. ESTIGONI[a],
J. RAYMOND[a] , G.M. DAVIS[a]
[a] *Faculty of Health Sciences, The University of Sydney, Australia*
[b] *University of Campinas, Brazil*

Abstract. The purpose of this study was to identify relationships between energy expenditure (EE) derived from an arm-mounted multi-sensor device versus indirect calorimetry in wheelchair users undertaking treadmill exercise. Six individuals with SCI performed two different wheelchair treadmill protocols, one at a constant grade but 6 different velocities, and the other with a constant velocity but at 6 variable grades. EE was measured concurrently from breath-by-breath measures of VO_2 and a 4-sensor arm-mounted commercial device (SenseWear). To assess internal validity of the SenseWear armband and its equations employed to transform skin temperature, GSR, heat flux and accelerometry to EE, the estimated submaximal EE and VO_2 were contrasted using each system. Across all treadmill velocity and gradient combinations (n=84), SenseWear overpredicted mean VO_2 (680±322 ml•min^{-1}) and mean EE (at 14.3±6.8 kJ•min^{-1}) when compared to calorimetry (VO_2=521±173 ml•min^{-1}; EE=11.3±3.9 kJ•min^{-1} [R^2=0.76 and R^2=0.73, respectively]). Algorithms utilised by the SenseWear armband apparently overestimated the metabolic demand of wheelchair propulsion, a finding previously demonstrated utilising other types of accelerometry that have compared able-bodied versus spinal cord injured individuals.

Keywords. spinal cord injury, energy expenditure, SenseWear armband, indirect calorimetry.

1. Introduction

Reductions in energy expenditure (EE) over time may be caused by both loss of lean tissue and physical inactivity [1]. In fact, regular participation in physical activity (PA) has the potential to increase exercise capacity and physical fitness, which can lead to numerous health benefits [2]. PA and/or EE have traditionally been studied under supervised laboratory conditions, and the quantification of EE in daily physical activities has been not well investigated. Accordingly, a better understanding of valid and reliable measures to accurately assess PA and/or EE in a SCI population may contribute to the determination of daily energy needs and exercise prescription in this population.

---

[1] Corresponding Author. Ricardo A. Tanhoffer, Rehabilitation Research Centre, Faculty of Health Sciences, The University of Sydney, Australia; Email: r.tanhoffer@usyd.edu.au

The purpose of this study was to compare direct measures of energy expenditure to those derived from a commercially-available 4-sensor arm-mounted device (SenseWear Armband) during speed- and grade-variable wheelchair propulsion.

2. Methods

Six individuals with SCI performed two different wheelchair treadmill protocols – one at a constant grade (0.5%) but 6 different velocities (1, 2, 3, 4, 5 and 6 km•h^{-1}), and the other with a constant velocity (2 km•h^{-1}) but at 6 variable grades (0.5%, 1%, 1.5%, 2%, 2.5% and 3%). EE was measured concurrently from: (i) breath-by-breath measures of oxygen uptake (VO$_2$) via indirect calorimetry (CPXD Measurement Cart; Medical Graphics Corporation, St Paul, Minnesota, USA), and, (ii) a 4-sensor arm-mounted commercial device (SenseWear Armband, BodyMedia Inc, Pittsburgh, PA, USA). Heart rate (HR) was measured continuously via 3-lead ECG. VO$_2$ and HR data were displayed in real-time on a personal computer using commercially available software. To assess the internal validity of the SenseWear Armband (SW) and its equations employed to transform skin temperature, galvanic skin response (GSR), heat flux and accelerometry into EE, estimated submaximal EE and VO$_2$ were contrasted using indirect calorimetric and SWA approaches.

3. Results

Across all treadmill velocity and gradient combinations (n=84), SWA over predicted mean VO$_2$ (680±322 ml•min^{-1}) and mean EE (at 14.3±6.8 kJ•min^{-1}) when compared to calorimetry (VO$_2$=521±173 ml•min^{-1}; EE=11.3±3.9 kJ•min^{-1} [R^2=0.76 and R^2=0.73, respectively]).

When speed- and grade- variable wheelchair propulsion tests were analysed separately, SW overestimated EE and VO$_2$. The range of over prediction varied from -6% to 41% as treadmill velocity increased and from 1% to 38% as the treadmill gradient was increased (Figure 1). However, the linear regression for the constant grade test was better for indirect calorimetry and SWA-derived EE (R^2=0.84) than for the constant speed test (R^2=0.68).

4. Discussion

SWA is a portable device that monitors different physiological responses (e.g. heat flux, skin temperature, galvanic skin response and near-body temperature) and movement (accelerometer) during physical activity or exercise [3]. Accelerometers are useful tools for PA assessments, however, upper-body movements such as cycling, swimming or wheelchair propulsion, do not seem to be adequately measured nor accurately quantified by algorithms used to effect accurate predictions of energy costs by this technique [4]. In contrast, EE can be accurately measured by indirect calorimetry, but this is cumbersome to do for free-living activities measurement. SWA is a portable device, which has good potential for the assessment of EE after SCI, but our preliminary results did not reveal a strong relationship between indirect calorimetry and SWA. Further research is needed to

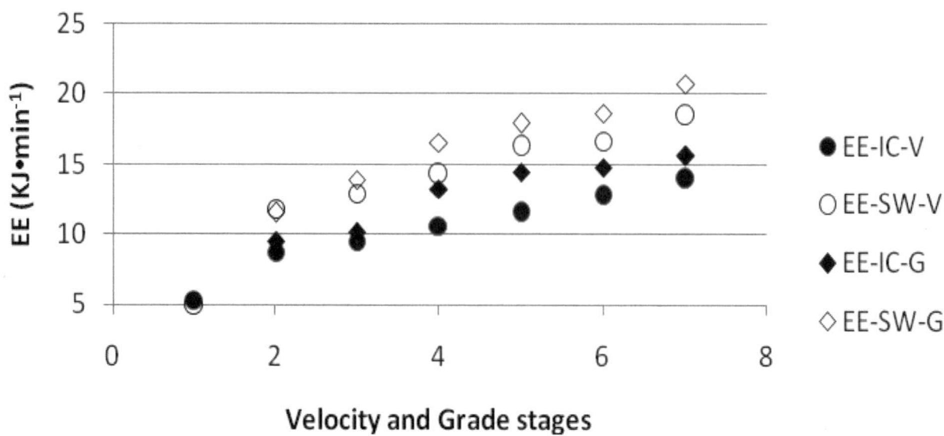

Figure 1. Energy expenditure assessed from indirect calorimetry (IC) and and SenseWear Armband (SW). Linear correlation between IC and SW for constant grade was R^2=0.84 and for constant velocity was R^2=0.68. EE-IC-V refers to energy expenditure assessed by indirect calorimetry during incremental velocity test. EE-SW-V refers to energy expenditure assessed by SenseWear Armband during incremental velocity test. EE-IC-G refers to energy expenditure assessed by indirect calorimetry during incremental grade test. EE-SW-G refers to energy expenditure assessed by SenseWear Armband during incremental grade test. Data are kJ•min^{-1}.

develop appropriate prediction equations from the physiological inputs to the SWA device in the derivation of predicted EE and VO_2 during wheelchair propulsion. Some problems to be overcome include the influence of rate coding of the accelerometers (reflecting push rim strike rate), how terrain gradient might influence energy expenditure, and key biomechanical factors such as wheelchair rolling resistance, and the variable energy costs of hand grasp versus hand strike upon the push rims.

5. Conclusion

This study revealed that an arm-mounted multi-sensor device developed for upright ambulation overestimates VO_2 and EE compared to indirect calorimetry during wheelchair propulsion. When analysed separately, SWA overestimated EE for both speed- and grade-variable treadmill tests, although the SWA was well correlated to calorimetry during constant grade variable speed wheelchair propulsion.

References

[1]   M.B. Monroe et al., Lower daily energy expenditure as measured by a respiratory chamber in subjects with spinal cord injury compared with control subjects. *American Journal of Clinical Nutrition,* **68** (1998), 1223-1227.

[2]   A.E. Latimer et al., The physical activity recall assessment for people with spinal cord injury: Validity. *Medicine and Science in Sports and Exercise,* **38** (2006), 208-216.

[3]   J.M Jakicic, et al., Evaluation of the SenseWear Pro Armband (TM) to assess energy expenditure during exercise. *Medicine and Science in Sports and Exercise,* **36** (2004), 897-904.

[4]   L. Vanhees et al., How to assess physical activity? How to assess physical fitness? European Journal of Cardiovascular Prevention & Rehabilitation, **12** (2005), 102-114.

Rehabilitation: Mobility, Exercise and Sports
L.H.V. van der Woude et al. (Eds.)
IOS Press, 2010

doi:10.3233/978-1-60750-080-3-233

Inactive lifestyle in adults with bilateral spastic cerebral palsy

C. NIEUWENHUIJSEN[a,1], W.M.A. VAN DER SLOT[a,b], M.E. ROEBROECK[a],
H.J. STAM[a], H.J.G. VAN DEN BERG-EMONS[a]
[a]*Erasmus Medical Center, Department of Rehabilitation, Rotterdam, The Netherlands*
[b]*Rijndam Rehabilitation Center, Rotterdam, The Netherlands*

Abstract. Purpose: To quantify level of everyday physical activity (PA) in adults with bilateral spastic cerebral palsy (CP), and to study associations with personal and CP-related characteristics. Methods: Fifty-six adults with bilateral spastic CP (mean age 36.4 (SD 5.8 years), 62% male) participated. About 75% had high gross motor functioning (GMFCS level I or II). Level of everyday PA was measured with an accelerometry-based Activity Monitor and was characterized by 1) duration of dynamic activities (composite measure, percentage of 24-hours; 2) intensity of activity (motility, in gravitational acceleration [g]); and 3) number of periods of continuous dynamic activity. We compared outcomes in adults with CP to able-bodied age-mates. Results: Duration of dynamic activities was 8.1(SD 3.7)% (116 minutes per day), and intensity of activity was 0.020 (SD 0.007)g; both outcomes were significantly lower compared to able-bodied age-mates. Of adults with CP, 39% had at least one period of continuous dynamic activities lasting longer than 10 minutes per day. Gross motor functioning was significantly associated with level of everyday PA (Rs: –0.34 to –0.48; $p \leq .01$). Conclusion: Adults with bilateral spastic CP, especially those with low-level gross motor functioning, are at risk for an inactive lifestyle.

Keywords. cerebral palsy, physical activity, accelerometry.

1. Introduction

Cerebral palsy (CP) is one of the most frequently occurring conditions in childhood [1] and is defined as "a group of permanent disorders of the development of movement and posture, causing activity limitation, that are attributed to non-progressive disturbances that occurred in the developing fetal or infant brain".[2]

Many adults with CP return to rehabilitation care for treatment of worsening symptoms such as contractures, pain and fatigue.[3] This deterioration over time may lead to difficulties in performing daily activities and consequently to an inactive lifestyle [4]. The limited number of studies performed on level of everyday PA in persons with CP indicate that children [5] and adolescents with certain forms of CP [6] are less physically active than able-bodied age-mates. To our knowledge, no objective data are available regarding level of everyday PA for adults with bilateral spastic CP. The aim of this study was therefore to quantify the level of everyday PA in adults with bilateral spastic cerebral palsy and to study associations with personal and CP-related characteristics.

---

[1] Corresponding Author: C. Nieuwenhuijsen. Erasmus MC, Department of Rehabilitation Medicine. P.O. Box 2040, 3000 CA Rotterdam, The Netherlands. Email: c.nieuwenhuijsen@erasmusmc.nl

2.   Methods

Study sample

We recruited eligible participants from ten rehabilitation centers throughout the western and central regions of the Netherlands and via the Association of Physically Disabled Persons and Their Parents (BOSK). From 226 eligible subjects, 56 adults agreed to participate (response rate 25%). Participant characteristics are listed in **Table 1**.

Table 1. Personal and CP-related characteristics

	Participants (n=56)	
Age in years, mean (SD)	36.4	(5.8)
Gender, n (%) male	35	(62)
Limb distribution, n (%)		
Diplegia	30	(54)
Quadriplegia	26	(46)
Gross motor functioning, n (%)*		
Level I	13	(23)
Level II	28	(50)
Level III	11	(20)
Level IV	4	(7)
Level V	0	(0)
Educational level, n (%)		
Low	15	(27)
Medium	24	(43)
High	17	(30)

* Level of gross motor functioning is classified according to the Gross Motor Functioning Classification System (GMFCS), which identifies five levels ranging from 'walks without restrictions'(level I) to 'self-mobility is severely limited even with the use of assistive technology'(level V).

Measurements

We measured level of everyday PA with an Activity Monitor (AM) (Temec Instruments BV, Kerkrade, The Netherlands), which is based on long-term ambulatory monitoring of signals from four to six body-fixed accelerometers.[8] Stationary activities such as lying and sitting can be distinguished from dynamic activities such as walking and cycling. Furthermore, the variability of the acceleration signal (motility) can be measured as an indicator of body-segment movement intensity. Participants wore the AM for 48 continuous hours on randomly selected weekdays and were instructed to perform their ordinary activities (except swimming or bathing). To avoid measurement bias, we explained the principles of the AM to the participants after the measurement. We measured the following data per 24-hour period: 1) duration of dynamic activities as a percentage of a 24-hour period (composite measure of walking, wheelchair propulsion, running, cycling, and general movement); 2) intensity of activities (mean motility (in gravitational acceleration [g])); and 3) periods with continuous dynamic activity (1 to 5 minutes and greater than 5 minutes). We compared outcomes in adults with CP with able-bodied age-mates.

3.   Level of everyday physical activity

On average, participants had a mean dynamic activity duration of 8.1 (SD 3.7)%, which corresponds to one hour and 56 minutes of dynamic activities per day (Table 2). With regard to intensity of activities, we found a mean motility of 0.020 (SD 0.007)g. Both dynamic activity duration (8.1% versus 10.9%, respectively; $p \leq .01$) and mean motility (0.020g versus 0.027g; $p \leq .01$) were significantly lower in adults with CP than in able-bodied age-mates. Participants with lower levels of gross motor functioning (GMFCS III/IV) had a lower level of everyday PA than those with better gross motor functioning (Table 2).

Table 2. Level of everyday PA, by level of gross motor functioning. Values are presented as means (SD).

		Level of gross motor functioning		
	All *(n=56)*	GMFCS I *(n=13)*	GMFCS II *(n=28)*	GMFCS III-IV *(n=15)*
Duration of dynamic activities (% of 24-h)	8.1 (3.7)	10.3 (2.6)[a]	8.3 (3.7)[c]	5.7 (3.1)
Mean motility (g)*	0.020 (0.037)	0.024 (0.006)[a]	0.020 (0.007)[c]	0.015 (0.005)
Periods of continuous dynamic activities (1-5 min)	16 (11)	21 (7)	17 (13)	12 (9)
Periods of continuous dynamic activities (> 5 min)	1 (1)	2 (2)[b]	1 (2)	1 (1)

* Mean motility was assessed for ambulators only (n=49) and is expressed in g (1 g = 9.81 m/s^2).
[a] Significant difference between GMFCS level I and GMFCS level III-IV at $p \leq .01$
[b] Significant difference between GMFCS level I and GMFCS level III-IV at $p \leq .05$
[c] Tendency for difference between GMFCS level II and GMFCS level III-IV at $p \leq .10$

4.   Conclusion

In this study, we have demonstrated that adults with bilateral spastic CP, and particularly those with low-level gross motor functioning, have inactive lifestyles when compared to able-bodied age-mates. Personal and CP-related characteristics other than gross motor functioning were not related to level of everyday PA.

References

[1]   SCPE. Surveillance of cerebral palsy in Europe: a collaboration of cerebral palsy surveys and registers. Surveillance of Cerebral Palsy in Europe (SCPE). Dev Med Child Neurol 2000; 42: 816-824.

[2]   Rosenbaum P, Paneth N, Leviton A, Goldstein M, Bax M, Damiano D, et al. A report: the definition and classification of cerebral palsy April 2006. Dev Med Child Neurol Suppl 2007; 109: 8-14.

[3]   Andersson C, Mattsson E. Adults with cerebral palsy: a survey describing problems, needs, and resources, with special emphasis on locomotion. Dev Med Child Neurol 2001; 43: 76-82.

[4]   van den Berg-Emons HJG, Bussmann JB, Meyerink HJ, Roebroeck ME, Stam HJ. Body fat, fitness and level of everyday physical activity in adolescents and young adults with meningomyelocele. J Rehabil Med 2003; 35: 271-275.

[5]   van den Berg-Emons HJ, Saris WH, de Barbanson DC, Westerterp KR, Huson A, van Baak MA. Daily physical activity of schoolchildren with spastic diplegia and of healthy control subjects. J Pediatr 1995; 127: 578-584.

[6]   Maher CA, Williams MT, Olds T, Lane AE. Physical and sedentary activity in adolescents with cerebral palsy. Dev Med Child Neurol 2007; 49: 450-457.

[7]   van der Slot WM, Roebroeck ME, Landkroon AP, Terburg M, Berg-Emons RJ, Stam HJ. Everyday physical activity and community participation of adults with hemiplegic cerebral palsy. Disabil Rehabil 2007; 29: 179-189.

[8]   Bussmann JB, Martens WL, Tulen JH, Schasfoort FC, van den Berg-Emons HJ, Stam HJ. Measuring daily behavior using ambulatory accelerometry: the Activity Monitor. Behav Res Methods Instrum Comput 2001; 33: 349-356.

6.2

Poster Presentations

Rehabilitation: Mobility, Exercise and Sports
L.H.V. van der Woude et al. (Eds.)
IOS Press, 2010

doi:10.3233/978-1-60750-080-3-239

Factors determining the self-assessed wheelchair mobility in individuals with spinal cord injury

V. ANNEKEN[a,1], T. SCHEUER[b], S. HIRSCHFELD[c], P. RICHARZ[d]

[a] *Research Institute for Disability and Sport at the German Sports University Cologne and the Lebenshilfe NRW e.V. (FiBS e.V.)*
[b] *Institute of Rehabilitation and Sport for the Disabled, German Sport University Cologne*
[c] *Spinal Cord Injury Centre of the BG Hospital Hamburg*
[d] *German Wheelchair Sports Federation*

Abstract: Purpose: Wheelchair mobility is preconditioning for wheelchair dependent individuals with SCI to participate in activities required for daily living. The focus was to identify factors which distinguish good wheelchair mobility throughout daily life. Methods: Postal, retrospective and anonymous data was collected based upon a self developed questionnaire including questions for self-assessment of wheelchair mobility, sociodemographic and lifestyle data. Inclusion criteria comprised subjects with acquired SCI, age > 16 years, complete wheelchair dependency and a lesion level lower C5. Results: 287 persons aged 17 to 74 years (Mean = 42.8) were included. Statistical analysis showed that a good self-assessed wheelchair mobility is correlated with a lower lesion level, accidental SCI, male gender and younger age. Furthermore a low or normal BMI, employment, participation in leisure activities and athleticism distinguish good wheelchair mobility. Conclusion: To improve self-determination and independence in daily living of individuals with SCI the factors which were shown to be positively correlated with increased wheelchair mobility require intensive attention in the rehabilitation process. Many of these factors are already integrated into the inpatient rehabilitation program, however, greater consideration is required in the life-long aftercare. Hence, providing a perspective and support for the vocational situation and leading to a more active lifestyle in leisure time can help prevent social isolation and health risk factors such as obesity and depression.

Keywords: wheelchair mobility, vocational situation, active lifestyle, spinal cord injury.

1. Introduction

For individuals with SCI requiring a wheelchair in everyday life the abilities of wheelchair handling decide on the degree of mobility in different environments and situations [1]. A sufficient wheelchair mobility presupposes an intensive training in the first rehabilitation phase, which trains correct wheelchair handling in daily life-relevant exercises [2]. Apart from wheelchair training the mobility of individuals with SCI is

---

[1] Dr. Volker Anneken, FIBS e.V., Römerstr. 100, 50226 Frechen, Germany, anneken@fi-bs.de

affected by several socio-demographic and personal data [3], which might provide important indicators to improve the rehabilitation process.

2. Purpose

Wheelchair mobility is preconditioning for wheelchair dependent individuals with SCI to participate in activities required for daily living. The focus was to identify factors which distinguish good wheelchair mobility throughout daily life.

3. Methods

Data collection was based on a questionnaire of 44 questions. As no suitable standardised questionnaire for the examination of self-assessed wheelchair mobility, sociodemographic data and lifestyle data for wheelchair-dependent individuals with SCI exists, all questions were specifically developed and designed for our investigation by experts from the medical, sports science and social sciences field. 11 items are related to wheelchair mobility (see table 1).

Table 1. Items of the self-assessed wheelchair mobility – The scale ranges from 0 (low mobility) to 4 (high mobility).

items	
1. forward drive, brake, curves drive	7. curb (10-15cm) backward down
2. backward drive	8. ramp (6%) forward up and down
3. overcome rough ground surface	9. ramp (20%) forward up and down
4. staicase with more than 2 steps forward down	10. get in and out of bus/tram
5. curb (10-15cm) forward up	11. use an escalator
6. curb (10-15cm) forward down	

Subjects with acquired SCI older than 16 years with a complete wheelchair dependency in everyday life and a lesion level below C5 were included. 918 patients who have been treated at the SCI Centre of the BG Trauma Hospital Hamburg between January 1997 and July 2007 (first treatments or readmissions), as well as of 445 individuals listed in the national data base of the German wheelchair sport federation (DRS e. V.) fulfilled the above mentioned criteria and were contacted via postal mail. The investigation period extended from September 2007 until January 2008.
Statistical analysis was accomplished by SPSS 17.0 containing frequencies, mean values and comparing mean values (t-test, variance analysis).

4. Results

287 persons (77% male, 23% female) aged 17 to 74 years (mean = 42.8) were included. In most cases, the subjects suffered from a complete paralysis (61.7%). In individuals with paraplegia deep lesion levels (below Th7, 56,8%) dominated in comparison to high lesion levels (Th1-Th6, 22,6%). Individuals with tetraplegia (C5-C8) amounted to 20.6% of all subjects in this study. In 78% of all cases the injury was caused by an accident (22% disease/other).

At the time of investigation, 15.8% of all subjects were employed full-time, 13.6% were part-time workers and 6.2% worked in casual position or irregularly. Overall, 60.7% were unemployed. 10 subjects were involved in a vocational rehabilitation.

The sample group had a mean self-assessed wheelchair mobility of 2.3 ($\pm$ 1.1).

Statistical analysis showed that good self-assessed wheelchair mobility is correlated with male gender, younger age, low or normal Body Mass Index (BMI) and employment. Furthermore a lower lesion level, accidental SCI, participation in leisure activities and athleticism distinguish good wheelchair mobility.

The distinction of wheelchair mobility according to kind of lesion shows that individuals with tetraplegia (N=59; 1.6 $\pm$ 0.8) exhibit an accepted significantly worse self-assessed mobility compared to subjects with paraplegia (N=228; 2.6 $\pm$ 1.0). No significant mobility differences show up between high (Th1-Th6; N=65; 2.6 $\pm$ 1.0) and lower paraplegia (below Th7; N=163; 2.5 $\pm$ 1.0).

5. Discussion and conclusion

To improve self-determination and independence in daily living of individuals with SCI the factors gender, age, BMI, employment, kind and cause of lesion, leisure activity and athleticism which were shown to be positively correlated with increased wheelchair mobility require intensive attention in the rehabilitation process. It's not possible to change factors like age, gender, kind and cause of lesion, but vocational reintegration and participation possibilities in leisure time and sports might lead to improved wheelchair mobility in individuals with SCI. Many of these factors are already integrated in the inpatient rehabilitation program, however, greater consideration is required in the life-long aftercare. Especially individuals with lower paraplegic lesion level should focus more on their wheelchair mobility improving their better functional possibilities compared to individuals with higher lesion level. Hence, providing a perspective and support for the vocational situation and leading to a more active lifestyle in leisure time can help prevent social isolation and health risk factors such as obesity and depression [4,5].

References

[1]　Donnelly C, Eng JJ, Hall J, Alford L, Giachino R, Norton K, Kerr DS, Client-centred assessment and the identification of meaningful treatment goals for individuals with a spinal cord injury, *Spinal Cord*, **42(5)** (2004), 302-307.

[2]　Kilkens OJ, Post MW, Dallmeijer AJ, van Asbeck FW, van der Woude LH, Relationship between manual wheelchair skill performance and participation of persons with spinal cord injuries 1 year after discharge from inpatient rehabilitation, *Journal of rehabilitation research and development*, **42(3 Suppl 1)** (2005a), 65-73.

[3]　Kilkens OJ, Dallmeijer AJ, Angenot E, Twisk JW, Post MW, van der Woude LH, Subject- and Injury-Related Factors Influencing the Course of Manual Wheelchair Skill Performance During Initial Inpatient Rehabilitation of Persons With Spinal Cord Injury, *Archives of Physical Medicine and Rehabilitation*, **86(11)** (2005b), 2119-2125.

[4]　Chen Y, Obesity intervention in persons with spinal cord injury, *Spinal Cord*, **44(2)** (2006), 82-91.

[5]　Jain NB, Sullivan M, Kazis LE, Tun CG, Garshick E, Factors associated with health-related quality of life in chronic spinal cord injury, *American journal of physical medicine & rehabilitation*, **86(5)** (2007), 387-396.

Rehabilitation: Mobility, Exercise and Sports
L.H.V. van der Woude et al. (Eds.)
IOS Press, 2010
© *2010 The authors and IOS Press. All rights reserved.*
doi:10.3233/978-1-60750-080-3-242

The availability of desired physical activity following spinal cord injury

R. BASSETT[a], K.M. GINIS[a], A.E. LATIMER[b], D.L. WOLFE[c]
[a]*McMaster University, Hamilton, Ontario Canada*
[b]*Queen's University, Kingston, Ontario Canada*
[c]*University of Western Ontario, London, Ontario Canada*

Abstract. Purpose: To determine the discrepancy between the types of leisure time physical activity (LTPA) people with spinal cord injury (SCI) desire and the types of LTPA available. A secondary objective was to determine the relationship between this discrepancy in desired and available LTPA and participants' thoughts and feelings towards LTPA. Methods: Questionnaires were completed during a telephone interview. People with SCI (n=259; 75% male, 63% quadriplegic) reported their current LTPA and were classified as active or inactive. The most desired LTPA and its availability was reported. Participants' thoughts and feelings toward LTPA were measured. Results: The most desired LTPA were sports and swimming. Only 54% stated their desired LTPA was available with no difference in availability between active and inactive people. This suggests it is possible to be active when ideal activities are unavailable. However, among inactive people attitudes, intentions and self-efficacy were higher among those who believed the desired LTPA was available versus those who did not (p<.05). Conclusion: Among inactive individuals, increasing LTPA availability may positively influence thoughts and feelings toward LTPA. LTPA initiatives should focus on improving the availability of desired PA such as sports and swimming. Inactive individuals with access to desired PA must be encouraged to participate.

Keywords: physical activity, spinal cord injury, theory of planned behaviour.

1. Introduction

The benefits of leisure time physical activity (LTPA) for people with spinal cord injury (SCI) are well established. LTPA offers health benefits including reduced risk of secondary complications, improved fitness, and reduced pain [1]. Despite the recognized benefits, approximately 50% of people with SCI engage in no LTPA [2].

Understanding and modifying factors that influence theory-based social cognitive predictors of LTPA [3] may improve LTPA rates in the SCI population. As such, there is a growing body of research examining predictors of LTPA among people with SCI. Still, we know little about the types of LTPA desired and the availability of these LTPA. A lack of availability of accessible LTPA may be a barrier for this population [4]. Further, access to desired LTPA may be related to predictors of LTPA such as attitudes, intentions and perceived behavioural control (PBC). According to the theory of planned behaviour (TPB; [5]), individuals may have more favourable attitudes toward LTPA if they believe LTPA will be enjoyable or valuable. Likewise, the availability of LTPA could influence individuals' PBC for LTPA. Understanding

LTPA desirability and availability in relation to social cognitions may aid in developing theory-based interventions.

The current research aimed to determine: (1) What is the discrepancy between desired and available LTPA? (2) Is the discrepancy related to (a) TPB-based predictors of LTPA, and (b) LTPA? It was hypothesized that: (1) A discrepancy would exist between desired and available LTPA such that many desired LTPA would be unavailable, (2) individuals who reported their desired LTPA to be available would have more favourable cognitions toward LTPA and (3) would engage in greater LTPA vs. those who did not.

2. Method

Participants

Participants (*M* age = 46 ± 12) were 194 men and 65 women with SCI. The sample was 63% people with tetraplegia and 37% people with paraplegia. Participants were recruited from a larger study of health and LTPA among people with SCI (i.e., SHAPESCI; [6]).

Measures

LTPA was measured using a 3-day physical activity recall for people with SCI (i.e., PARA-SCI; [7]). Participants were classified as *active* or *inactive* based on their self-reported LTPA. Desired LTPA was measured by participants reporting LTPA that they would like to, but do not currently, participate in. Next, participants reported if the desired LTPA was available in their community. Finally, selected TPB-based social cognitive predictors of LTPA (i.e., attitudes, intentions and PBC) were measured.

3. Results

Sixty-seven percent of participants were *inactive* and 33% *active*. Wheelchair sports (29%), swimming (18%), and cardiovascular training activities (17%; e.g., arm ergometery, aerobics) were most desired. Only 54% of the participants stated their desired LTPA was available. Since mean scores for the social cognitive predictors of LTPA differed between *active* and *inactive* individuals (*p* <.05), separate ANOVAs were conducted on each group to examine these constructs as a function of LTPA availability. For *active* individuals, there were no significant differences in attitudes, intentions, PBC, or LTPA between those who stated their desired LTPA was available vs. unavailable. Among *inactive* individuals, attitudes (p<.10), intentions (p<.05) and PBC (p<.05) were higher among individuals who reported their desired LTPA was available compared to those who did not.

4. Discussion

Sports, swimming and cardiovascular LTPA were most desired. Yet only 54% of the sample stated that their desired LTPA was available. Clearly, many desired LTPA are not available to individuals with SCI.

Among *inactive* individuals only, LTPA availability was related to social cognitive predictors of LTPA. In particular, *inactive* participants who believed their desired LTPA were available had more favourable LTPA attitudes, intentions and PBC than those who did not. These findings are consistent with the tenets of the TPB [5]. A lack of available desirable LTPA may be demotivating for individuals who are not currently active. For example, if a person believes that the only accessible LTPA options are not particularly desirable, these beliefs could in turn prompt negative attitudes towards LTPA and poor intentions to engage in LTPA [5]. Further, PBC for engaging in LTPA may be lacking among *inactive* individuals who believe that desirable LTPA are unavailable. Improved availability of desired LTPA could improve social cognitions regarding LTPA among *inactive* individuals with SCI. Alternatively, when desired LTPA cannot be made readily available, extra effort may be required to improve social cognitions that predict LTPA for *inactive* people with SCI (e.g., interventions to change attitudes towards available LTPA).

There was no relationship between LTPA availability and TPB predictors of LTPA among *active* individuals. These individuals reported desirable LTPA that they would like to do *in addition* to current LTPA. As such, their LTPA attitudes, intentions, and PBC were probably based on beliefs associated with LTPA that they could do, rather than unavailable LTPA. LTPA did not vary between those who reported their desired LTPA to be available vs. unavailable suggesting that LTPA is possible when ideal activities are unavailable.

One limitation of the current study was the subjective and self-report nature of LTPA and LTPA availability. Future research should examine the relationship between actual availability of LTPA, and objective measures of LTPA. Nevertheless, the results of the current study suggest that availability of desired LTPA is an important predictor of attitudes, intentions and PBC for LTPA among *inactive* individuals with SCI.

References

[1]   K.A Martin Ginis & A. L Hicks. Considerations for the development of a physical activity guide for Canadians with physical disabilities. *Applied Physiology, Nutrition and Metabolism,* **32** (2007), S135-S147.

[2]   T. Tasiemski, E. Bergstrom, G. Savic, & B. P. Gardner. Sports, recreation and employment following spinal cord injury - a pilot study. *Spinal Cord,* **38**, (2000), 173-184.

[3]   L. R. Brawley. The practicality of using social psychological theories for exercise and health research and intervention. *Journal of Applied Sport Psychology,* **5**, (1993), 99-115.

[4]   J. H. Rimmer, B. Riley, E. Wang, A. Rauworth, & J. Jurkowsi. Physical activity participation among persons with disabilities: barriers and facilitators. *Am. J.Prev. Med.* **26,** (2004), 419-425.

[5]   Azjen From intentions to action: A theory of planned behavior. In J. Kuhl & J. Beckmann (Eds.), *Action- control: From cognition to behavior* (pp. 11–39). New York: Springer. 1985.

[6]   K. A. Martin Ginis, A. E. Latimer, A. C. Buchholz, S. R. Bray, B. C. Craven, K. C. Hayes, et al. Establishing evidence-based physical activity guidelines: methods for the study of health and activity in people with spinal cord injury. *Spinal Cord,* **46**, (2008), 216-221.

[7]   K. A. Martin Ginis, A. E. Latimer, A. L. Hicks, & B. C. Craven. Development and evaluation of an activity measure for people with spinal cord injury. *Medicine and Science in Sports and Exercise,* **37,** (2005), 1099- 1111.

Rehabilitation: Mobility, Exercise and Sports
L.H.V. van der Woude et al. (Eds.)
IOS Press, 2010

doi:10.3233/978-1-60750-080-3-245

245

Validity of an activity questionnaire in persons with a physical disability

A.A.M.H.J. L'ORTYE[a,b], H.J.G. VAN DEN BERG-EMONS[a], L.M. BUFFART[a], C. NIEUWENHUIJSEN[a], M.P. BERGEN[b], H.J. STAM[a], J.B.J. BUSSMANN[a]

[a] *Department of Rehabilitation Medicine, Erasmus Medical Center, Rotterdam, The Netherlands*
[b] *Rijndam Rehabilitation Center, Rotterdam, the Netherlands*

Abstract. Purpose: To determine the criterion validity of the Physical Activity Scale for Individuals with Physical Disabilities (PASIPD) to assess the level of everyday physical activity (PA) in persons with a physical disability. Methods: In a total of 124 ambulatory and non-ambulatory subjects with cerebral palsy, meningomyelocele or spinal cord injury, we assessed level of everyday PA using the PASIPD, a recall questionnaire, and using an accelerometry-based activity monitor (AM), which served as reference method. Results: Significant (p $\leq$ 0.05) spearman correlation coefficients between the outcome parameters of the PASIPD and AM ranged between 0.22 and 0.37. The PASIPD significantly (p<0.0001) overestimated the duration of PA (3.9 (2.9) versus 1.48 (0.90) hours per day by AM). There was a significant correlation (spearman's rho -0.74, p<0.0001) between the level of everyday PA and the discrepancy between the methods, indicating higher overestimation with increasing level of everyday PA. Conclusion: The PASIPD is poorly correlated with objective PA measurements using the AM in people with a physical disability. Although similar low correlations between objective and subjective PA measurements have been found in the general population, users of the PASIPD should be cautious for overestimating physical activity levels.

Keywords. questionnaire, accelerometry, cerebral palsy, meningomyelocele, spinal cord injury.

1. Introduction

Persons with a physical disability are often restricted in their performance of everyday physical activities and are more at risk for developing hypoactive lifestyles compared to the general population. Previous research has focused on measurement instruments to assess everyday physical activity in persons with a physical disability. For example, an activity monitor (AM) with body-fixed accelerometers has been used to assess body postures and physical activities in persons with bilateral spastic cerebral palsy (CP), meningomyelocele (MMC) and spinal cord injury (SCI). These studies demonstrated subnormal everyday physical activity levels [1-3]. Although an AM provides objective, detailed, and valid data on everyday physical activity for ambulatory and wheelchair-dependent persons [4], measurements are time-consuming and relatively expensive. Therefore, the AM is less useful in large population studies and alternatives are needed.

The Physical Activity Scale for Individuals with Physical Disabilities (PASIPD) is a seven-day physical activity recall questionnaire designed to evaluate physical activity levels in persons with physical disabilities [5]. Overall, little is known about the validity of the PASIPD because few studies have been performed, and external criteria validity is questionable. The aim of our study, therefore, was to determine the criterion validity of the PASIPD to assess everyday physical activity levels in a large group of persons with a physical disability, including wheelchair-dependent persons. As external criterion, we used the extensively validated AM.

2. Methods

We studied 124 participants, including 51 (41%) who were wheelchair-dependent. The subjects were aged 13 to 65 years, and each had a diagnosis of spastic bilateral CP (n=56), MMC (n=47) or SCI (n=21). The subjects were identified from three studies focusing on everyday physical activity level and physical fitness conducted at the Department of Rehabilitation, Erasmus Medical Center or Rijndam Rehabilitation Center (both in Rotterdam, The Netherlands).

Instruments: The PASIPD [5] is a 13-item, seven-day recall questionnaire, that solicits information about: leisure activities performed for purposes other than exercise (including walking and wheeling outside the home); light, moderate and strenuous sports and recreation; exercise to increase muscle strength and endurance; light and heavy household activity; home repair; lawn work; outdoor gardening; caring for another person; and occupational activity. We used the Dutch version of the PASIPD, which integrates lawn work and outdoor gardening into one item about gardening. For the external criterion, we used an AM, an instrument that uses long-term (greater than 24 hours) ambulatory accelerometry to measure body postures and physical activities [4]. For the measurement, a small portable data recorder is worn on a belt around the waist and connected to four accelerometers that are fixed at the upper legs and trunk. In wheelchair-dependent subjects, an additional sensor is attached to each wrist. Each participant wore the AM for 48 hours (on two randomly selected, consecutive weekdays) under their normal living conditions.

3. Analysis

We calculated total PASIPD scores according to the method of Washburn et al. [5]. This method multiplies the metabolic equivalent (MET) value for each activity by the average number of hours per day spent on each activity, then sums all activities. We report this total PASIPD score as *PASIPD intensity* (in MET-hrs/day). In addition, we summed the average activity durations, without multiplying by MET values, and report this as the *PASIPD duration* (in hrs/day).

We chose two AM measures that best reflect the outcome measures of the PASIPD. One outcome measure was *AM duration*, in hours per day, that subjects performed physical activities. *AM duration* was a composite measure of walking (including walking stairs and running), cycling, driving a wheelchair, (including hand-biking) and general non-cyclic movement. The second outcome measure, *AM intensity*, was calculated as mean body motility over a 24-hour period (in gravitational acceleration [g], 1 g = 9.81 m/s^2), representing intensity of everyday physical activity.

We calculated Spearman correlation coefficients between outcome measures of the PASIPD and the AM. In addition, we compared the average number of hours per day that physical activities were performed as measured by the PASIPD (*PASIPD duration*), to the average number of hours as measured by the AM (*AM duration*). We also calculated the relationship (Spearman correlation) between the number of hours per day spent on physical activities (assessed as the average of the *PASIPD duration* and *AM duration*) and the difference in number of hours between methods.

4. Results

Significant (p≤0.05) spearman correlation coefficients between the outcome parameters of the PASIPD and AM ranged between 0.22 and 0.37. The PASIPD significantly (p<0.0001) overestimated the duration of PA (3.9 (2.9) versus 1.48 (0.90) hours per day by AM). There was a significant correlation (spearman's rho -0.74, p<0.0001) between the level of everyday PA and the discrepancy between the methods, indicating higher overestimation with increasing level of everyday PA (Figure 1).

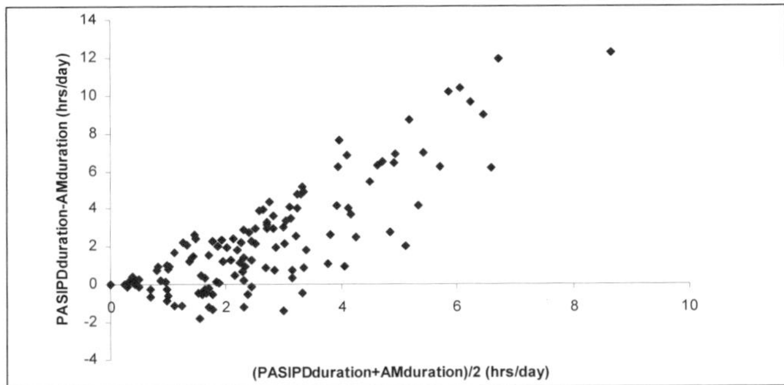

Figure 1. Bland-Altman plot comparing the average number of hours per day of physical activity, as assessed by PASIPD (*PASIPD duration*) and the Activity Monitor (*AM duration*) (x-axis), to the difference between both methods (y-axis)

5. Conclusion

The PASIPD is poorly correlated with objective PA measurements using the AM in people with a physical disability. Although similar low correlations between objective and subjective PA measurements have been found in the general population, users of the PASIPD should be cautious for overestimating physical activity levels. The PASIPD may be useful in assessing the contribution of specific activity domains (such as sports, household or work-related activities), to total physical activity. The PASIPD may also be useful in measuring perceived physical activity.

References

[1]   van den Berg-Emons RJ, Bussmann JB, Haisma JA, Sluis TA, van der Woude LH, Bergen MP, Stam HJ. Prospective study on physical activity levels after spinal cord injury during inpatient rehabilitation and the year after discharge. Arch Phys Med Rehabil 2008;89:2094-2101.

[2]   Buffart LM, Roebroeck ME, Rol M, Stam HJ, van den Berg-Emons RJ. Triad of physical activity, aerobic fitness and obesity in adolescents and young adults with myelomeningocele. J Rehab Med 2008;40(1):70-75.

[3]   Nieuwenhuijsen C, van der Slot WM, Beelen A, Arendzen JH, Roebroeck ME, Stam HJ, van den Berg-Emons HJ & the Transition Research Group South-West Netherlands. Inactive lifestyle in adults with bilateral spastic cerebral palsy. J Rehabil Med [in press].

[4]   Bussmann JB, Martens WL, Tulen JH, Schasfoort FC, Berg-Emons van den HJ, Stam HJ. Measuring daily behavior using ambulatory accelerometry: the activity monitor. *Behav* Res Methods Instrum Comput. 2001;33(3):349-356.

[5]   Washburn RA, Zhu W, McAuley E, Frogley M, Figoni SF. The physical activity scale for individuals with physical disabilities: development and evaluation. Arch Phys Med Rehabil. 2002;83(2):193-200.

Rehabilitation: Mobility, Exercise and Sports
L.H.V. van der Woude et al. (Eds.)
IOS Press, 2010

doi:10.3233/978-1-60750-080-3-248

Implementation of a physical activity programme for cancer patients

E. CANONNE[a], J. BONNETERRE[b], V. WIECZOREK[a], A. THEVENON[a]
[a]*Lille Université Club, Lille, France*
[b]*Centre Oscar Lambret, 3 Rue Frédéric Combemale, F-59020 Lille Cedex, France*

Abstract. We present a collaboration between the Regional Cancer Centre and a sports club for providing a specific physical activity programme for cancer patients during and after therapy. A promotional brochure was created in order to advertise the programme and inform patients of the value of physical activity, which reduces the side effects of cancer therapies, improves the quality of vie and may prolong life expectancy. To date, the programme has attracted 15 participants.

Keywords. cancer, adapted physical activity, health.

Physical activity is beneficial for cancer patients, both during and after therapy [1,2]. During the acute treatment phase (chemotherapy and radiotherapy), physical activity helps improve quality of life on the physical, psychological and social levels. In fact, greater muscle strength leads to better functional capacity and facilitates the activities of daily living. Physical activity also decreases chronic fatigue [1,3] and improves sleep quality. After the acute treatment phase [2], physical activity results in better physical fitness, which influences chronic fatigue and favours social and professional reinsertion. Physical activity decreases the risk of comorbidities and cardiovascular diseases and has a preventive effect on cardiovascular risk factors: diabetes, arterial hypertension, dyslipidaemia and osteoporosis - all diseases that cancer patients are more likely to develop. Very few studies have looked at this matter with respect to the progression of cancer. Hence, the sole objective is to improve quality of life and the well-being via specialized care according to the individual's needs and abilities. There may also be a decrease in the risk of relapse (between 26% and 40%) for breast cancer and colon cancer, although there are not enough data at present to confirm this unambiguously. Physical activity may decrease the risk of a second cancer (only those for which physical activity is preventive).

In conclusion, physical activity is beneficial in cancer patients at all stages of the disease. This observation prompted us to develop a physical activity program for cancer patients in northern France in collaboration with the "Lille Université Club" multisports club.

1. The "Physical Activity and Cancer" project: (methods)

Initiation

The Lille Regional Cancer Centre and the Lille Université sports club have set up a collaborative "Physical Activity and Cancer" project, aimed at getting participants back into shape after cancer therapy, rebuilding self-confidence and increasing "socialisation" via the performance of physical activity in a club setting. The goal is also to encourage participants to continue a sports activity when they feel able stop attending the special sessions.

Implementation of the project required funding and equipment. The latter was provided by Lille Université Club, with a hall and additional equipment (steps, mats, "Swiss ball" exercise balls, an instructor, etc.). In terms of funding, grant applications were submitted to the Regional Public Health Programme and the Nord Pas de Calais Regional Council.

So that cancer patients would hear about the project, a promotional campaign was initiated. It was centred on a brochure that summarized the benefits of physical activity, the cost of the training sessions, where the sessions were to take place and the contact person for registration. The brochure was circulated to patients by physicians: Professor Bonneterre at the Oscar Lambret Cancer Centre (coordinator of the cluster cancer) and Professor Triboulet at Lille University Hospital (cancer federation). The project also linked up with the Northern France Cancer League, which handled the provision of information to patient associations and publication of the brochure so that it could be circulated in northern France. In addition, the League subsided part of the programme cost for participants.

The activity started in March 2008.

Project content

The project consists of the implementation of a suitable physical activity programme for people with or having had cancer, regardless of their age or gender. The physical activity sessions were performed individually in a group setting, that is to say that the exercises were adapted to suit each participant but sessions were performed as part of a group. The 60-minute sessions were supervised by a specialist adapted physical education teacher. Each session comprised a warm-up phase, a physical conditioning phase, a "discovery" phase (step, dance, tai chi, etc.) and a relaxation/stretching phase.

So that the activity was appropriate for each participant, a sport physician performed an individual medical check-up before the first session in order to review the person's medical history and any contraindications. The check-up featured a 6-minute gait test, an electrocardiogram and (for breast cancer patients) arm measurements checking for lymphoedema. The participant also had to fill out the SF36 quality of life questionnaire, the Piper fatigue scale and the Hospital Anxiety and Depression scale. A report on indications for physical activity was sent to the programme teacher, who then designed sessions with individually appropriate muscle exercises. In order to monitor the participants' progress, the check-up was scheduled every 6 months.

2. The participants: (results)

Fifteen people participated in the programme (13 women and 2 men). Three were on chemotherapy, one was receiving radiotherapy and 11 were in remission from cancer. Other than 2 women with uterine cancer, all the female participants had breast cancer. Two of the breast cancer patients had lymphoedema of the arms. One of the men had mantle cell lymphoma and the other had pancreatic cancer. The mean age was 54±12.

On average, participants attended 80% of the sessions. Two participants had to stop for 6 weeks due to chemotherapy (in a breast cancer patient) and a hernia operation (in a pancreatic cancer patient). One of the participants is a member of a rambling club.

Four patients were referred by their oncologist, 6 were referred by patient associations and 5 learned about the programme through brochures at pharmacies and the town hall.

Table 1. Muscle status and change over the duration of 3-month programme (percentage increase).

	Endurance (abdominal muscles)	Endurance (quadriceps)	Finger-floor distance	Lumbar crunches	Trunk exercise on both elbows
Mean	+ 15%	+24%	+88%	+67%	+90%

3. Conclusion

In terms of the promotional campaign, participant recruitment should have involved the medical profession and patient associations to a greater extent. The project is going to be extending to the city of Lens in the Pas de Calais county. Children and adolescents suffering from cancer will also be able to benefit from a physical activity programme with a specific promotional approach.

References

[1]   B. Hoerni, G. Kantor, A. Mortureux, (2005). Cancérologie et hémopathies. Masson
[2]   Collen Doyle, Lawrence H. Kushi, Tim Byers, Kerry S. Courneya, American cancer society. "Nutrition and physical activity during and after cancer treatment: an American cancer society guide for informed choices", *A cancer Journal for Clinician* **56** (2006), 323-353.
[3]   Labourey. (2007) « Place de l'activité physique dans la prise en charge de la fatigue cancéreuse induite par les traitements oncologiques. » Annales de réadaptation et de médecine physique 50. 445-449.

Rehabilitation: Mobility, Exercise and Sports
L.H.V. van der Woude et al. (Eds.)
IOS Press, 2010

doi:10.3233/978-1-60750-080-3-251

251

Using SenseWear® armband to evaluate energy expenditure in manual wheelchair users with SCI

D. DING[1], S. HIREMATH, A. KELLEHER, R. COOPER
Dept. of Rehabilitation Science and Technology, University of Pittsburgh
Human Engineering Research Laboratories, VA Pittsburgh Healthcare System
Pittsburgh, PA, USA

Abstract. Accelerometry-based devices have been studied in measuring activities and predicting energy expenditure (EE) for ambulatory populations. The purpose of the study is to examine the validity of SenseWear® Armband (SenseWear), a multi-sensor activity monitor, in assessing EE in manual wheelchair (MWC) users. This paper presents the preliminary data obtained from five subjects (n=5) with spinal cord injury (SCI) performing wheelchair propulsion, arm-ergometer exercise, and deskwork. Wheelchair propulsion and arm-ergometer exercise involved three trials at different intensities. The EE estimated from the SenseWear was compared with the EE measured from a metabolic cart, used as the criterion measure. It was found that the SenseWear was relatively accurate when estimating EE for resting, but overestimated EE for wheelchair propulsion (+87.48%, +47.14%, and +124.77%), arm-ergometer exercise (+57.64%, +30.50%, and +42.94%) and deskwork (+10.12%). In future raw data and extracted features from multiple sensors of the SenseWear will be utilized to model EE for MWC users with SCI.

Keywords: energy expenditure, spinal cord injury, activity monitor

1. Introduction

In the recent times, there has been a growing interest in the assessment of physical activity and energy expenditure (EE, kilocalories expended) using various activity monitors ranging from pedometers to multi-sensor based monitors. Accelerometry-based devices have been studied in measuring activities and predicting EE for ambulatory populations [1-3]. Researchers have assessed the validity of a uniaxial accelerometer worn on the wrists as a measure of EE during wheelchair propulsion at three different speeds and found significant associations between the accelerometer readings from both wrists and EE over the three pushing speeds [4]. Warms and Belza assessed the suitability and validity of a uniaxial accelerometer and found that Pearson correlation coefficients between the activity counts and self-reported activity intensity varied from .30 to .77 for wheelchairs users with SCI [5]. The purpose of this study is to examine the validity of the SenseWear® Armband, a multi-sensor monitor, in assessing EE in manual wheelchair (MWC) users with spinal cord injury (SCI). This paper describes the preliminary data obtained from five subjects (n=5) performing wheelchair propulsion, arm-ergometer exercise and deskwork.

---

[1] Corresponding Author.

2.   Methods

Participants

The study was approved by the Institutional Review Board at the University of Pittsburgh and the VA Pittsburgh Healthcare System. Subjects were recruited based on the inclusion criteria that they were between 18 and 60 years of age, MWC users, have a SCI of T1 or below and are at least six months post-injury. Subjects were asked to obtain a physician release form before participating in the study. The subjects were consented on their arrival, following which they participated in resting and three activity sessions including wheelchair propulsion, arm-ergometer exercise, and desk work. The activity sessions were counterbalanced and the trials in the activity session were randomized to counter order effects. Subjects wore a SenseWear on the upper right arm and a portable metabolic cart while performing the activities. The subjects performed each activity trial for a maximum period of eight minutes and rested between each trial and activity sessions. In the wheelchair propulsion activity the subject's wheelchair was restrained on a stationary dynamometer with a speed feedback display in front. The subjects propelled their wheelchair for two trials of 2 miles per hour (mph) (2mph Dyno) and 3 mph (3mph Dyno), respectively. In the third trial, the subjects propelled their wheelchair at 3 mph on a tiled floor (3mph on tile). The arm-ergometer exercise included three trials of 20 watts (W) resistance at 60 rpm (20W at 60rpm), 40W resistance at 60 rpm (40W at 60 rpm) and 40W resistance at 90 rpm (40W at 90rpm), respectively. The desk work involved the subjects to use a computer and read a book retrieved from a shelf for four minutes each.

Data Collection

The SenseWear and metabolic cart were synchronized before use. The data collected from the metabolic cart included volume of oxygen consumed in mL/kg, EE in kcal per minute, and heart rate data at each breath. The data collected from the SenseWear included average transverse and longitudinal accelerations, EE in kcal per min, heat flux, galvanic skin response and skin temperatures sampled every minute.

Data Analysis

The energy costs in kcal/min from the SenseWear were compared with those obtained from the metabolic cart obtained after the response stabilized. The percent difference ($\Delta EE\%$) between the EE measured (EE_{MET}), using the metabolic cart, and the EE estimated (EE_{SW}), by the SenseWear, was obtained by the following equation.

$$\Delta EE\% = \frac{EE_{SW} - EE_{MET}}{EE_{MET}} * 100$$

3.   Results

Participants were five Caucasian men with a mean (SD) age of 41.8 (12.23) years, weight of 87.8 (17.34) kg, height of 184.36 (10.20) cm, and body mass index of 25.73 (4.10) kg/m^2. The mean (SD) EE measured using a metabolic cart for each activity is shown in Table 1. The SenseWear underestimated EE (Figure 1) for resting (-0.49%), overestimated EE for wheelchair propulsion (+87.48%, +47.14%, and +124.77%), arm-ergometer exercise (+57.64%, +30.50% and +42.94%) and deskwork (10.12%).

Table 1. EE measured using metabolic cart per each activity.

Activity	Trial	Mean in kcal/min	SD in Kcal/min
Resting	Resting	1.58	0.33
Wheelchair propulsion	2mph on Dynamometer	4.99	1.73
	3mph on Dynamometer	6.32	2.36
	3mph on Tile surface	3.26	1.05
Arm-ergometer exercise	20W at 60 rpm	3.6	0.51
	40W at 60 rpm	4.48	0.45
	40W at 90 rpm	5.79	0.68
Deskwork	Deskwork	1.61	0.19

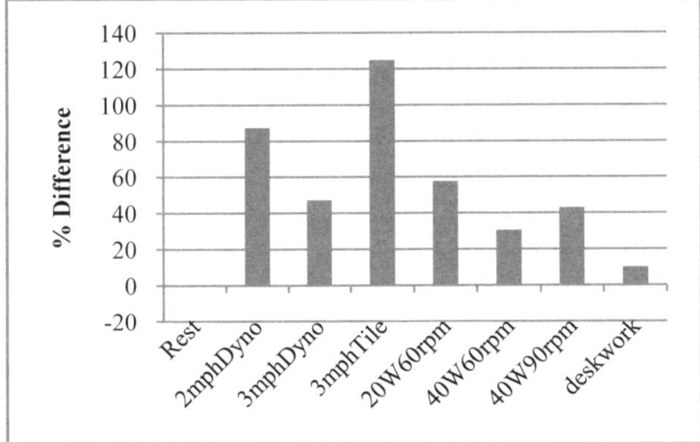

Figure 1: The plot of %EE predicted by SenseWear with respect to the EE measured versus activity.

4. Conclusion

Our preliminary analysis has shown that SenseWear was able to predict the resting EE very closely (0.49%) to criterion measure by the metabolic cart. However, it significantly overestimated the EE in other activity trials, especially for the overground wheelchair propulsion. We are in the process of recruiting more subjects and will develop an EE model based on multi-sensor data available in SenseWear to provide an effective tool for MWC users with SCI to gauge their physical activity and energy expenditure in free living conditions.

References

[1]   Chen KY, Sun M. Improving EE estimation by using a triaxial accelerometer. *Journal of Applied Physiology.* 83 (1997) 2112-2122.

[2]   Choi JH, Lee J, Hwang HT, Kim JP. Estimation of Activity EE: Accelerometer Approach. 2005 IEEE Engineering in Medicine and Biology Conference; (2005) 3830-3833.

[3]   Hendelman D, Miller K, Baggett C, Debold E, Freedson P. Validity of accelerometry for the assessment of moderate intensity physical activity in the field. Medcine & Science in Sports & Exercise. (2000) 442-449.

[4]   Washburn RA, Copay AG. Assessing physical activity during wheelchair pushing: validity of a portable accelerometer. Adapted Physical Activity Quarterly. 16(3) (1999) 290-299.

[5]   Warms CA, Belza BL. Actigraphy as a measure of physical activity for wheelchair users with spinal cord injury. Nursing Research. 53(2) (2006) 136-143.

Rehabilitation: Mobility, Exercise and Sports
L.H.V. van der Woude et al. (Eds.)
IOS Press, 2010
© 2010 The authors and IOS Press. All rights reserved.
doi:10.3233/978-1-60750-080-3-254

The physical activity scale for individuals with physical disabilities: limited validity in people with spinal cord injury

S. DE GROOT[a,b,1], M.W.M. POST[c], C.A.J. SMIT [a], L.H.V. VAN DER WOUDE[b]
[a] *Rehabilitation Center Amsterdam*
[b] *Centre for Human Movement Sciences, University Medical Centre Groningen,*
University of Groningen
[c]*Rehabilitation Center De Hoogstraat and Rudolf Magnus Institute for Neuroscience,*
Utrecht

Abstract. The purpose of this study was to determine the construct and divergent validity of the Physical Activity Scale for Individuals with Physical Disabilities (PASIPD) in people with spinal cord injury (SCI). The construct validity was examined by relationships between PASIPD and measures of fitness (peak oxygen uptake, peak power output, muscular strength) and activities (wheelchair skills, Utrecht Activity List, mobility range and social behaviour subscales of the SIP68) in 139 persons with SCI 1 year after discharge from inpatient rehabilitation. Divergent validity was determined by comparing PASIPD scores of people with different personal (age, gender, body mass index) and lesion characteristics (paraplegia/tetraplegia, completeness, time since injury). PASIPD scores showed low correlations with fitness parameters (0.25-0.36, p<0.05) and low to moderate correlations with activities (0.36-0.51, p<0.01). Persons with a tetraplegia or longer time since injury had significantly lower PASIPD scores compared to those with a paraplegia (p<0.02; effect size: 0.17) or those with a short time since injury (p<0.03; effect size: 0.30). It can be concluded that the PASIPD showed weak to moderate relationships with fitness and activity parameters. This construct validity is comparable to self-report questionnaires from the general population. The divergent validity of the PASIPD was low. Therefore, the PASIPD should be used with caution in persons with SCI.

Keywords. spinal cord injuries, exercise, leisure activities, validation study.

1. Introduction

Being physically active and fit appears to be associated with several health benefits in persons with spinal cord injury (SCI). Therefore, it is important to promote a physical active lifestyle in people with SCI to prevent secondary complications such as cardiovascular disease [1], pain, fatigue and depression [2]. To determine the level of active lifestyle, a reliable and valid measure of physical activity for people with SCI is necessary.

The Physical Activity Scale for Individuals with Physical Disabilities (PASIPD) was developed to assess the physical activity level of individuals with a disability [3]. The purpose of the present study is to determine the construct and divergent validity of the PASIPD in people with SCI.

---

[1] Corresponding Author: Sonja de Groot; s.d.groot@rcamsterdam.nl

2. Methods

Participants

The study was part of the Dutch Research Project 'Physical Strain, Work Capacity, and Mechanisms of Restoration of Mobility in the Rehabilitation of Persons with a Spinal Cord Injury'[2]. 139 Persons with SCI 1 year after discharge from inpatient rehabilitation participated.

Variables

The following variables were measured:
- Main outcome variable: The PASIPD was filled out to obtain a total physical activity score, according to Washburn et al. [3].
- Construct validity variables: Physical capacity was determined by the peak oxygen consumption, peak power output, and muscle strength. Activity measures were determined by the wheelchair skills performance time and ability score, the Utrecht Activity List and the subscales Mobility Range and Social Behavior of the SIP68.
- Divergent validity variables: Personal (age, gender, body mass index (BMI)) and lesion (level, completeness, time since injury (TSI)) characteristics.

Statistics

Construct validity was determined with a Spearman correlation coefficient between the PASIPD and physical capacity and activity measures. To determine the divergent validity, PASIPD scores of people with different personal and lesion characteristics were compared with a Mann-Whitney test (p<0.05).

3. Results

Construct validity

PASIPD scores showed low correlations with physical capacity (0.25-0.36, P<0.05) and low to moderate correlations with activities (0.36-0.51, p<0.01).

Divergent validity

Persons with a tetraplegia or long time since injury had a significantly lower PASIPD score compared to those with paraplegia (p=0.02) or a shorter time since injury (p=0.03) (Table 1).

---

[2] www.scionn.nl

Table 1. Mean (M) and standard deviations (S) of the PASIPD scores of people with different personal and lesion characteristics. * = significant difference at $p<0.05$.

	Age (years)		Gender		BMI (kg/m^2)		Lesion level*		Completeness		TSI (days)*	
	≤40.8	*>40.8*	*Men*	*Women*	*≤24.7*	*>24.7*	*Tetra*	*Para*	*Compl*	*Incompl*	*≤672*	*>672*
M	21.1	15.0	17.7	18.1	18.6	17.2	15.7	18.9	18.0	18.7	20.7	15.1
S	20.9	15.8	18.9	18.0	19.2	18.5	21.0	17.6	18.2	20.9	19.3	17.5

4. Conclusion

The PASIPD showed a weak relationship with fitness measures and a moderate relationship with activity parameters in people with SCI. This construct validity is comparable to well established self-report questionnaires of physical activity for the general population. The divergent validity of the PASIPD was low. Therefore, the PASIPD should be used with caution in persons with SCI. Other measures for physical activity in SCI should be considered.

References

[1]   Wartburton D et al., Cardiovascular Health and Exercise Rehabilitation in Spinal Cord Injury. *Top Spinal Cord Inj Rehabil* **13** (2007), 98-122.
[2]   Tawashy AE et al., Physical activity is related to lower levels of pain, fatigue and depression in individuals with spinal-cord injury: a correlational study. *Spinal Cord* (2008) Epub.
[3]   Washburn RA et al., The physical activity scale for individuals with physical disabilities: development

Rehabilitation: Mobility, Exercise and Sports
L.H.V. van der Woude et al. (Eds.)
IOS Press, 2010

doi:10.3233/978-1-60750-080-3-257

Compliance with a physical activity programme: comparison of an obese group with a low back pain group

M. PREUD'HOMME-MAURICE[a], B. LERICHE[a,b], C. BOURON[a,b], V. TIFFREAU[a], A. THEVENON[a,b]

[a]*Physical Medicine and Rehabilitation Department, Lille University Hospital, Lille, France*
[b]*Lille University Club, Lille, France*

Abstract. Purpose: although regular physical activity is recommended for low back pain (LBP) and obesity, compliance with exercise programmes is a critical problem. Here, we compared compliance with group exercises for these two conditions. Methods: we performed a cohort survey from January 2003 until June 2007. The Lille University sports club provides specific exercise programmes for LBP and for obesity. This programme has been designed as a transitional stage to help people start taking regular physical activity in a normal environment. Results: 154 LBP patients (104 females) and 41 obese patients (33 females) were included. Obese patients participated for longer than the LBP patients (16.49±12.9 months vs. 13.16±8.4 months, p< 0.04). 15% of the LBP patients and 29.3% of the obese subjects attended for over two years. Conclusion: it is unclear whether participants stayed in our programmes because they have a positive opinion or because they are afraid to exercise in ordinary settings.

Keywords. exercise, low back pain, obesity.

1. Introduction

Sedentariness has a major role in the occurrence or aggravation of various diseases, including low back pain (LBP) and obesity. Many different physical training programmes have been proposed for these two diseases and scientific studies have confirmed the benefits of such initiatives. However, most of these programmes have taken place in a protected environment (in hospital, in particular) and have been proposed for a limited duration (coinciding with the study schedule)[1,2]. Maintenance of physical activity in the aftermath of these targeted actions is rarely addressed. It is known that compliance with personal exercise programmes decreases rapidly over time. Furthermore, sport clubs tend to hesitate to welcome people with healthcare problems, for fear of an accident. Conversely, patients dread participating with healthy people and so many do not dare join a club.

Lille University Hospital therefore contacted one of the city's largest multisports clubs (the Lille University Club, LUC) in order to organize physical activity sessions for homogeneous groups of patients - notably obese and LBP groups. These patients had already participated in a functional retraining programme in hospital. The transitional sessions offered by the LUC were meant to last 6 months and prepare registered participants for continuation of their physical activity programme in an ordinary setting. Here, we present results on the patients' compliance with the programme. Participants had to pay a subscription fee (€120 for the LBP group and €70 for the obese group, since the latter programme was subsidized).

2. Method

We examined the medical files of patients having registered between January 2003 and June 2007. The patient's age, the number of weekly sessions in which he/she participated (between 1 and 3) and the duration of attendance at the programme were recorded. The LBP group was compared with the obese group using an analysis of variance and Bartlett's test. The significance threshold was set to 0.05.

3. Results

154 LBP patients and 41 obese patients participated in our programme during the study period. The mean age was 45.49 in the LBP group and 48.56 in the obese group (the difference was not significant). The distribution in terms of the number of sessions attended was comparable in the two groups. 82.5% of the LBP patients attended only one session a week, 16.2% attended 2 sessions a week and 1.3% (2 patients) attended 3 sessions a week. 85.4 % of the obese patients attended a single session a week and 14.6% (6 patients) attended two sessions a week.

Only 6.5% of the LBP patients and 12.2% of the obese withdrew from the programme before the end of the planned 6 months. Indeed, 79.9 % of the LBP patients and 85.3% of the obese patients wanted to renew their registration. 15% of the LBP patients and 29% of the obese patients even stayed in the programme for over 2 years. On average, the LBP patients attended the programmes for 13.16 ± 8.4 months and the obese patients attended for 16.49 ± 12.9 months; this difference was significant.

4. Discussion and Conclusion

The creation of physical activity sessions suited to specific pathologies appears to be a good way of maintaining compliance with exercise programmes for LBP patients and obese patients in an ordinary setting. The early withdrawal rate is low - on the contrary, most of the patients register for several successive programmes. However, it is unclear whether people stick to our programmes because they have a positive opinion or because they are afraid of exercising in ordinary settings.

We are currently investigating the level of physical activity that our patients maintained after leaving our programme.

This work is part of a Regional Health Programme and was funded by CRAM Nord Picardie.

References

[1] Tresierras MA, Balady GJ., Resistance Training in the Treatment of Diabetes and Obesity: MECHANISMS AND OUTCOMES. J Cardiopulm Rehabil Prev. 29(2009):67-75.
[2] Henchoz Y, Kai-Lik So A. Exercise and nonspecific low back pain: a literature review. Joint Bone Spine. 75(2008):533-9.

Rehabilitation: Mobility, Exercise and Sports
L.H.V. van der Woude et al. (Eds.)
IOS Press, 2010
© 2010 The authors and IOS Press. All rights reserved.
doi:10.3233/978-1-60750-080-3-259

Return to work after spinal cord injury: Is it related to wheelchair capacity at discharge from clinical rehabilitation?

J.M. VAN VELZEN[a,1], S. DE GROOT[b,c], M.W.M. POST[d], H.R. SLOOTMAN[e],
C.A.M. VAN BENNEKOM[a,e], L.H.V. VAN DER WOUDE[b]

[a] *Heliomare Research and Development, Wijk aan Zee*
[b] *Center for Human Movement Sciences, University Medical Center Groningen,
University of Groningen, Groningen*
[c] *Rehabilitation Center Amsterdam, Amsterdam*
[d] *Rehabilitation Center De Hoogstraat, Utrecht*
[e] *Rehabilitation Center Heliomare, Wijk aan Zee, The Netherlands*

Abstract. The purpose of the study is to evaluate whether return to work (RTW) can be predicted from wheelchair capacity (WC) at discharge from inpatient rehabilitation, after correction for confounders. 118 Subjects with recent spinal cord injury (SCI) from 8 Dutch rehabilitation centers participated. Main outcome measure was RTW ($\geq$1hr/wk). Outcome variables of WC were peak oxygen uptake ($VO2_{peak}$), peak aerobic power output (PO_{peak}), and wheelchair skill scores (ability, performance time and physical strain). Possible confounders were age, gender, lesion level and completeness. Where necessary, corrections were made for education level. 33% of the subjects returned to work. PO_{peak} (persons with a 10 Watt higher PO_{peak} were 1.37 times more likely to RTW), ability score (persons with a one-point higher score were 2.22 times more likely to RTW) and performance time (an increase, or worsening, of one second gave an odds ratio of 0.87, so persons with lower and therefore better scores were more likely to RTW) were significant predictors of RTW after correction for confounders and education level. It can be concluded that RTW was successful in 33% of the subjects. Outcomes for WC were independently related to RTW. Therefore it is recommended to train WC in the context of RTW.

Keywords. employment, spinal cord injuries, rehabilitation, wheelchairs, physical fitness.

1. Introduction

The quality of life of people with spinal cord injury (SCI) is known to be influenced by the ability to be actively involved in paid employment [1]. Returning to work is therefore important. Different studies investigated return to work (RTW) of people with SCI [1], but little has been published on the relationship between wheelchair capacity (WC), determined by the physical capacity (PC) and manual wheelchair skill

---

[1] Corresponding Author: Judith van Velzen, Heliomare research & development, Relweg 51, 1949 EC Wijk aan Zee, The Netherlands; E-mail: j.van.velzen@heliomare.nl

performance (WSP), and RTW although it is known that a relationship exists between PC, WSP and other domains of participation [2, 3].

The aims of the study are: 1) to describe the number of people with SCI that return to work, one year after discharge from inpatient rehabilitation, and 2) to investigate whether successful RTW can be predicted one year after discharge from the PC and WSP at discharge from inpatient rehabilitation.

2. Methods

Participants

Analyses were based on data of 118 subjects who were working before the occurrence of SCI and of whom it was known whether they were working or not one year after discharge from inpatient rehabilitation. All subject were admitted to inpatient rehabilitation because of an acute SCI and were wheelchair dependent. The study was part of the Dutch Research Project 'Physical Strain, Work Capacity, and Mechanisms of Restoration of Mobility in the Rehabilitation of Persons with a Spinal Cord Injury'.

Variables

The following variables were involved in the study:
- Main outcome measure: Return to work, determined one year after discharge from inpatient rehabilitation with the help of a questionnaire. RTW was classified as either successful (RTW group, $\geq$1hr/wk) or not successful (non-RTW group).
- Independent variables: Wheelchair capacity, determined by the PC (described by peak oxygen uptake ($VO2_{peak}$) and peak aerobic power output (PO_{peak})) and WSP (described by the ability score, performance time score and physical strain score on a wheelchair circuit) [3,4].
- Personal and lesion characteristics: age at the time of injury, gender, level and completeness of the lesion and education level were registered in order to control their influence on RTW and WC.

Statistics

To describe the number of people returning to work, descriptive statistics were used. To answer the second research question multilevel multiple regression analysis was used. The effect of education level on RTW was investigated first by including education level in the model. The possible confounding effect of the personal and lesion characteristics was evaluated and, if necessary, controlled.

3. Results

The number of subjects that returned to work

33% Of the subjects returned to work one year after discharge from inpatient rehabilitation. The mean number of hours working before injury was 40.6 (range: 3-100 hours) while after SCI the mean number of hours was 20.7 (range: 3-50 hours).

Wheelchair capacity

- $VO2_{peak}$: After correction for the confounders, $VO2_{peak}$ was not a significant predictor on RTW (p=0.44).
- PO_{peak}: After correction for the confounder, PO_{peak} was a significant predictor for RTW (p=0.02): persons with a 10 Watt higher PO_{peak} were 1.37 times more likely to return to work.
- Ability score: After correction for the confounders, a significant effect of the ability score on RTW was found (p=0.02). Persons with a one-point higher ability score were 2.22 times more likely to RTW.
- Performance time score: After correction for the confounders, performance time was found to be a significant predictor for RTW (p=0.01). An increase, or worsening, of one second on the performance time gave an odds ratio of 0.87, so persons with lower, or better, performance time scores were more likely to RTW.
- Physical strain score: Physical strain score was not found to be a predicting variable after correcting for the confounders (p=0.11).
- Education level turned out to strongly influence RTW and was, therefore, included in all statistical models.

4. Conclusions

In the current study 33% of the included participants successfully returned to paid work ($\geq$1hr/wk) one year after discharge. It would be interesting to investigate RTW after a longer follow-up time since the vocational rehabilitation process can take more than one year if, for example, education is necessary. From the current study it can be concluded that RTW one year after discharge is associated to PO_{peak}, ability score and performance time at discharge from inpatient rehabilitation. Therefore, it is recommended to optimize wheelchair capacity during and after rehabilitation.

References

[1] S .Yasuda, Return to work after spinal cord injury: a review of recent research. *NeuroRehabilitation* **17** (2002), 177-186.

[2] O.J. Kilkens, The Wheelchair Circuit: Construct validity and responsiveness of a test to assess manual wheelchair mobility in persons with spinal cord injury. *Archives of Physical Medicine and Rehabilitation* **85** (2004), 424-431.

[3] O.J. Kilkens, The longitudinal relation between physical capacity and wheelchair skill performance during inpatient rehabilitation of people with spinal cord injury. *Archives of Physical Medicine and Rehabilitation* **86** (2005), 1575-1581.

Rehabilitation: Mobility, Exercise and Sports
L.H.V. van der Woude et al. (Eds.)
IOS Press, 2010

doi:10.3233/978-1-60750-080-3-262

Ambulatory sensing of the dynamic interaction between the human body and the environment

P.H. VELTINK[a,1], H.M. SCHEPERS[a]
[a]*University of Twente, Enschede, the Netherlands*

Abstract. This paper presents a method to estimate power transfer between the human body and the environment during short interactions and relatively arbitrary movements using a combination of inertial and force sensing. The work performed was estimated for varying movements with net displacement and varying loads (mass and spring), and appeared to be accurate within 4%.

Keywords. ambulatory sensing, forces sensing, inertial movement sensing, power estimation, work estimation.

1. Introduction

Study of the dynamic interaction with the environment and loading of the human body is important in ergonomics, sports and rehabilitation. This paper presents a method to estimate power transfer between the human body and the environment during short interactions and relatively arbitrary movements using a combination of inertial and force sensing, and illustrates the feasibility of this method. The full feasibility study has been published elsewhere [1].

2. Methods

Estimation of Power and Work

Power transfer between two bodies is given by:

$$P = \vec{F} \cdot \vec{v} + \vec{M} \cdot \vec{\omega} \tag{1}$$

Performed work follows by integrating power over time. Angular velocity $\vec{\omega}$ can be measured using rate gyroscopes, velocity $\vec{v}$ can be estimated from accelerometers after rotation to the inertial coordinate system, subtraction of gravitational acceleration, integration and applying adequate start and end conditions. Force $\vec{F}$ and moment $\vec{M}$ can be sensed by a 6 DOF force/moment sensor system [2]

---

¹ Corresponding Author.

Estimation of Power and Work

Mass and spring loads were moved by hand over a fixed height difference via varying free movement trajectories. Kinematic and kinetic quantities were measured in the handle between the hand and the load (figure 1). 3D force and moments were measured using a six degrees of freedom force/moment sensor module, 3D movement was measured using 3D accelerometers and angular velocity sensors.

The estimated performed work was compared to the potential energy difference corresponding to the change in height of the loads.

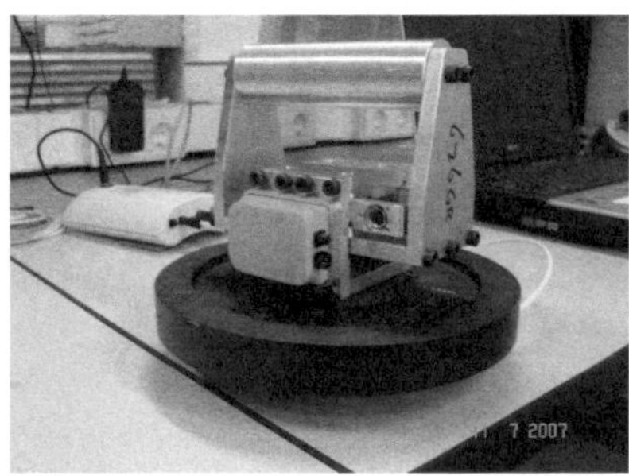

Figure 1. Experimental setup of a handle connected to a mass load, with 3D inertial and force/moment sensors.

3. Results

An example result is shown in figure 2. The mass is transferred from the ground to a 75 cm high table, accounting for a potential energy change of 69 J. The estimated performed work in this case is 70 J.

The work performed was estimated for varying movements with net displacement and varying loads (mass and spring), and appeared to be accurate within 4%.

4. Discussion

The feasibility of the presented method has been demonstrated (see also [1]). The method also allows partial characterization of the dynamic characteristics of unknown loads. After miniaturization, the sensors will be incorporated in gloves and shoes, and applications of this method in ergonomics, rehabilitation and sports will be investigated.

Acknowledgement

This research is supported by the Dutch Technology Foundation STW, applied science division of NOW and the Technology Program of the Ministry of Economic Affairs

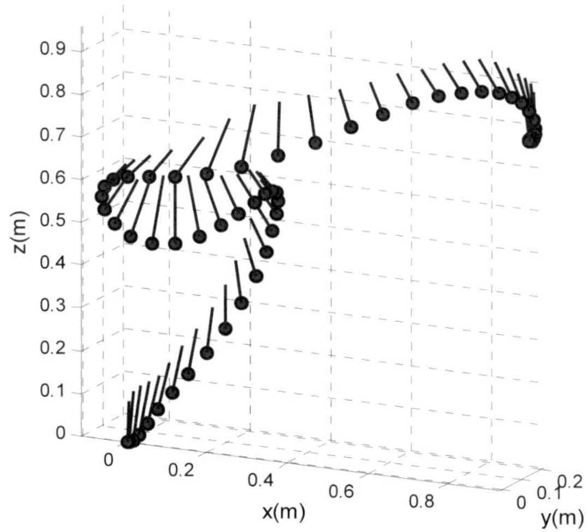

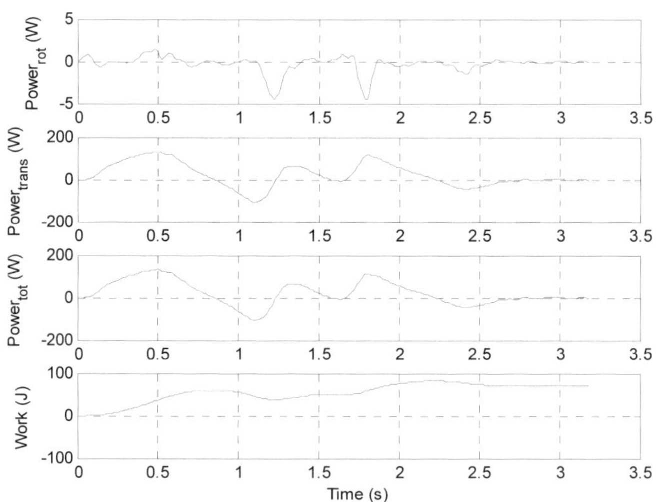

Figure 2. Example measurement: Upper: reconstructed position and force directions;
Lower: Estimated power transfer and work done.

References

[1] P.H. Veltink, H. Kortier, H. Martin Schepers, Sensing Power Transfer between the Human Body and the Environment, *IEEE Transactions on Biomedical Engineering* (2009), in press.
[2] H.M. Schepers, H.F.J.M. Koopman, P.H. Veltink, Ambulatory Assessment of Ankle and Foot Dynamics, IEEE Trans. Biomedical Engineering **54** (2007), 895-902.

Chapter 7

Training Strategies

7.1

Keynote

Rehabilitation: Mobility, Exercise and Sports
L.H.V. van der Woude et al. (Eds.)
IOS Press, 2010

doi:10.3233/978-1-60750-080-3-267

Lokomat: automated electromechanical gait training in neurological patients

K.H. GERRITS[a,1]

[a] *Research Institute MOVE, Faculty of Human Movement Sciences, VU University Amsterdam*
[b] *Duyvensz-Nagel Research Laboratory, Rehabilitation Centre Amsterdam (RCA)*

Abstract. Neurological disorders such as stroke and (incomplete) spinal cord injury (SCI) usually lead to difficulties in performing locomotor activities, such as walking or climbing stairs. Therefore, an important part of rehabilitation programs is aimed at restoration of gait function. To improve walking ability it seems important to include task-specific repetitive training with focus on higher intensities of walking practice. These concepts have lead to the development of various automated electromechanical gait-training devices, such as the Lokomat, which assist walking practice. Although it is claimed that such devices may be highly beneficial owing to the intense practice possible in non-ambulatory patients, scientific evidence which could justify their relatively high cost is scarce. Recently, within our research institute in collaboration with the Rehabilitation Centre Amsterdam, we have started a randomized controlled clinical trial investigating the effectiveness of Lokomat-training in patients after stroke and SCI on gait performance, quality of life and neuromuscular and cardiovascular properties. This lecture will give an overview on the existing literature concerning the efficacy of electromechanical assisted training for walking and the concepts which would favor the use of these devices will be discussed. In addition, developments and preliminary results from our study will be presented and discussed.

Keywords. robot assisted treadmill training, stroke, cardiovascular accident, spinal cord injury.

1. Introduction

Over the last decades the use of robotic devices has entered the field of rehabilitation medicine. Usually, these devices are used by rehabilitation centers to assist physical therapists improving/restoring mobility in patients with neurological injuries such as stroke or spinal cord injury (SCI). Many neurological patients have difficulties performing locomotor activities such as walking or stair climbing so restoration of gait function is an important purpose of their rehabilitation program. One of the different robots developed for this purpose, is the Lokomat. This automated electromechanically controlled gait orthosis combines a treadmill with body weight support (BWS) and robotic arms that attach to the subjects leg, thereby allowing assisting or inducing gait. The Lokomat is now used by various rehabilitation centers across the world and in 2006 the first in the Netherlands was introduced in the Rehabilitation Centre Amsterdam.

---

[1] Corresponding Author. k_gerrits@fbw.vu.nl

2.   Why use treadmill training in neurological patients?

Stroke and SCI are neurological disorders which lead to severe motor disabilities. Many patients suffer from partial or complete paralysis or paresis leading to difficulties in, for instance, walking ability. The majority of these patients have to rely on walking aids or even become wheelchair dependent for the rest of their lives. In persons with SCI the motor impairment originates from a (partial) interruption of descending and ascending pathways within the spinal cord and in stroke damage to brain areas involved in motor control lead to disturbed gait.

It has been demonstrated that the largest improvement in motor function in stroke patients occurs in the first months after stroke and is associated with spontaneous (partial) recovery of the damaged brain areas. In addition, there is some evidence suggesting that intensive task-specific training such as with robot assisted treadmill training can promote supraspinal plasticity in the motor centers known to be involved in locomotion[1]. In addition, intensive daily locomotor training in persons with chronic SCI can lead to improved corticospinal tract function and motor recovery[2].

Most chronic diseases like neural disorders will ultimately lead to deconditioning of other biological systems such as the musculoskeletal and cardiovascular system as well as metabolism, thereby further limiting functional performance. For instance, we recently observed that stroke not only leads to impaired voluntary control of the affected lower limb muscles but also to reduced 'intrinsic' strength capacity of these muscles, most likely due to muscle atrophy. There is still no direct evidence for a beneficial effect of strength training to improve gait function. However, we suggest that rehabilitation strategies of stroke and SCI patients should target the neuroplastic capacity of brain and descending/ascending neural pathways as well as the secondary adaptations in, for instance, the musculoskeletal and cardiovascular system. Automated robot assisted treadmill training devices such as the Lokomat allow intense repetitive gait training even in the early rehabilitation period. Therefore, this rehabilitation device may have a great potential for targeting both primary (neural) and secondary (musculoskeletal and cardiovascular) adaptations.

3.   Efficacy of (robot assisted) treadmill training

Over the last decade, there has been growing scientific support for the use of (manually assisted) treadmill training as a task-specific rehabilitation approach in various neurological populations such as after stroke[3] and SCI[4]. Reported beneficial effects include improved gait[5], balance[6], muscle strength[7], and endurance[6], reduced spasticity[7] and enhanced cardiovascular fitness[8]. In addition, it was suggested that this type of locomotor training can lead to higher return to functional walking ability than conventional gait training[6]. Nevertheless, a systematic review reported inconclusive results on the efficacy of treadmill training, with or without body weight support, although it was suggested that specific patients may benefit from the treatment[9].

More recently, owing to advanced technology, automated (i.e. robot-assisted) gait training has been introduced to combat some of the limitations associated with manually assisted treadmill training such as the high physical demand on the therapists. An additional advantage is that it allows gait training even in patients with severe disabilities. Further, the gait patterns imposed by the robot can be more easily and consistently adjusted and optimized for each patient. Over the past few years some studies have been performed investigating the efficacy of this innovative rehabilitation strategy. For instance, beneficial effects of Lokomat therapy were reported in stroke patients[10] and people with SCI[11] although others could not confirm this[12]. Importantly, a recent systematic review suggests that stroke patients who receive electromechanical-assisted gait training in combination with physiotherapy are more likely to achieve independent walking than patients receiving gait training without these devices[13]. Literature is, however, somewhat less optimistic, with respect to its potential to be more effective for gait improvement when compared to other locomotor training strategies in the SCI population[14]. This may be due to lack of large RCT's.

Collectively, despite the lack of conclusive evidence the results of the limited studies reporting beneficial effects of treadmill training on gait function in stroke as well as in SCI patients seem promising. Robot-assisted treadmill training may be a valuable new therapeutic approach in the development of task-specific training strategies. Because this treatment is also feasible for severely disabled patients with only limited or no gait function, it may be used for a more extensive population of neurological patients and expedite the rehabilitation process, which may result in better or earlier participation and improvement of quality of life.

References

[1]   P. Winchester et al. Changes in supraspinal activation patterns following robotic locomotor therapy in motor-incomplete spinal cord injury. *Neurorehabil Neural Repair* **19** (2005) 313-324.

[2]   S.L. Thomas et al. Increases in corticospinal tract function by treadmill training after incomplete spinal cord injury. *J Neurophysiol* **94** (2005) 2844-2855.

[3]   H. Barbeau. Locomotor training in neurorehabilitation: emerging rehabilitation concepts. *Neurorehabil Neural Repair* **17** (2003) 3-11.

[4]   H. Barbeau et al. Walking after spinal cord injury: evaluation, treatment, and functional recovery. *Arch Phys Med Rehabil* **80** (1999) 225-235.

[5]   S. Hesse et al. Treadmill training with partial body weight support compared with physiotherapy in nonambulatory hemiparetic patients. *Stroke* **26** (1995) 976-981.

[6]   M. Visintin et al. A new approach to retrain gait in stroke patients through body weight support and treadmill stimulation. *Stroke* **29** (1998) 1122-1128.

[7]   G.V. Smith et al. "Task-oriented" exercise improves hamstring strength and spastic reflexes in chronic stroke patients. *Stroke* **30** (1999) 2112-2118.

[8]   R.F. Macko et al. Treadmill exercise rehabilitation improves ambulatory function and cardiovascular fitness in patients with chronic stroke: a randomized, controlled trial. *Stroke* **36** (2005) 2206-2211.

[9]   A.M. Moseley et al. Treadmill training and body weight support for walking after stroke. *Cochrane Database Syst Rev* (2005) .

[10] A. Mayr et al. Prospective, blinded, randomized crossover study of gait rehabilitation in stroke patients using the Lokomat gait orthosis. *Neurorehabil Neural Repair* **21** (2007) 307-314.

[11] M. Wirz et al. Effectiveness of automated locomotor training in patients with chronic incomplete spinal cord injury: a multicenter trial. *Arch Phys Med Rehabil* **86** (2005) 672-680.

[12] J. Hidler et al. Multicenter randomized clinical trial evaluating the effectiveness of the Lokomat in subacute stroke. *Neurorehabil Neural Repair* **23** (2009) 5-13.

[13] J. Mehrholz et al. Electromechanical-assisted training for walking after stroke. *Cochrane Database Syst Rev* (2007) .

[14] J. Mehrholz et al. Locomotor training for walking after spinal cord injury. *Cochrane Database Syst Rev* (2008)

7.2

Oral Presentations

Rehabilitation: Mobility, Exercise and Sports
L.H.V. van der Woude et al. (Eds.)
IOS Press, 2010

doi:10.3233/978-1-60750-080-3-273

A preliminary evaluation of a community-based exercise program for people with mobility impairments

M.L. KASPERAVICIUS[a], A.E. LATIMER[a, 1], S.P. HETZ [a], M.A. McCOLL[a], M. McGUIRE[b], K. SMITH[b]

[a] *Queen's University, Kingston, Ontario, Canada*
[b] *St. Mary's of the Lake Hospital, Providence Care, Kingston, Ontario, Canada*

Abstract. Individuals with mobility impairments face numerous barriers to exercise participation. Offering a community-based exercise program has been suggested as a strategy for reducing these barriers. The purpose of this study was to identify the factors that facilitate ongoing participation and the barriers that persist in a community-based exercise program for people with mobility impairments. Eleven members of a community-based exercise program (M_{age}=45.64±12.75 years; spinal cord injury n=5; other n=6) took part in focus groups examining facilitators and barriers to program participation. The program being evaluated included volunteer-supervised, twice weekly strength and aerobic training. Focus group transcripts were coded and recurrent themes were identified. A framework identifying factors that promote and hinder program participation emerged. The beneficial changes in quality of life, the positive interaction with volunteers, and the program's ability to fill a niche were perceived as catalysts encouraging attendance. Remaining barriers included intrapersonal (e.g., feeling self-conscious) and systemic factors (e.g., transportation). These findings can be used to inform the optimal implementation of a community-based exercise program for people with mobility impairments.

Keywords. community exercise program, exercise barriers, spinal cord injury.

1. Introduction

Mobility impairment is the second most common type of disability in Canada; between 5 to 15% of adults (25-64 years of age) report having difficulty performing mobility activities[1]. Of concern, individuals with mobility impairments are at increased risk for chronic diseases and often experience a reduced quality of life. In this population, physical activity can reduce risk factors for many chronic diseases, and contribute to symptom management, functional independence, and improved quality of life[1].

In spite of these benefits, adults with mobility impairments tend to be less active than adults in the general population; only 44% of Canadians with disabilities are active, compared to 65% of the general population[1]. Low physical activity participation rates among adults with a disability are the result of the numerous barriers

---

[1] Amy E. Latimer, School of Kinesiology and Health Studies, Physical Education Centre, 69 Union Street, Queen's University, Kingston, ON, Canada, K7L 3N6, amy.latimer@queensu.ca

impeding participation. Common obstacles include intrapersonal factors (e.g., lack of motivation or energy) and systemic barriers (e.g., lack of accessible facilities, lack of knowledgeable health professionals)[2]. Providing a targeted community-based exercise program in an accessible facility is a suggested strategy for addressing these barriers. The purpose of this study was to identify factors that both facilitate ongoing participation and barriers that persist in a community-based exercise program for people with mobility impairments.

2. Methods

Participant and Program Description

The 11 study participants were drawn from Kingston Revved Up (M_{age}=45.64±12.75 years; spinal cord injury n=5; other n=6; male n=6, female n=5; $M_{participation}$=6.7 months). Revved Up is a twice-weekly community-based exercise program for adults (18-65 years of age) with mobility impairments. The program is offered at fully equipped rehabilitation centre. Participants follow a prescribed endurance and strength training program. Each participant is matched with a volunteer trainer who assists setting up exercise equipment and monitors participants' exercise technique and progress. Volunteers are primarily undergraduate kinesiology students.

Data Collection and Analysis

A trained facilitator led three in-depth, open-ended focus groups each lasting 1 hour with 3-5 people attending. Participants' responses to the following questions were tape-recorded: 1) Have you noticed differences in your physical functioning since beginning Revved Up? 2) How satisfied are you with the social interaction at Revved Up? 3) Overall, do you enjoy attending? 4) Has Revved Up adequately met your needs?

Each interview was transcribed verbatim and confirmed for accuracy. The author read the transcripts and coded the text. Recurrent themes were identified and a framework was developed.

3. Results

Figure 1 presents the categories of enablers and barriers to participation that emerged.

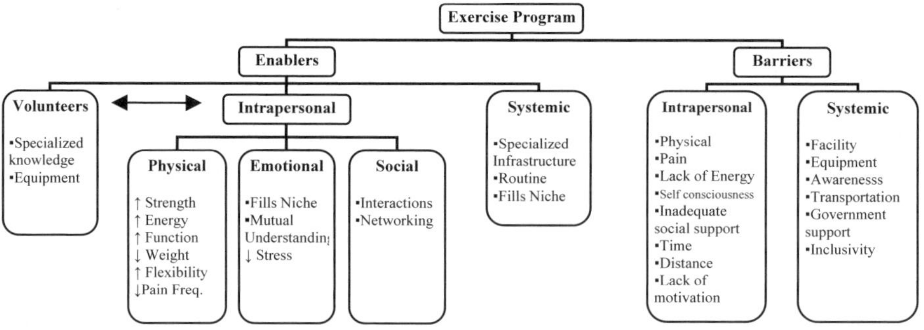

Figure 1. Enablers and barriers to participation; ↑ = Increased, ↓ = Decreased

Overall, enablers to participation included intrapersonal, volunteer, and systemic factors. Barriers to participation were divided into intrapersonal factors and systemic factors. Participants identified factors that occasionally discouraged their own attendance and elaborated on reasons why others may to attend.

4. Discussion

Participants were overwhelmingly positive in their discussions of Revved Up; however, barriers remain. These findings can be used to help similar programs address barriers and target enablers during program development and implementation. Careful program design will ensure equitable access to physical activity and optimal participation.

Factors that emerged as enabling participation included improvements in the physical, social, and emotional components of quality of life. These factors reinforcing participation are similar to those found in previous studies[1]. In addition to promoting exercise as safe and efficacious, program coordinators should emphasize the less tangible but equally important social and emotional benefits of community programs.

The participant-volunteer relationship emerged as a factor integral to program success. Lack of social support is a common barrier to exercise, thus pairing participants with a volunteer seems to be a potential strategy to increase motivation, satisfaction and attendance, especially for new clients[1]. Furthermore, volunteer-participant benefits are bidirectional. Volunteers gain invaluable knowledge and experience that will contribute to future professional success.

Systemic factors were the third category of enablers. Many participants stated that the program fills a niche. Unlike the public health care system, Revved Up emphasizes self management (i.e., taking responsibility for personal health) and preventative medicine. Furthermore, the accessible infrastructure offered by Revved Up provides a unique advantage over other fitness facilities in the area. The segregated environment made participants more comfortable and less self-conscious. When designing a community-based program, program coordinators should attend to systemic factors ensuring the program promotes health in an accessible and welcoming environment.

While a number of factors enabling participation emerged, participants indicated that intrapersonal and systemic barriers to participation remained. Intrapersonal barriers varied across participants and likely would be best addressed on an individual basis. Systemic barriers were related to facility and equipment limitations. Having additional equipment would ease this program demand. Lack of awareness of the program within the community, a limited definition of mobility impairment, and transportation were identified as barriers limiting program uptake. When developing a community-based exercise program, program coordinators should choose a central location and ensure that the program is visible and can be accessed via public transit.

Limitations to this study included small sample size. Future studies should be conducted as larger, multi-location initiatives.

References

[1]   K.A. Martin-Ginis & A.L. Hicks, Considerations for the development of a physical activity guide for Canadians with physical disabilities, *Applied Physiology, Nutrition, and Metabolism* **32** (2007), S135-S147.
[2]   J.H. Rimmer, B. Riley, E. Wang, A. Rauworth, & J. Jurkowski, Physical activity participation among persons with disabilities, *American Journal of Preventative Medicine* **26** (2004), 419–425.

Rehabilitation: Mobility, Exercise and Sports
L.H.V. van der Woude et al. (Eds.)
IOS Press, 2010

doi:10.3233/978-1-60750-080-3-276

Endurance training and improved aerobic capacity after traumatic brain injury

K.A. MOSSBERG[a,1], B.E. MASEL[b]
[a] *University of Texas Medical Branch at Galveston*
[b] *Transitional Learning Center at Galveston*

Abstract. The purpose of this study was to assess the feasibility and effectiveness of an endurance training program in patients who had sustained a traumatic brain injury (TBI) and were in the post-acute recovery phase. Methods: Thirteen patients gave written consent. Inclusion criteria were: ability to ambulate safely on a treadmill at a minimal speed of 1.6kph (1.0mph), no overt cardiovascular disease, ability to follow 2-step commands, and compliance with the expired gas collection apparatus. A modified Balke protocol was used. Speed was gradually increased to the safest possible speed in the first two minutes at 1% incline. Incline was then increased 2% per minute until two of three peak criteria (O_2 plateau, HR >90% age-predicted max, respiratory exchange ratio (RER) >1.15) or ambulation became unsafe. Multivariate comparisons were performed (alpha=0.05). Results: Peak O_2 improved (23.1sd7.6 vs 30.3sd6.9 mL/min/kg) (p<0.01). Peak HR and RER did not change. Submaximal ventilatory equivalents decreased. Conclusions: Despite the cognitive and behavioral challenges, patients were found to be compliant with properly prescribed aerobic exercise. Further randomized controlled trials are warranted in this population. TBI is a chronic disease and increased physical activity should be encouraged early in the rehabilitation process.

Keywords. head injury, cardiorespiratory fitness, oxygen consumption.

1. Introduction

The incidence and prevalence of traumatic brain injury (TBI) is relatively high when compared to other permanent disabling conditions[1, 2]. Complaints of fatigue are extremely common in persons with TBI even long after the original injury[3, 4]. The causes of fatigue are multifactorial but one of the factors may be a reduced aerobic capacity and impaired cardiorespiratory fitness. It has been shown that cardiorespiratory fitness is reduced 60-70% in patients after TBI compared with healthy sedentary controls[5]. A number of studies have been performed examining the effects of aerobic training programs on patients with TBI[6-8] with mixed results.

We hypothesized that if patients were trained appropriately in the post acute phase of recovery that improvement in cardiorespiratory fitness would occur even with the high prevalence of cognitive and behavioral impairments. Therefore, the purpose of this study was to assess the feasibility and effectiveness of an endurance training program in patients who sustained a TBI and were in the post-acute recovery phase.

---

[1] Corresponding Author: Kurt A. Mossberg, PT, PhD, Department of Physical Therapy / SHP, 301 University Blvd., Galveston, TX 77555-1144, USA; E-mail: kmossber@utmb.edu

2. Methods

Subjects

Subjects were patients in a post-acute residential treatment facility and were receiving comprehensive rehabilitation. Twenty-two individuals (17m, 5f) gave written informed consent to participate. Thirteen subjects (11m, 2f) completed at least 10 weeks of endurance training (Table 1). All subjects were capable of independent ambulation (minimal safe treadmill speed was 1.6kph (1.0mph)), able to follow two step commands and tolerant of the expired gas collection requirements for testing.

Table 1. Characteristics of the 13 subjects who completed at least 10 weeks of training.

	Mean ± SD	Range
Age at injury (years)	29.6 ± 9.5	19 - 49
Recovery time (months)	11.0 ± 9.5	2.4 - 33.2
Training duration (weeks)	14.8 ± 4.6	10 - 23

Procedures

Subjects were tested using a modified Balke protocol[9] during which EKG was monitored; expired gases were collected and analyzed by an automated metabolic cart. Speed was gradually increased to the safest possible speed in the first two minutes at 1% incline. Incline was then increased 2% every minute until the subject met two of three peak criteria (O_2 plateau, HR >85-90% age-predicted maximum, respiratory exchange ratio (RER) >1.15) or ambulation became unsafe. Training sessions were performed 2-3x per week on a treadmill for a minimum for 20-30 minutes. Subjects were monitored throughout and coached. Intensity was maintained at 60-80% of peak HR achieved during the pre-training aerobic capacity test by changing speed and/or incline.

Paired samples t-tests were performed on all peak responses. Two-way analyses of variance were performed on all submaximal responses. All analyses were performed at an alpha level of 0.05.

3. Results

Peak responses before and after training are shown in Table 2. Submaximal O_2 uptake did not change while submaximal heart rates decreased after training. These results translated into an increase in submaximal O_2 pulse (estimate of cardiac stroke volume) shown in Figure 1. In addition, the submaximal ventilatory equivalent for O_2 decreased after training suggesting an improvement in the efficiency of ventilation.

Table 2. Peak responses before and after cardiorespiratory fitness training (n=13; * $p<0.01$).

Variable	Pre-training Mean ± SD	Post-training Mean ± SD
Oxygen uptake (mL/kg/min) *	23.1 ± 7.6	30.3 ± 6.9
Heart rate (beats/min)	166 ± 24	176 ± 19
Minute ventilation (L/min) *	76.2 ± 27.8	95.7 ± 31.5
Respiratory exchange ratio	1.25 ± 0.12	1.22 ± 0.11
Oxygen pulse (mL/beat) *	10.2 ± 2.8	12.8 ± 2.8

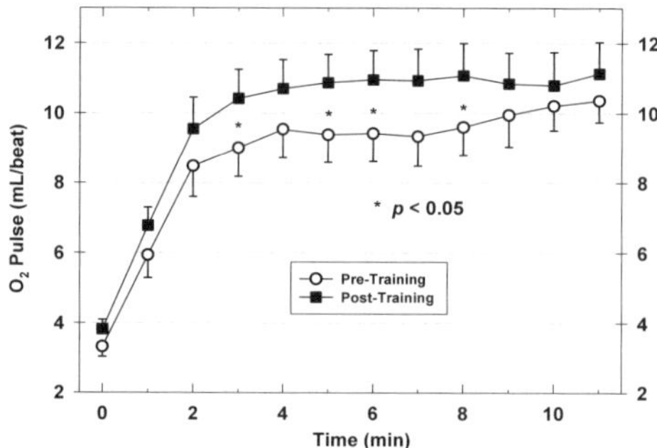

Figure 1. Submaximal oxygen pulse (all values are mean ± SE)

Nine subjects were unable to complete program; three were withdrawn due to lack of motivation to sustain duration and intensity requirements. Six were discharged from the facility prematurely.

4. Discussion and conclusions

Despite the motivational challenges that many subjects experienced, we observed a 30% increase in peak aerobic capacity. However, these subjects were, on average, only in the 10th percentile of fitness level for their age after training[10].

Given the high likelihood of leading a sedentary lifestyle, diseases of inactivity will increase burden and further decrease functional independence. Rehabilitation specialists should be more proactive educating patients on the beneficial effects of an active lifestyle in the early phases of TBI rehabilitation. Further randomized controlled trials and longitudinal studies are warranted.

References

[1]   E. Finkelstein, *et al*, *The Incidence and Economic Burden of Injuries in the United States*. Oxford University Press, New York, 2006.

[2]   Traumatic Brain Injury in the United States: Emergency department visits, hospitalizations, and deaths, J. Langlois, et al. National Center for Injury Prevention and Control, Atlanta, GA, 2004.

[3]   T. Bushnik, *et al*, Patterns of fatigue and its correlates over the first 2 years after traumatic brain injury, *J Head Trauma Rehabil* **23** (2008), 25-32.

[4]   J. Olver, *et al*, Outcome following traumatic brain injury: a comparison between 2 and 5 years after injury, *Brain Inj* **10** (1996), 841-848.

[5]   K. Mossberg, *et al*, Aerobic capacity after traumatic brain injury: comparison with a nondisabled cohort, *Arch Phys Med Rehabil* **88** (2007), 315-320.

[6]   Y. Bhambhani, *et al*, Effects of circuit training on body composition and peak cardiorespiratory responses in patients with moderate to severe traumatic brain injury, *Arch Phys Med Rehabil* **86** (2005), 268-276.

[7]   A. Bateman, *et al*, The effect of aerobic training on rehabilitation outcomes after recent severe brain injury: a randomized controlled evaluation, *Arch Phys Med Rehabil* **82** (2001), 174-182.

[8]   L. Jankowski, *et al*, Aerobic and neuromuscular training: Effect on the capacity, efficiency, and fatigability of patients with traumatic brain injuries, *Arch Phys Med Rehabil* **71** (1990), 500-504.

[9]   K. Mossberg, *et al*, Reliability of graded exercise testing after traumatic train injury: submaximal and peak responses, *Am J Phys Med Rehabil* **84** (2005), 492-500.

[10]   M. Pollock, *et al*, *Exercise in Health and Disease*. 2nd ed. WB Saunders Co, Philadelphia, PA, 1990.

Rehabilitation: Mobility, Exercise and Sports
L.H.V. van der Woude et al. (Eds.)
IOS Press, 2010

doi:10.3233/978-1-60750-080-3-279

Effectiveness of robot-assisted gait training in persons with spinal cord injury: a systematic review

E. SWINNEN[1], S. DUERINCK, E. KERCKHOFS
[a] Faculty of Physical Education and Physiotherapy, ARTS (Advanced Rehabilitation, Technology and Science), ALTACRO (Automated Locomotor Training using an Actuated Compliant Robotic Orthosis), Vrije Universiteit Brussel, Belgium

Abstract. This systematic review summarizes studies concerning the effectiveness of robot-assisted gait training in persons with spinal cord injury. Although promising results have been reported in case studies and small cohort studies, but there is insufficient evidences to draw firm conclusions.

Keywords. spinal cord injury, robot-assisted gait training, driven gait orthosis.

1. Introduction

Different kinds of gait rehabilitation are used in the domain of neurological rehabilitation, such as manually assisted over-ground and treadmill training, both with or without body-weight support (BWS). Robot-assisted gait training (RAGT) was introduced in the late nineties. The 'Lokomat' and the 'Gait trainer' are commercial available robots, 'Lopes' is a research-robot. RAGT seems to improve the independent walking and walking capacity in stroke patients, in multiple sclerosis patients there is insufficient evidence. We aim to investigate what the actual evidence is about RAGT in spinal cord injured (SCI) patients.

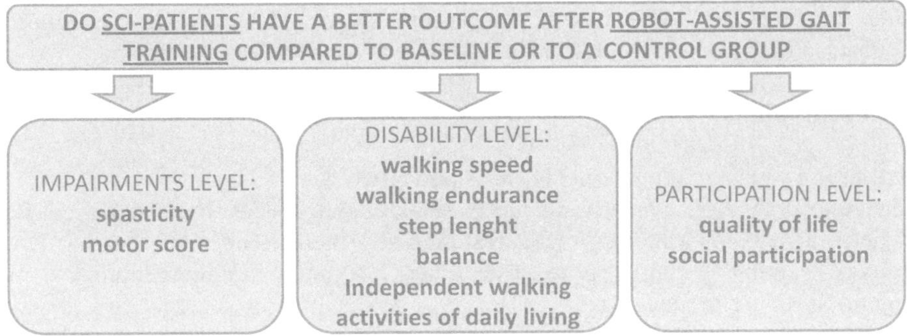

Figure 1. Research-questions

---

[1] Corresponding Author: Eva Swinnen, Vrije Universiteit Brussel, Department KINE, Laarbeeklaan 103, 1090 Brussels, Belgium; E-mail: eswinnen@vub.ac.be

2. Methods

A computerized search was conducted for English, French, German and Dutch articles in Medline (Pubmed), Web of Knowledge, Cochrane Library, PEDro and DAREnet (1990 to 2008). Key-words like 'spinal cord injury', 'quadriplegia', 'robot-assisted gait training' and 'locomotor training' were used.

Articles were included when acute or chronic incomplete adult SCI-patients were involved in a RAGT intervention study with outcome on walking speed, walking endurance, walking independence, step length, balance, spasticity, activity of daily living, quality of life and/or social participation. Excluded studies are studies about functional electrical stimulation or surgery. Studies with outcome on physical capacity, electromyography activity or cardio-respiratory functioning are excluded. Animal studies or studies on children are also not included in this review.

3. Results

722 titles appeared after key-word search. After screening title and abstract, hand-search and scanning reference lists and narrative reviews for relevant publications, and removing duplicates 37 papers remained. After extraction full texts for more detailed application of in- and exclusion criteria, 31 papers are excluded by two researchers (70% consensus). The descriptive analysis of the ultimately six included studies is presented in table 1 (1-6). The methodological quality was rated with the 'van Tulder quality assessment score' (RCTs) or the 'Evaluation of quality of an intervention study'.

There is a great variability in the outcome measures On the level of impairments: (Modified) Ashworth Scale, Spinal Cord Assessment Tool for Spasticity, Motricity Index and Lower Extremity Motor Score. On the level of disability: (Over-ground) walking speed, 10-meter walk test, 6-minutes walk test, step length, step symmetry, balance tests, (Modified sitting) Functional Reach Test, Rivermead Mobility Index, Functional Independence Measure, Walking Index for Spinal Cord Injury-II, Functional Ambulation Category, assistive device usage and Timed Up & Go test. No studies with outcome on the level of participation were found.

One RCT compared RAGT with three other BWS therapy modalities and reported that all the forms of locomotor training are associated with improved walking performance (walking speed) and that there are no obvious differences between groups. The other RCT compared RAGT with therapist-assisted BWS gait training and over-ground ambulation with a mobile suspension system. There were no significant differences in the extent of motor or functional recovery between the groups.

4. Conclusion

There are promising improvements measured after RAGT, but there is insufficient evidence to draw firm conclusions due to small samples sizes, methodological flaws and heterogeneity of training procedures. Actually there is no evidence that RAGT improves walking function more than other locomotor training strategies. Well designed RCTs are needed.

REF.	STUDY-DESIGN	POPULTATION				INTER-VENTION	COMPARIS ON GROUPS	OUTCOME
author (year)	category/ Meth. quality	lesion level / ASIA (I/C)	time after injury	sam ple size	robot / training freq.	patients / therapy		results
Field-Fote (2005)	True-exp. / van Tulder score: 12/19	C4, C5, C6, T2, T7, T10 (I)	1y, 1.8y, 4.4y, 10y, 11.4y, 23.4y	6	Lokomat / 60', 5x/w for 12w (27-54 sessions)	3x7 SCI / BWS TT+ phys.assist. - BWS TT+ stimul.- BWS OT+ stimul.		Walking speed: ↑57% (slow walkers), ↓19% (fast walkers) Step length:↓1% in stronger and 22% in weaker legs Step symmetry: ↑24%
Hornby (2005) b	True-exp./ van Tulder score: 11/19	above T10 / B/C/D (I)	14d-180d	10	Lokomat / 30', 3x/w for 8w	2x10 SCI / BWS TT + phys. assist. - BWS OT		FIM-L, WISCI and LEMS: sign ↑ Ambulate without manual assistance: ±50%
Wirz (2005)	Pre-exp./ Quality score: 28/48	2xC3, 5xC5, 2xC6, 2xC7, 1xT1, 2xT8, 1xT9 2xT10, 3xL1 / C/D (I)	5x2y, 5x3y, 3x4y, 2x6y, 1x8y, 1x10y, 1x13y, 1x16y, 1x17y	20	Lokomat / 45', 3-5x/w for 8w (24-37 sessions)			WISCI II: ↑ 10MWT: ↑(mean 0.11±10m/s, 56%±60%) 6MWT: ↑(mean 32.3±37,5m, 53%±50%) Timed up & go test: ↑(mean 25±30s, 32%±19%) LEMS**: ↑(mean 2.5 - initially: 32, finally: 35) Ashworth scale**: no changes SCATS**: ↓extensor spasm score
Freivogel (2008)	Pre-exp./ Quality score: 25/48	T12 / C(I)	16m	1	LokoHelp / 30', 3-5x/w for 6w (20 sessions)			FAC: initially: 0, finally: 3 10MWT: initially: unable, finally: 0,2 Motricity Index: initially: 67, finally: 73 Berg Balance Scale: initially: 13, finally: 13 Modified Ashworth scale: initially: 0, finally: 0 Rivermead mobility index: initially: 5, finally: 7
Winchest er (2005)	Pre-exp./ Quality score: 24/48	2xC5, 2xC6 / C/D (I)	14w, 6m, 1y, 4y	4	Lokomat / 60' (≥ 20min as + OT), 3x/w for 12w			WISCI II: ↑ Gait speed: ↑ Assistive device: P1: stand with assistance → ambulating+single-tip cane P2: walker+AFO+manual assistance → single tip cane+AFO P3: unable to stand → ambulate+walker+manual assistance P4: unable to stand → unable to stand
Hornby (2005) a	Pre-exp./ Quality score: 20/48	C6, T2 / C (I)		2	Lokomat / 60', 1-3x/w for 7-9w (20-27 sessions) *			LEMS: initially: 19-31, finally: 46-30 FIM: initially: 0-5, finally: 5-6 WISCI II: initially: 0-13, finally: 13-13 Gait speed: initially: 0.11m/s (p2), finally: 0.36-0.14m/s Gait endurance: initially: 100ft (p2), finally: 460-179ft Functional Reach Test: initially: >10 (p2), finally: >10->10 Modified Sitting FRT: initially: 10 (p2), finally: 6-7

Table 1: Legend: TT: treadmill training, OT: overground training, FIM-L: Functional Independence Measure-Locomotor subscale, LEMS: Lower extrimity motor score, 10MWT: 10 meter walk test, 6MWT: 6 minutes walk test, SCATS: Spinal cord assessment tool for spasticity, WISCI: Walking index for spinal cord injury, FAC: Functional ambulation categories. *Only this study describe co-interventions (physical and occupational therapy), **n=10, in 1 of the 4 centers.

References

[1] Field-Fote E, Lindley S & Sherman A. *Locomotor training approaches for individuals with spinal cord injury: a preliminary report of walking-related outcomes.* Journal of neurological physical therapy 2005; 29(3): 127-37

[2] Freivogel S, Mehrholz J, Husak-Sotomayor T & Schmalohr D. *Gait training with the newly developed 'lokohelp'-system is feasible for non-ambulatory patients after stroke, spinal cord and brain injury. a feasibility study.* Brain Inj 2008; 22(7-8): 625-32

[3] Hornby TG, Zemon DH & Campbell D. *Robotic-assisted, body-weight-supported treadmill training in individuals following motor incomplete spinal cord injury.* Phys Ther 2005; 85(1): 52-66

[4] Hornby TG, Campbell DD, Zemon DH & Kahn JH. *Clinical and quantitative evaluation of robotic-assisted treadmill walking to retrain ambulation after spinal cord injury.* Top Spinal Cord Inj Rehabil 2005; 11(2): 1-17

[5] Winchester P, McColl R, Querry R, Foreman N, Mosby J, Tansey K et al. *Changes in supraspinal activation patterns following robotic locomotor therapy in motor-incomplete spinal cord injury.* The American Society of Neurorehabilitation 2005; 19(4): 313-24

[6] Wirz M, Zemon DH, Rupp R, Scheel A, Colombo G, Dietz V et al. *Effectiveness of automated locomotor training in patients with chronic incomplete spinal cord injury: a multicenter trial.* Arch Phys Med Rehabil 2005; 86: 672-80

7.3

Poster Presentations

Rehabilitation: Mobility, Exercise and Sports
L.H.V. van der Woude et al. (Eds.)
IOS Press, 2010
© 2010 The authors and IOS Press. All rights reserved.
doi:10.3233/978-1-60750-080-3-285

285

Therapeutic activities in 3 Dutch SCI rehabilitation centers recorded with the Spinal Cord Injury – Interventions Classification System (SCI-ICS)

A.H.B. VAN LANGEVELD[a,b], M.W.M. POST[a,b], F.W.A. VAN ASBECK[a], K. POSTMA[c], J. LEENDERS[a], P. TER HORST[c], H. RIJKEN[d], E. LINDEMAN[a,b]

[a] *Rehabilitation Center De Hoogstraat, Utrecht*
[b] *Rudolf Magnus Institute for Neuroscience, Utrecht*
[c] *Rijndam Rehabilitation center, Rotterdam*
[d] *Rehabilitation center St. Maartenskliniek, Nijmegen*
Utrecht

Abstract. The purpose of this study was. to examine the contents of therapy directed at self-care and mobility for patients with a spinal cord injury (SCI) in inpatient rehabilitation. Therapists from 3 Dutch rehabilitation centers used the SCI-ICS to record treatment sessions of patients with a SCI over a period of 4 weeks.The SCI-ICS consists of 25 categories at 3 levels of functioning (body functions, basic activities, and complex activities) and 139 different interventions. Time spent on different levels, categories, and types of interventions, was used to describe similarities and differences between the centers. Therapists (n=53) recorded 1640 treatment sessions of 48 patients. Most time was spent on interventions to improve muscle power, walking and wheelchair propulsion. Although differences were found, over-all the findings indicate that the 3 Dutch centers provided similar therapy programs.

Keywords. spinal cord injuries, rehabilitation, interventions.

1. Introduction

Research on spinal cord injury (SCI) rehabilitation has emphasized the contributions made by therapeutic activities involving physical therapy (PT), occupational therapy, (OT) and sports therapy to the improvement of physical performance and capacity regarding mobility and self-care by SCI patients. [1] To correlate the complex and broad range of rehabilitation interventions with outcomes, specification of the many treatments is required. Describing the contents of interventions, by means of uniform concepts and language would enable us to create a basis to correlate interventions with rehabilitation outcomes. Since no such classification system was available for therapeutic interventions in SCI rehabilitation, we developed the spinal cord injury-interventions classification system (SCI-ICS) for the main domains of SCI rehabilitation, mobility and self-care. [2-4]

The purpose of the present study is to compare therapy provided to patients with SCI in 3 different centers in the Netherlands.

2. Methods

Design

Therapists from rehabilitation center St. Maartenskliniek, Nijmegen, Rijndam, Rotterdam, and The Hoogstraat, Utrecht, used the SCI-ICS to record interventions provided to patients with SCI in their initial rehabilitation after acquiring SCI over a period of 4 weeks. Preset minimum of number of recorded treatment sessions was set at 250 per center.

Participants

Therapists
Twenty PT, 16 OT, 4 sports therapists, 9 PT assistants, 3 PT students and 1 sports therapy student from 3 Dutch specialized rehabilitation centers.

Patients
Eleven patients with motor complete paraplegia (Asia impairment Scale (AIS) A, B), 15 with motor incomplete paraplegia (AIS C, D, E), 9 with motor complete tetraplegia, and 13 patients with motor incomplete tetraplegia were included.

Instrumentation

Therapists were asked to record each treatment session on a separate recording form. The recording form allowed users to record 5 different interventions with 4 or 5 digit codes from the SCI-ICS and to record the time spent on each intervention, in 5-minute increments. The percentage of time spent on interventions at (1) the 3 levels (body functions, basic activities and complex activities), (2) the 25 categories (e.g. muscle power, transfers), and (3) the types of interventions (exercises, assessment, education, equipment and unspecified) was used to describe similarities and differences in treatment sessions between the 3 centers.

Statistics

Descriptive statistics were used for the distribution and time spent on the SCI-ICS interventions.

3. Results

Therapists recorded 1640 treatment sessions with a total of 2596 interventions and a total time of 45925 minutes. The total number of recorded treatment sessions and total therapy time varied by center ($p=>0.05$). The mean number of treatment sessions per patient per week and the mean time per treatment session per patient differed by center ($p=<0.05$). The total time per patient per week did not differ significantly ($p=>0.05$).

All patients received PT, 93.8 % (45/48) received OT, and 56.3% (27/48) received sports therapy. The percentage of provided therapy by discipline varied by center. In all 3 centers the highest percentage of treatment sessions was delivered by the PT, and the lowest percentage by the sports therapists. The PT spent most time on the categories Walking , Muscle power and Joint mobility, the OT on the on Arm and hand use,

Muscle power and Using or driving of transportation. The sports therapists spent most time on the categories Using or driving a hand rim wheelchair, handcycle or bicycle, Swimming, and Cardiovascular system. Highest mean time for all 3 centers was found in the categories Muscle Power, Walking, and Using or driving a hand rim wheelchair, handcycle or bicycle. In the centers the least time was spent on interventions in the categories Neuropathic pain, Eating and drinking, and Toileting. The distribution of time spent on interventions in the categories differed by center and by discipline. In all 3 centers together, most time (84%) was spent on exercise interventions. The percentage of time spent on the types of interventions varied by center and by discipline.

4. Conclusion

In this study we described the contents of therapy provided to patients with a SCI in different specialized SCI rehabilitation centers. The results demonstrated differences and similarities in contents of therapy between centers. Over-all, the 3 Dutch SCI rehabilitation centers provide similar therapy to patients with a SCI.

References

[1]   Noreau L et al, Spinal cord injury, exercise and quality of life *Sports Med. 20* (1995); 227-250.
[2]   Langeveld SA van et al, Development of a classification system of physical, occupational, and sports therapy interventions to document mobility and self-care in spinal cord injury rehabilitation. *J Neurol Phys Ther* **32** (2008); 2-7.
[3]   Langeveld SA van et al, Feasibility of a Classification System for Physical Therapy, Occupational Therapy, and Sports Therapy Interventions for Mobility and Self-Care in Spinal Cord Injury Rehabilitation. *Arch Phys Med Rehabil* **89** (2008); 1454-1459.
[4]   Langeveld SA van et al, Reliability of a new classification system for mobility and self-care in spinal cord injury rehabilitation: the Spinal Cord Injury- Interventions Classification System. *Arch Phys Med Rehabil* (2009). In press.

Rehabilitation: Mobility, Exercise and Sports
L.H.V. van der Woude et al. (Eds.)
IOS Press, 2010
© *2010 The authors and IOS Press. All rights reserved.*
doi:10.3233/978-1-60750-080-3-288

Benefits of virtual sports, Wii-Sport activity for children with cerebral palsy in the Pető Institute

Z.S. SARINGER-SZILARD
Pető Institute, Budapest, Hungary

Abstract. Would you have thought that a person with Cerebal Palsy (CP) – no matter how severe the injury is –can play tennis, golf, and box and can achieve the same results like their healthy fellows, can break out in sweat, develop muscle fatigue and fight to win a point? All this, despite the fact that people with cerebral palsy characteristically have little muscle on them, are overweight beyond their teenage years, have coordination problems, and can have sensory injuries, which may impede locomotory experiences as well as a lack of attention and concentration. We have used the virtual world to assist us. Using the Wii console we studied the effects of play on 10-18 year old children with CP (N=19) over a period of 30 weeks. The physical, psychological and mental tests we conducted at the outset and the end of the study has provided a good evidence of the changes we have observed. The results of the work we have performed have shown well that playful exercise tasks had a beneficial impact on the psychological status; children experienced a sense of success, which motivated them to work on, to develop while playing, and to become more active, while practice and play also resulted in muscle development. Their cognitive function was also positively influenced (attention, memory and concentration). There was development of the locomotory condition of even the very gravely injured children with CP, their injured side became more active, in the case of atetotic children there was improvement in their targeted movements, whereas the endurance of diplegic and the fine motorics of the tetraparetic children also improved.

Keywords. cerebral palsy, adapted PE, virtual sport, activity, leisure time, sports experience, conductive education .

1. Introduction

Research has shown that one third of 10-18 year old boys and one fifth of the girls nowadays have some sort of a game console in their rooms. The attractiveness of the virtual world is supported by the fact that computer games are in a leading position when it comes to all game categories sold. Adolescent children with disabilities show the same kind of attraction to computer games as their healthy peers.

This attraction to the virtual world is rooted in the fact that here the players can realise dreams and desires, can fulfil needs that they cannot in the real world. Virtual reality is built up in such a way that it can cater for needs that the natural environment cannot or does not wish to fulfil. It can help to momentarily change the state of our mind, to forget daily problems, since an imaginary world does not need to be as depressing as reality is sometimes. We are attracted to such types of games, because here we have the opportunity more often to experience a feeling or a mood that we miss or lack. Play transports the player from the real time situations to virtual worlds, however excessive virtual gaming can lead to an addiction. The question is, whether such games are harmful for children or not?

2. About the research project

The project I am conducting now, aims to present a new, completely safe side of the virtual world and to present how exercise and play can be combined. The virtual world can help those with disabilities to adopt and even practice a healthy lifestyle that is possible for others in the real world.

Up until the autumn of 2006, many were on the opinion that people with disabilities had little or no opportunities for leisure sports. I too shared this opinion to some extent. Thanks to the advances of computer technology, this was the first computer game which was not about pushing buttons to move a virtual player, but instead the player actually has to perform the same movements that he/she wants the virtual player to do. Thus at least for the duration of the game, a player can become a real tennis player. For all sports on the console, the movements to perform copy the real movements of the real sports discipline (hit a ball with a racket, roll a ball etc.)

For the first time in Hungary, cerebral paretic children, adolescents and adults have the possibility to get acquainted and to practice with 5 sport disciplines (tennis, boxing, golf, bowling and baseball) with the help of a virtual game console. Virtual games allows the players to transport themselves from the real world into a virtual one, where they can play and execute sports movements with their hands (Wii Sports), with their feet (Wii Fit) when playing ball games (tennis, golf, bowling), winter sports (ski jumping, snowboarding, skiing), contact sports (boxing) and even fun games (like hullahoop) or balancing games, which can all play an important role in adopting and leading a healthy life-style.

This year we measured personal factors of children between 7-18 years, did physical, psychological and mental tests with them on three occasions. We carried out an initial survey in September 2008, which provided a good basis for us to obtain an overall picture of the general conditional and psychological status of 10-18 year old children (N=19). We also included a control group in the survey (N=18). Two-third of the children involved in the work are boys, the majority of them (63%) suffering from tetraparesis spastica, while 10-10% have diplegia spastica and athetosis. In the period that followed we had two groups of upper elementary school students play Wii Sports and Wii Fit with weekly regularity (one hour sessions) under professional supervision.

Virtual games allow children to test themselves in different sports disciplines. We allowed the children to decide themselves, which sports discipline they wanted to play regularly after having tried all the different sports and ability games. On the first and the last occasion we also recorded data (BPFT) on general physical stamina (abdomen, back, arm, balance, flexibility) which were adapted to take note of their physical disabilities. We used a questionnaire to keep track of psychological changes. We were in continuous contact with conductors and recorded the changes they saw and we also distributed a questionnaire among them.

3. Results

During the course of the study children not only had the opportunity to practice and play different sports games, but at the same time, they also learned the rules of the given sport. It became evident during the duration of the play, that when play started the atmosphere changed, the children became preoccupied with what they were doing; it was evident that they lived their part and enjoyed the sports exercise. Children with CP, thanks to this program experienced the joy of sports and exercise, the feeling of exhaustion, competition and the possibility of relieving tension through sports. One hour of exercise does not satisfy the needs of children with disabilities, yet we saw that even this much exercise resulted in a change. Thanks to this play they showed changes in their psychological status, which also had an influence on their motor status. Play allowed them to freely articulate their feelings, sentiments while they could also ease any tension they had in them.

Measurement results have shown that all those who carried out some sort of sports activities have developed more perseverance (75%) and 38% have shown an improvement in their conditional status, with improved coordination capabilities, reaction time and sense of rhythm. We have also seen that some children with severe disabilities (4 children) showed an outstanding improvement in their ability to play. During the course of the play we saw significant changes in improved movements and motor performance of moves required for play. The Wii console counts and keeps track of the results, which proved to be a further source of feedback and motivation for the children. 58% of those surveyed had doubled their initial scores, while by the end of the study 18% of the children achieved results which were two-thirds better than their initial scores. There were some children (N=4) who because of the severity of their injury (typically impaired coordination in the upper limbs) could only play with Wii Fit. The duration of play was always the same (60 minutes) but the quality of play improved continuously, which was evidenced by increased scores and decreased level of mistakes.

4. Conclusion

Results have shown that the main objectives of the research have been achieved. Regular physical activity and playful sports had a positive effect on adolescent children with disabilities. Increasing the time of play may even result in better results. The virtual world offering the possibility of sports provides a good opportunity for people with disabilities to be engaged in active sports exercise, to acquire skills and abilities which are important in sports, to be willing to play for victory, to learn endurance and to be able to fight for a result or an objective. Sports activity has brought about changes in circulation and breathing, the feeling of playing together, the notion of fair play as an important pattern of behaviour are all important results. The computer has become an integral part of the life of 10-18 year olds, thus this console has combined play, sports exercise and amusement to develop the children. We wish to continue our work in the future and to extend it to other forms of disability.

References

[1]   Zsuzsanna Saringer Szilard, 2009. Wi(i)nning is easy! Would you have thought that a person with Cerebral Palsy could play tennis, golf, or box? Research in sport science. Data2win LtD. UK 271-275 p.

[2]   Sáringerné Dr. Szilárd Zsuzsanna – Nádasi Zsófia *Virtuális sport, mint szabadidős tevékenység a Pető Intézetben Magyar Sporttudományi Szemle 10. évfolyam. 37. szám. 2009/1. 28-29. o.*

Rehabilitation: Mobility, Exercise and Sports
L.H.V. van der Woude et al. (Eds.)
IOS Press, 2010
© 2010 The authors and IOS Press. All rights reserved.
doi:10.3233/978-1-60750-080-3-291

The influence of patient values on the adjustment of the inclusion criteria for a low back stabilizing exercise program: a case report

H.P.L.M. VOSSEN[a], K. BARTHOLOMEEUSEN[b], P. HUISMAN[c]

[a] *Fysio/manueeltherapeut Heliomare revalidatie te Wijk aan Zee.Docent (minikliniek) opleiding Master Manuele Therapie, SOMT te Amersfoort. Bestuurslid Nederlandse Vereniging voor Manuele Therapie (NVMT), beroepsinhoud en wetenschap*
[b] *Tutor opleiding Master Manuele Therapie SOMT te Amersfoort. Sportfysio/manueeltherapeut Bartholomeeusen te Lier, België Praktijkvaardigheidsdocent ReVaKi, Universiteit Gent*
[c] *Paul Huisman, Fysio/manueeltherapeut Praktijk Fysio-Manuele Therapie Huisman te Eelde-Paterswolde*

Abstract. The authors discuses the influence of a patient of the inclusion criteria for a low back stabilizing exercise program. If you have any questions regarding this case, please contact the Rehabilitation Centre Heliomare by e-mail: *h.vossen@heliomare.nl*.

Keywords. [MeSH]: chronic back pain, multidisciplinary back training , motor control impairments, program evaluation.

1. Introduction

Multidimensional factors contribute to the manifestation of chronic low back pain and the treatment. The results of the standardized program as used in our setting is moderate and it's unclear whether the inclusion criteria meet the requirements for a better outcome. The authors tried to investigate the influence of patient values on the adjustment of the inclusion criteria for a low back stabilizing exercise program.

2. Objective

Enhancing the outcome of a standardized exercise program used for chronic low back pain patients classified with lumbar segmental instability by adjustment of the inclusion criteria.

3. Methods

A 50 year old woman sub classified as lumbar segmental instability was treated in our centre with the standardized back exercise program during 12 weeks. See figure 1 and

2. The study was evaluated on inclusion criteria in relation to patient values and the perceived effect.

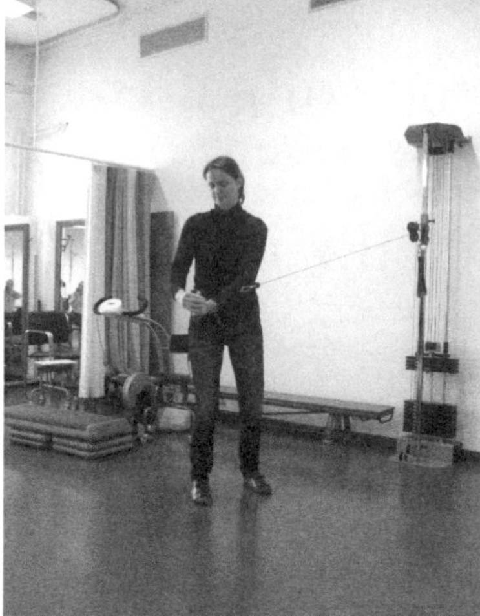

Figure 1. Patient in Rehabilitation Center Heliomare with Pully®..

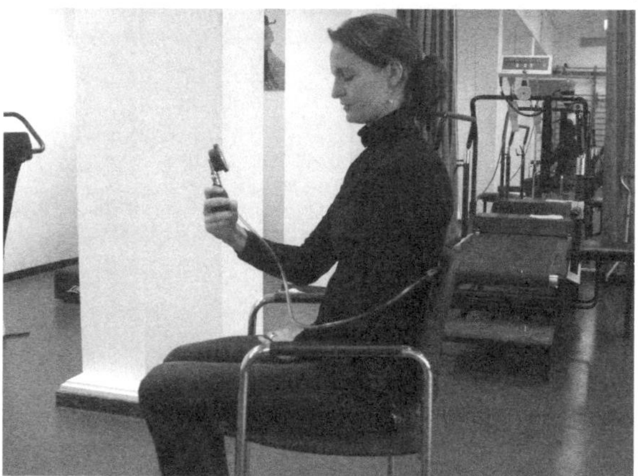

Figure 2. Patient in Rehabilitation Center Heliomare with Stabiliser®.

4. Results

At the level of impairment, the outcome was satisfactory but no results on activity level could be obtained. See figure 2. The fear of "give way" in the low back persisted. In a second part of the treatment, exercises were focused "Graded Exposure". There was a relevant improvement on activity level.

Measurements	Baseline	After 1e intervention	After 2e intervention	Range
VAS -pain	43	30	0	0-100
VAS –activity	42	29	15	0-100
TSK	33	22	18	17-68
RDQ	14	5	4	0-24
PSK	348	321	12	0-500

Figure 3. Patient in Rehabilitation Center Heliomare

- VAS-pain: Visual Analoge Scale -pijn
- VAS-act. : Visual Analoge Scale –activiteiten
- PSK: Patient Specific Complaints

5. Conclusion

The results of this case report suggest that current used inclusion criteria aren't sufficient. Further research is needed focused on the additional value of patient values or the use of a two track policy.

References

[1]   *Tulder JA van, Koes BW, Bouter LMA*. Cost-of illness study of backpain in the Netherlands. Pain. 1995; 62:232-240.

[2]   *Skouen SJ, Grasdal AL, Haldorsen EMH, Ursin H*. Relative Cost-Effectiveness of Extensive and Light Multidisciplinary Treatment Program Versus Treatment as Usual for Patients With Chronic Low Back Pain on Long-Term Sick Leave. Randomised Controled Study. Spine. 2002; 27(9):901-910.

[3]   *World Health Organization (WHO)*. Het ICF-model. Nederlandse vertaling WHO-FIC Collaborating Centre in the Netherlands. RIVM, Bilthoven. 2002.

[4]   *Vossen HPLM*. Evaluatie multiprofessioneel revalidatieprogramma.Tijdschrift Manuele Therapie (TMT). 2007; 4(2)18-26.

[5]   *O'Sullivan P*. Clinical instability of the lumbar spine: its pathological basis, diagnosis and conservative management. Grieve's modern manual therapy. Boyling, Elsevier; 2004; 7:311–31.

[6]   *Dankaerts W, O'Sullivan PB, Burnett AF, Straker LM*. The use of a mechanism-based classification system to evaluate and direct management of a patient with non-specific chronic low back pain and motor control impairment--a case report. Manual Therapy. 2007; 12(2):181-91.

[7]   *Fritz JM, Erhard RE, Hagen BF*. Segmental instability of the lumbar spine. Physical Therapy, 1998; 78(8): 889-895.

[8]   *Hicks GE, Fritz JM, Delitto A, Mishock J*. Interrater reliability of clinical examination measures for identification of lumbar segmental instability. Arch Phys Med Rehabil. 2003; 84:1858-1864.

[9]   *Panjabi MM*. Clinical spinal instability and low back pain. Journal of Electromyography and Kinesiology 2003;13:371-379.

[10] *Panjabi M*. The stabilizing system of the spine, part I and II. Journal of spinal disorders, 1992; 5(4): 383-397.

[11] *Hicks EG, Fritz M, Delitto A, McGill SM*. Preliminary Development of a Clinical Predicion Rule for Determining Wich Patients With Low Back Pain Will Respond to a Stabilization Exercise Programm. Arch Phys Med Rehabil. 2003; 84:1858-1864.

[12] *Cook C Brismee, JM, Sizer PS jr*. Subjectieve and objectieve descriptors of clinical lumbar spine instability: A Delphi study. Manual Therapy 2006 ;11(1):11-21.

[13] *Hides JA, et all*. Effect of stabilization training on multifidus muscle cross-sectional area among young elite cricketers with low back pain. J Orthop Sports Phys Ther. 2008 Mar;38(3):101-8.

[14] *Ferreira PH, Ferreira ML, Maher CG, Herbert RD, Refshauge K*. Specific stabilisation exercise for spinal and pelvic pain: a systematic review. Aust J Physiother. 2006;52(2):79-88.

[15] *Standaert CJ, Weinstein SM, Rumpeltes. J*. Evidence-informed management of chronic low back pain with lumbar stabilization exercises. Spine J. 2008 Jan-Feb;8(1):114-20.

[16] *O' Sullivan PB*. Lumbar segmental "instability": clinical presentation and specific stabilizing exercise management. Manual Therapy. 2000; 5(1): 2-12.

[17] *Cholewicki J, McGill SM*. Mechanical stability of the in vivolumbar spine: implications for injury and chronic low back pain. Clin Biomech (Bristol, Avon) 1996;1 l:l-15.

[18] *Vlaeyen JW, et al*. Graded exposure in vivo in the treatment of pain-related fear: a replicated single-case experimental design in four patients with chronic low back pain. Behav Res Ther. 2001; 9(2):151-66.

Rehabilitation: Mobility, Exercise and Sports
L.H.V. van der Woude et al. (Eds.)
IOS Press, 2010

doi:10.3233/978-1-60750-080-3-294

Muscle activity patterns during robotic walking and overground walking in patients with stroke

G. VAN WERVEN[a,b,1], P. COENEN[a,b], M.P.M. VAN NUNEN[a,b]
H.L. GERRITS[a,b], T.W.J. JANSSEN[a,b]
[a] *Duyvensz-Nagel Research Laboratory, Rehabilitation Centre Amsterdam,*
The Netherlands
[b] *Research Institute MOVE, Faculty of Human Movement Sciences,*
VU University Amsterdam, The Netherlands

Abstract. The aim of the present study was to examine the muscle activity of patients with stroke during robotic walking. In the robotic walking condition (RWC), subjects (n=10) walked in a robotic walking device with minimal support and a walking speed of 2.2 km/h. In the overground walking condition (OWC), subjects walked without any assistance on their preferred walking speed. The results showed significant differences between conditions in individual phases of the gait cycle. Thereby, a significant lower EMG amplitude was found in the RWC compared to the OWC. Furthermore, significant interaction effects were found indicating a higher activity of the paretic semitendinosus and gastrocnemius muscle during the RWC compared to the OWC, supporting the use of robot treadmill training after stroke.

Keywords. robotic orthosis, gait, stroke, EMG, rehabilitation.

1. Introduction

Often reported results of stroke are a decreased walking speed and stride length as well as an asymmetric walking pattern [1]. Since the improvement of walking ability is a major determinant to become independent in daily functioning, it is an important aim in rehabilitation after stroke. A method to improve walking ability is robot assisted treadmill training, which assists the lower limbs by providing a normal walking pattern. Whether this training method has an effect on the muscle activity is unknown in patients with stroke. Therefore, the purpose of the present study is to investigate the muscle activity of the lower limb muscles during robot assisted treadmill walking compared to overground walking in patients with stroke.

---

[1] Corresponding Author: G.v.Werven@rcamsterdam.nl

2. Method

Subjects: Ten persons (6 males and 4 females) with chronic stroke, aged 55 ± 11 years with either a left (n=2) or a right (n=8) hemiparesis participated in this study. The mean time since trauma was 65 weeks and all subjects had a Functional Ambulation Category (FAC) score of 5, indicating they were able to walk without assistance.

Protocol: During the robotic walking condition (RWC), subjects walked in a robotic walking device (Lokomat, Hocoma AG) with minimal support (minimal body weight support and guidance force) and a walking speed of 2.2 km/h. In the overground walking condition (OWC), subjects walked without assistance at their preferred walking speed.

Data collection and statistics: In both conditions, electromyographic (EMG) data were collected from seven muscles in both legs: the rectus femoris, semitendinosus, adductor longus, gluteus maximus, gluteus medius, gastrocnemius and the tibialis anterior muscle. Data of ten gait cycles were collected in each condition. Data were subsequently high pass filtered (20 Hz), rectified, low pass filtered (4 Hz), normalized (%maximal EMG amplitude) and divided into seven phases of the gait cycle [2]. For the RWC these phases were determined by a footswitch and the percentages of the gait cycle, while for the OWC these phases were determined by video analysis. Differences in amplitude were investigated by a multifactor ANOVA and an additional t-test (p<.05).

3. Results

The results showed significant differences between conditions in individual phases in several muscles (table 1). Significant lower mean EMG amplitude in the RWC compared to the OWC was found for the rectus femoris, gluteus maximus and tibialis anterior muscle (figure 1). Thereby, significant interaction effects were found for the semitendinosus, gastrocnemius and tibialis anterior muscle.

Table 1. Differences between the RWC and the OWC of the paretic (upper panel) and non-paretic (lower panel) leg. + indicates a significantly higher value of OWC compared to RWC whereas − indicates a significantly lower value of OWC compared to RWC.

Muscle	Initial Loading	Mid Stance	Terminal Stance	Pre Swing	Initial Swing	Mid Swing	Terminal Swing
Rectus Femoris	+						
Semitendinosus			−	−			+
Adductor Longus	+						
Gluteus Maximus	+						+
Gluteus Medius	+	+		−			
Gastrocnemius							
Tibialis Anterior					+	+	+

Muscle	Initial Loading	Mid Stance	Terminal Stance	Pre Swing	Initial Swing	Mid Swing	Terminal Swing
Rectus Femoris							
Semitendinosus	+	+			+	+	+
Adductor Longus					+		
Gluteus Maximus	+						+
Gluteus Medius	+						
Gastrocnemius	+	+	+				
Tibialis Anterior	+				+	+	+

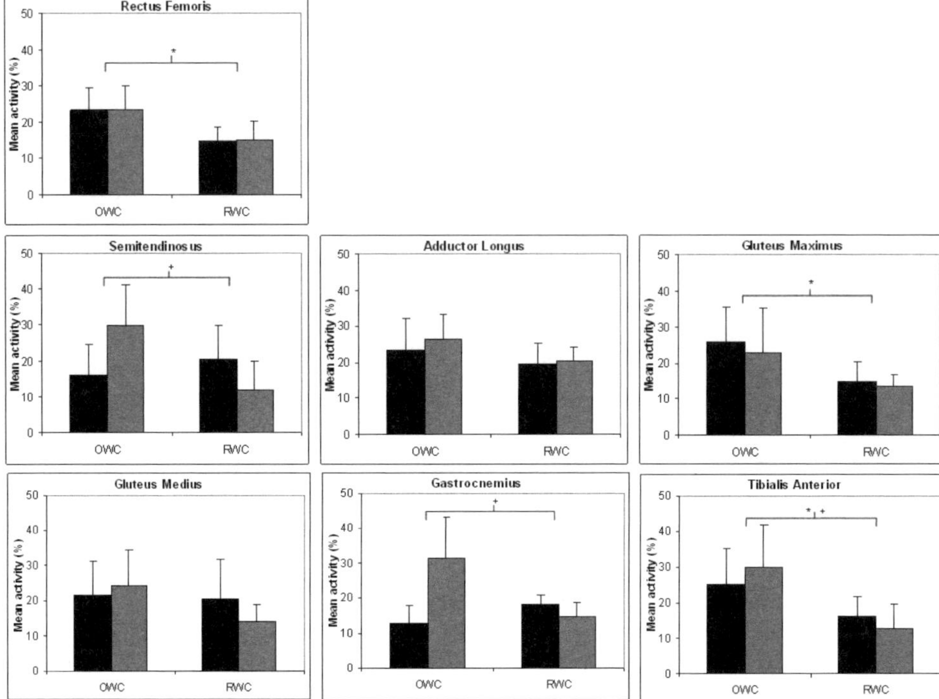

Figure 1. Mean muscle activity during the total gait cycle for the OWC and the RWC in both the paretic (black bars) and the non-paretic (grey bars) leg. * indicates a significant difference between conditions whereas + indicates a significant interaction effect.

4. Conclusion

Differences in muscle activity patterns between robotic walking and overground walking can be seen in individual phases in several muscles. These differences can be explained by both the support of the robotic orthosis and the restriction of leg movements in the saggital plane. The lower mean activity in the RWC compared to the OWC can be explained by the stabilisation of the gait orthosis reducing the co-activation of the lower limb muscles. Furthermore, the support of the gait orthosis reduces the effort of the legs during walking which reduces the muscle activity. However, the interaction effects suggest that although the overall activity of the muscles decreases during robotic walking, the activity of the paretic semitendinosus, gastrocnemius and tibialis anterior muscle have a lower decrease or even an increase during robotic walking, supporting the use of robot assisted treadmill training in rehabilitation after stroke.

References

[1] Giuliani, C.A., *Adult hemiplegic gait, gait in rehabilitation*, Churchill Living Stone, New York, 1990.
[2] Perry, J., *Gait Analysis, Normal and Pathological Function*, Slack Inc, Thorofare, 1992.

Rehabilitation: Mobility, Exercise and Sports
L.H.V. van der Woude et al. (Eds.)
IOS Press, 2010

doi:10.3233/978-1-60750-080-3-297

Body weight-supported gait training for restoration of walking in people with an incomplete spinal cord injury : a systematic review

M. WESSELS[a,1], C. LUCAS[b], I. ERIKS-HOOGLAND[a,c], S. DE GROOT[a,d]
[a] *Rehabilitation Center Amsterdam*
[b] *Department of Clinical Epidemiology and Biostatistics, Academic Medical Centre*
[c] *Swiss Paraplegic Research*
[d] *Centre for Human Movement Sciences, University Medical Centre Groningen, University of Groningen*

Abstract. The purpose of this study was to evaluate the effect of body weight-supported (BWS) gait training on restoration of walking, activities of daily living (ADL) and quality of life (QoL) in persons with an incomplete spinal cord injury (SCI). Datasources: Cochrane, MEDLINE , EMBASE, CINAHL, PEDro and DocOnline. Studies were assessed for methodological quality and described regarding population, training protocol and effects on walking ability, ADL and QoL. A descriptive and quantitative synthesis was conducted. 18 articles/17 studies were included. Two randomized controlled trials (RCTs) showed that subjects with American Spinal Injury Association Impairment Scale (AIS) C or D of less than one year duration reached higher scores on the locomotor item of the Functional Independence Measure (FIM-L, range 1-7) in the over-ground training group than in the BWS treadmill training group at the end of training, mean difference 0.80 (0.04-1.56). There were no differences regarding walking velocity and hardly data on ADL or QoL. Concluded was that subjects with subacute SCIs classified AIS C or D reached a higher level of independent walking after over-ground training compared to BWS treadmill training. More RCTs are needed to clarify the effectiveness of BWS gait training on walking, ADL and QoL for subgroups of persons with incomplete SCIs.

Keywords. spinal cord injuries, gait training, body-weight support, systematic review.

1. Introduction

Gait training techniques using partial body weight-support (BWS) seem to be promising in restoring walking function in people with incomplete spinal cord injuries (SCIs), but the effectiveness of these techniques is still to be determined. The objective of the present study was to evaluate the effectiveness of BWS techniques that facilitate gait training for the recovery of walking function in persons with incomplete SCI by a systematic review of the literature. We also considered its effect on level of

---

[1] Corresponding author. (Monique.Wessels@kpnplanet.nl)

performance of activities of daily living (ADL) and the experienced quality of life (QoL).

2.   Methods

Search strategy for identification of studies

The following databases were searched: Cochrane Central Register of Controlled Trials (Cochrane Library), MEDLINE (PubMed and OVID), EMBASE (OVID), Cumulative Index to Nursing and Allied Health Literature (CINAHL) through OVID, the Physiotherapy Evidence Database (PEDro) and DocOnline, a reference database of the Dutch Institute of Allied Health Professions, from 1980 (CINAHL: 1982) until September 2008. The search was conducted by the first author. Reference lists of all selected trials and of retrieved reviews over the past two years were screened.

Inclusion of studies

Participants: adults (over 18 years) with incomplete SCI classified as American Spinal Injury Association Impairment Scale (AIS) B, C or D.

    Intervention: BWS treadmill training, robotic-assisted BWS treadmill training or gait training in water.

    Comparison: conventional therapy and/or gait training without BWS techniques or no intervention.

    Outcomes: walking ability, ADL and QoL. Gait velocity, motor skills and walking independence were considered indicators of walking ability, and were the outcomes of primary interest.

Randomized controlled trials (RCTs), quasi RCTs and controlled trials were included. Initial exploration of the literature showed that RCTs in this field probably would be scarce. For studies with subjects that were in the chronic phase of injury (> 1 yr) uncontrolled trials were included as well.

Quality assessment

The quality of studies was assessed independently by two reviewers (MW and SdeG) with the checklist developed by Van Tulder (1997). A modified version of the 1997-list was used to assess the quality of uncontrolled trials.

Data analysis

A quantitative synthesis would be undertaken when homogeneity of data and trial design allowed. If a quantitative was not possible, because of clinical heterogeneity, heterogeneity of outcome measures and insufficient reporting of data, a descriptive and best-evidence synthesis was to be conducted rating evidence according to strength.

3.   Results

Study selection

The search retrieved 3022 articles. 18 articles were included in this review, including 3 articles concerning two RCTs.

Outcome of interventions

In this two RCTs, concerning people with subacute SCIs, a pooled mean difference 0.68 (0.09-1.26) was detected between the BWS treadmill training (BWSTT) and over-ground training group regarding walking independence on the locomotor item of the Functional Independent Measure (FIM-L , 1-7) at 8-12 weeks, in favour of over-ground training. Subgroup analysis revealed that the higher score on FIM-L for controls compared with BWSTT was only significant for subjects with AIS C or D, mean difference 0.80 (0.04-1.56), p=0.04. The uncontrolled trials all concerned people with chronic SCIs and presented a diverse picture of modest gains in walking ability.

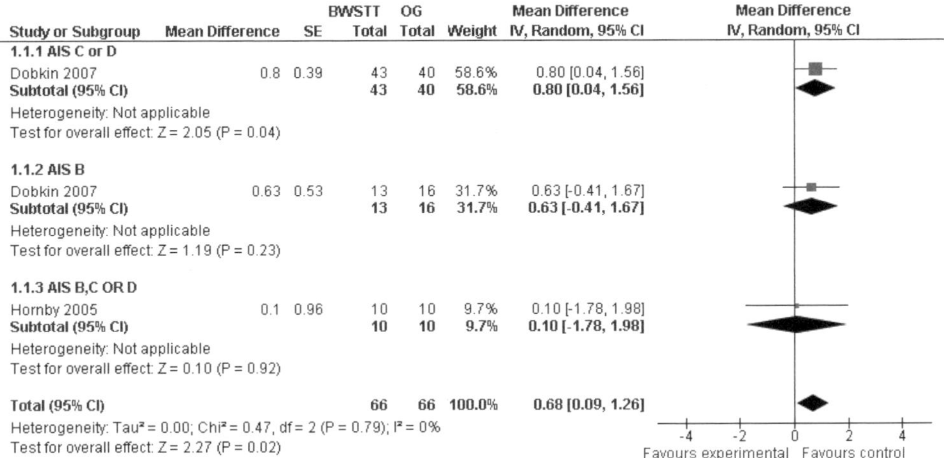

4.   Conclusion

Subjects with incomplete SCIs of less than one year duration reached a significantly higher walking independence (FIM-L) in the over-ground gait training group than subjects in the BWSTT group at the end of training. There were no differences regarding walking velocity and capacity. Subgroup analysis makes clear that this difference in gains in FIM-L were only significant for subjects with AIS C or D. For other BWS interventions or subgroups of participants study groups were too small. The studies did not provide enough data with respect to QoL and ADL.

References

[1]   Dobkin, B. et al. (2006). Weight-supported treadmill vs over-ground training for walking after acute incomplete SCI . Neurology, 66, 484-493.

[2]   Dobkin, B. et al. (2007).The evolution of walking-related outcomes over the first 12 weeks of rehabilitation for incomplete traumatic spinal cord injury: the multicenter randomized spinal cord injury locomotor trial Neurorehabil.Neural Repair, 21, 25-35.

[3]   Hornby, T. G. et al. (2005). Clinical and quantitative evaluation of robotic-assisted treadmill walking to retrain ambulation after spinal cord injury. Top.Spinal Cord Inj.Rehabil., 11, 1-17.

Rehabilitation: Mobility, Exercise and Sports
L.H.V. van der Woude et al. (Eds.)
IOS Press, 2010
© 2010 The authors and IOS Press. All rights reserved.
doi:10.3233/978-1-60750-080-3-300

Effect of 6-week CIMT of the upper extremity on motor function and quality of movement in persons with chronic stroke

N.I. ZIJP [a,1], C. BOERS[a], L. SWAAN[a], N.C. ROELSE[a], A. BLOKHUIS[a], M. TEN KATEN[a], K.N.G. NIENHUYS[a], S. DE GROOT [a,b]

[a] *Rehabilitation Center Amsterdam*
[b] *Centre for Human Movement Sciences, University Medical Centre Groningen, University of Groningen*

Abstract. The purpose of this study was to determine the effectiveness of 6-week constraint-induced movement therapy (CIMT) on motor function and quality of movement in persons with chronic stroke. Furthermore, the relationship between motor function and quality of movement was analyzed. 15 Persons with chronic stroke (time since stroke > 6 months) received 6-weeks of CIMT. Before and after the CIMT program the following tests were performed: Action Research Arm Test (ARAT), Motricity Index (MI), Dutch version of Motor Activity Log amount of use score (MAL-AOU) and quality of movement score (MAL-QOM), Nine-hole peg test (NHPT), and the Erasmus Modified Nottingham Sensory Assessment (EmNSA). Persons with a chronic stroke improved significantly on the ARAT (p=0.05), MI (p=0.02), MAL-AOU (p=0.01), MAL-QOM (p<0.001), NHPT (p=0.02) but not on the EmNSA (p=0.27). After CIMT, the quality of movement (MAL-QOM) was strongly correlated with the amount of use score (MAL-AOU, r=0.94) and the NHPT (r=0.81). Low correlations were found with ARAT (r=0.26), MI (r=0.05) and EmNSA (r=0.29). It can be concluded that a 6-week CIMT program is effective in improving motor function and quality of movement in persons with chronic stroke while sensory function did not improve. quality of movement is strongly related to the speed of task completion but not to strength or dexterity.

Keywords. stroke, CIMT, motor function, quality of movement, effectiveness, therapy-program.

1. Introduction

38% Of stroke survivors regain some dexterity in the paretic arm [1]. Constrained Induced Movement Therapy (CIMT) is an effective treatment for this group, if a person can show at least 10 degrees of finger extension in the affected limb. CIMT includes forced use (i.e. the patient is made to use the hemiparetic upper extremity through immobilization of the better limb in a sling and splint), repetitive task practice and adaptive task practice (also called "shaping") [2]. The CIMT-program of Rehabilitation Center Amsterdam is a 6 week group-therapy program. The purpose of the present study is to evaluate the effect of 6-week CIMT of the upper extremity on motor function and quality of movement in persons with chronic stroke. Furthermore the

---

[1] Corresponding Author: Nienke Zijp; n.zijp@rcamsterdam.nl

relationship between the subjective score of real life functional performance and motor function (e.g. strength, speed of task completion) is determined.

2. Methods

Participants

19 subject (4 male, 15 female) with chronic stroke (time since stroke > 6 months) received 6-weeks of CIMT; 3 days per week, 6 hours per day outpatient therapy, supplemented with home-work assignments. Each group consists of 4-6 patients. Subject characteristics are shown in Table1.

Table 1. Subject characteristics

	Age (yr) Mean (SD)	Time since onset (months) Mean (SD)	Paretic side (right/left)
	54.6 (13.3)	20.2 (17.3)	13/6

Variables

Before and after the CIMT program the following tests were performed: Action Research Arm Test (ARAT), Motricity Index (MI), Motor Activity Log-Amount of Use (MAL-AOU) and the subjective score of real life functional performance (Motor Activity Log -Quality of Movement, MAL-QOM), Nine-hole peg test (NHPT), and the Erasmus modified Nottingham Sensory Assessment (EmNSA).

Statistics

A paired sampled T-test was performed to determine differences between the test results before and after the CIMT program. The relationship between improvement of quality of movement and motor functions was investigated with Spearman correlation coefficient. Level of significance was set at $p<0.05$.

3. Results

Persons with a chronic stroke improved significantly on the ARAT ($p=0.05$), MI ($p=0.02$), MAL-AOU ($p=0.01$), MAL-QOM ($p<0.001$), NHPT ($p=0.02$) but not on the EmNSA ($p=0.27$) (Table 2).

Table 2. Mean (and standard deviation) of pre and post test outcomes.

	ARAT[*] (0-57)	NHPT[*] (pegs/sec.)	MI[*] (0-100)	EmNSA (0-32)	MAL-QOM[*] (0-5)	MAL-AOU[*] (0-5)
range						
Pre	38.9 (14.0)	0.2	77.7 (13.0)	27.7 (7.7)	1.3 (0.8)	1.5 (0.9)
post	44.2 (14.3)	0.3	84.1 (10.4)	28.2 (8.3)	2.1 (1.0)	2.2 (1.0)

ARAT: Action Research Arm Test, MI: Motricity Index, MAL-AOU: Motor Activity Log-Amount of Use, MAL-QOM: Motor Activity Log -Quality of Movement, NHPT: Nine-hole peg test , EmNSA: Erasmus modified Nottingham Sensory Assessment .
* = significant difference at $p<0.05$.

After CIMT, the quality of movement (MAL-QOM) was strongly correlated with the amount of use (MAL-AOU, r=0.94) (Figure 1) and the NHPT (r=0.81)(Figure 2). Low correlations were found with ARAT (r=0.26), MI (r=0.05) and EmNSA (r=0.29).

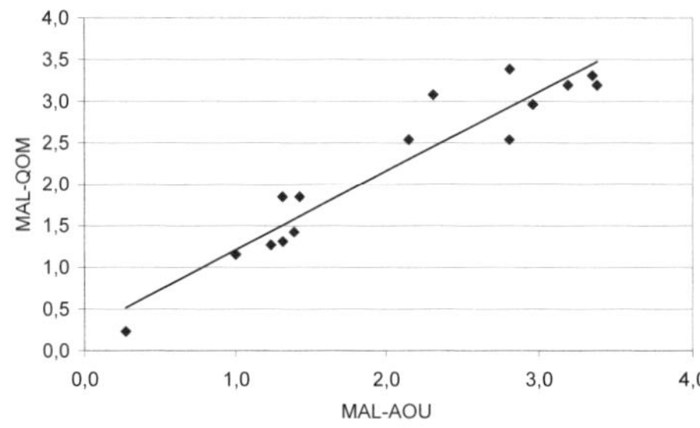

Figure 1. Relation amount of use (MAL-AOU) and quality of movement (MAL-QOM).

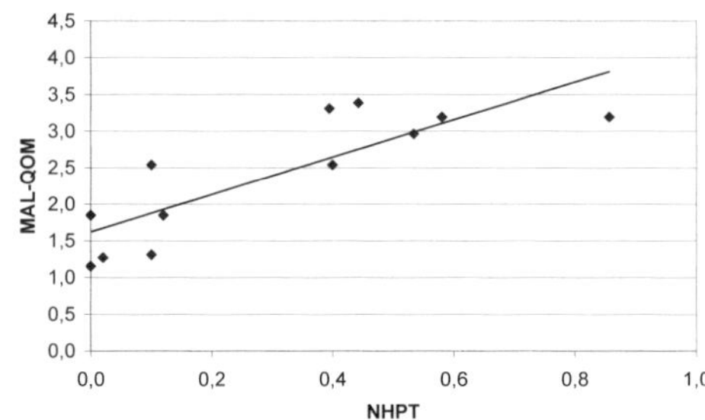

Figure 2. Relation speed of task completion (NHPT) and quality of movement (MAL-QOM).

4.   Conclusion

The CIMT-program of Rehabilitation Center Amsterdam is an effective outpatient-treatment program for chronic stroke-patients with some arm dexterity. An improvement in speed of task completion and amount of use during daily life activities are both related to the subjective score of the quality of real life functional performance.

References

[1]   Kwakkel G, et al. Probability of Regaining Dexterity in the Flaccid Upper Limb; Impact of Severity of Parasis and Time Since Onset in Acute Stroke *Stroke.* 2003; 34(9);2181-2186.
[2]   Wolf SL. Revisiting Contraint-Induced Movement Therapy: Are We Too Smitten With the Mitten? Is All Nonuse "Learned"? and Other Quanderies *Physical Therapy.* 2007;87(9);1212-1223.

Rehabilitation: Mobility, Exercise and Sports
L.H.V. van der Woude et al. (Eds.)
IOS Press, 2010
© 2010 The authors and IOS Press. All rights reserved.
doi:10.3233/978-1-60750-080-3-303

Effects of treadmill training on physical activity in infants at risk for neuromotor delay

R.M. ANGULO-BARROSO[a], L.C. CHEN[a], C.W. TIERNAN[a], M. LLOYD[a],
D.A. ULRICH[a]
School of Kinesiology & CHGD, University of Michigan, Ann Arbor, MI, USA

Abstract. Purpose: To examine the immediate and long term effects of pre-ambulatory treadmill training on the levels of physical activity (PAL) in infants at risk for neuromotor delay (ND). Relationships between PAL and walking onset (WO) were also examined. Method: Twenty eight infants with moderate risk for ND (9.4±1.3 mo) were randomly assigned to a treadmill training (Experimental group-E-TMT) or a control group (C). Infants were tested at home every two months until they walked independently, and 3 more visits at 1, 4, and 7 months of walking experience. Treadmill training was terminated at WO. PAL profiles were recorded using an activity monitor during the intervention and at the 3 follow-up visits. Results: Infants in both groups walked on average around 15 months corrected age. From 10 to 16 months, infants increased PAL (F(3,37)=2.91, p=0.047). However, the E-TMT group showed a suggestive larger amplitude of trunk activity compared to the C group during the intervention. During the follow-up phase, the E-TMT group showed significantly less time spent in high levels of PA at visit 1 compared to the C group (F(2,28)=5.41, p=0.01). PA and WO yielded significant relationships at 10,12, and 14 months for the E group and at 12 month for the C group. Conclusions: The treadmill intervention may facilitate high level of PA but the termination of the training at WO may be counterproductive. Apparently, infants who are more active in early development also show earlier WO. Therapeutic interventions should aim to improve the mobility of these infants at moderate risk for locomotor delay.

Keywords. pediatric rehabilitation, walking onset, treadmill intervention.

1. Introduction

Despite the recognized relevance of physical activity in the development and health of children, assessment of physical activity levels (PAL) in infancy are limited, especially in populations such as those with neuromotor delay (ND). Premature and/or small for gestational age infants with or without perinatal brain injuries are at a higher risk for ND. Research evidence suggests these infants have poorer motor repertoires and lower PAL (Bruggink, et al., 2008; Finn et al, 2002).

A treadmill training (TMT) intervention has been shown to promote motor skill in children with cerebral palsy (Schindl et al., 2000). Similarly, TMT enhanced walking onset (WO) and higher PAL in infants with Down syndrome compared to those without TMT (Angulo-Barroso, et al., 2008). Furthermore, levels of PAL were correlated to onset of independent walking (McKay & Angulo-Barroso, 2006; Lloyd et al., in press).

Objectives:
1. To examine the immediate and long term effects of pre-ambulatory treadmill training on the levels of physical activity (PAL) in infants at risk for neuromotor delay (ND).
2. To examine the relationships between levels of physical activity (PAL) and walking onset (WO) in this population.

2. Method

Participants
N = 28 infants at risk for ND
Randomly assigned to Experimental-TMT group (N=15) or Control group (N=13)
Procedures
Two phases: Intervention and Follow-up
- Intervention: E-TMT group = 8 minutes/day, 5 days/week, TM speed-.2m/s from   entry to WO
- Follow-up: 3 visits at 1, 4, 7 mo. of walking experience

PAL monitored every two months for 24 hours via Actiwatches placed in the trunk and right ankle
Dependent variables
Total and high activity; each with sum amplitude and duration; for both Trunk and Leg.
Statistics
- Repeated Measures ANOVA
- Intervention: (2 groups (E-TMT, C) x 4 months (10, 12, 14, 16 months)
- Follow-up: 2 groups (E-TMT, C) x 3 visits (1,4,7 Walking Experience)

3. Results

1- WALKING ONSET in both groups occurred at an average age of 15mo.
2- PAL – Trunk HIGH PA. Because the results of the leg parallel those of the trunk only the trunk data are shown. Also, the effects found in the total activity were mainly due to the high activity level as compared to the low level of activity; therefore, only trunk high PA is presented and discussed.

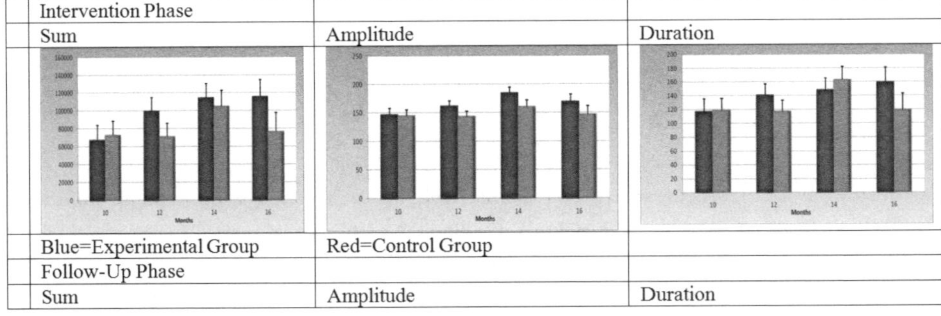

Intervention Phase		
Sum	Amplitude	Duration
Blue=Experimental Group	Red=Control Group	
Follow-Up Phase		
Sum	Amplitude	Duration

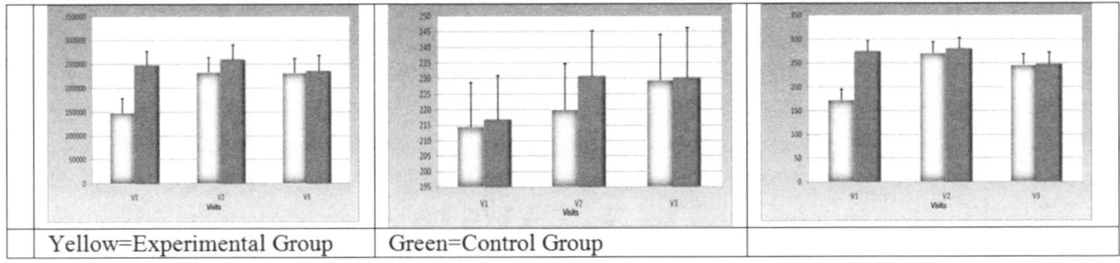

| Yellow=Experimental Group | Green=Control Group | |

3- RELATIONSHIP Trunk High PAL and Walking Onset (WO)

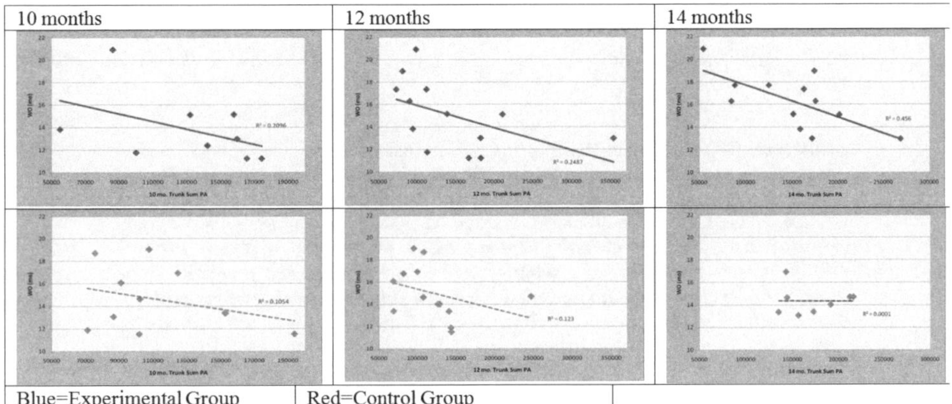

| Blue=Experimental Group | Red=Control Group |

4. Conclusions

The treadmill intervention did not enhance onset of walking since both groups achieved this milestone at similar ages.

However, the treadmill intervention facilitated high level of PA. In addition, the relationship between PA and walking onset was strengthened via the intervention.

The termination of the TMT intervention at WO may be counterproductive since levels of PA were lower in the E-TMT group than the control group at the beginning of the follow-up phase.

In general, infants who are more active in early development also show earlier WO. Overall, the present study suggests that therapeutic interventions should aim to improve the mobility (activity) of infants at moderate risk for neuromotor delay.

References

[3] Bruggink JLM et al. *Journal of Pediatrics,* 153(1):32-9, 2008.
[4] Finn K, et al. *Journal of Pediatrics*, 140:81-85, 2002
[5] Schindl MR, et al. *Arch Phys Med Rehabil.* 81:301-306, 2000
[6] Angulo-Barroso RM et al. *Gait & Posture,* 27:231-238, 2008
[7] McKay, SM & Angulo-Barroso, RM *Infant Behavior & Development,* 29, 153-168, 2006
[8] Lloyd M et al. *Adapted Physical Activity Quarterly,* in press

Acknowledgments: Financial support from the U.S. Office of Special Education & Rehabilitative Services and SteelCase are appreciated.

Rehabilitation: Mobility, Exercise and Sports
L.H.V. van der Woude et al. (Eds.)
IOS Press, 2010
© 2010 The authors and IOS Press. All rights reserved.
doi:10.3233/978-1-60750-080-3-306

Some insights in the metabolic energy cost of Nordic Walking

J.H.P. HOUDIJK

Research Institute MOVE, Faculty of Human Movement Sciences, VU University Amsterdam, The Netherlands
Heliomare Rehabilitation Research and Development, Wijk aan Zee, The Netherlands

Abstract. Purpose: To investigate the paradoxical increase in metabolic energy cost with a suggested decrease in mechanical load on the lower limbs in Nordic Walking compared to normal walking. We hypothesized that the increase in metabolic energy cost could originate from a difference in walking speed or could be attributed solely to the swinging movement of the arm. Methods: In three different sets of experiments subjects walked on a motorized treadmill while metabolic energy consumption and electro-myographical (EMG) activity of selected arm and leg muscles were measured. The effect of walking speed was assessed systematically for both normal and Nordic Walking. The effect of the swinging motion of the arms was assessed by having subjects walk without poles, with normal poles and with poles that were equipped with wheels at the bottom such that the normal arm motion of Nordic Walking was preserved while push off was prevented. Results: Metabolic load in Nordic Walking was significantly higher (20%) compared to normal walking, which was independent of walking speed. EMG of the arm muscles was significantly higher in Nordic Walking compared to normal walking, while only minor differences in leg muscle EMG were found. Simulating arm motion of Nordic Walking using wheeled poles significantly increased metabolic load compared to normal walking but this did not reach the level of unconstrained Nordic Walking. Similarly arm muscle EMG was increased but remained lower compared to normal Nordic Walking. Conclusion: Increased metabolic load of Nordic Walking cannot be accounted for by walking speed and is only partly explained by the swinging motion of the arms. Significant arm muscles action seems devoted to the push off during Nordic Walking although only moderate relief of leg muscle action is found.

Keywords. metabolic energy, energy cost, walking, exercise.

1. Introduction

Nordic Walking (NW) is a type of exercise often used within rehabilitation. It is believed to offer a higher metabolic load [1,2] with a concomitant lower mechanical load [3] on the lower extremities compared to normal walking. It is however unclear how such a paradox between increased metabolic and reduced mechanical load should be explained. When the mechanical load is transferred from the legs to the arms, where does the extra metabolic energy expenditure originate from?

We propose two hypotheses that could solve this paradox: 1) The higher metabolic energy expenditure is a side effect of the higher walking speed that is typically adopted during Nordic Walking, 2) The higher metabolic energy expenditure is accounted for solely by the swinging motion of the arms, which perform little push off work. This latter hypothesis would implicate that similar physiological responses could also be obtained when people walk with exaggerated arm swing without poles, and that the mechanical power for walking would still be generated by the leg muscles.

2. Methods

In three different sets of experiments subjects walked on a motorized treadmill while respiratory data (Oxycon Alpha, Jaeger, Germany) and electro-myographical activity (EMG, TMSi, The Netherlands) of selected arm and leg muscles were measured.

Experiment 1: 10 subjects (novice in NW) walked with and without poles at 4, 5, 6 and 7 km/h while metabolic energy consumption was analyzed.

Experiment 2: 12 subjects (experienced in NW) walked at 5 km/h with and without poles while EMG activity of 3 arm and 6 leg muscles was analyzed.

Experiment 3: 10 subjects (novice in NW) walked at 5 km/h without poles, with normal poles and with poles that were equipped with wheels at the bottom end, such that the normal arm motion of Nordic Walking was preserved while push off was prevented. Metabolic energy consumption and EMG activity of 4 arm muscles was analyzed. Range of motion of the arms was checked through video analysis.

3. Results

Metabolic energy cost per distance traveled (Emet in J/m) was on average 20% higher in Nordic Walking compared to normal walking. This difference was speed independent (Fig 1a).

EMG of the arm muscles was significantly higher in Nordic Walking compared to normal walking, while only minor differences in leg muscle EMG were found (Fig 1b).

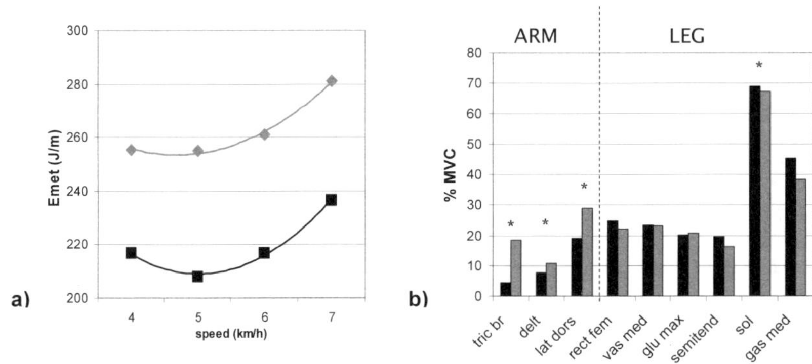

Figure 1. a) Metabolic cost during normal (black) and Nordic Walking (grey) at different walking speeds, b) Muscle activity in selected arm and leg muscles during Nordic Walking (grey bars) and normal walking (black bars). * denotes significant difference (p<0.05)

Simulating arm motion of Nordic Walking using wheeled poles significantly increased metabolic load compared to normal walking but this did not reach the level of unconstrained Nordic Walking. Similarly arm muscle EMG was increased in the wheeled poles condition but remained lower compared to Nordic Walking (Fig 2). The m. biceps brachii could be classified as a pure arm swing muscle and the m. deltoideus as a push off muscle. The m. triceps brachii and latissimus dorsi showed intermediate EMG activity between normal and Nordic Walking in the wheeled poles condition and therefore seem to assist both arm swing and push off.

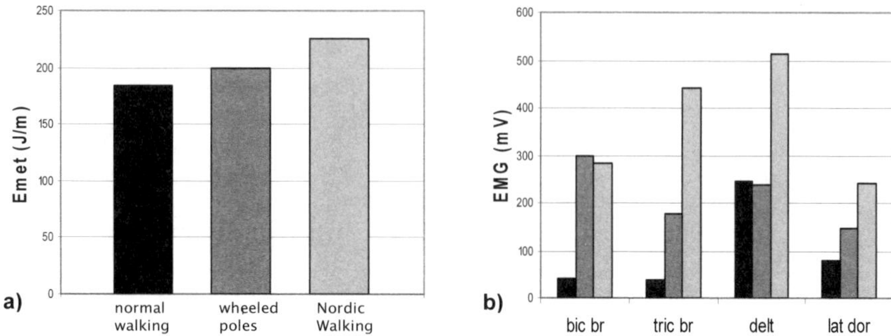

Figure 2. Metabolic load (a) and arm muscle activity (b) in normal walking (black), walking with wheeled poles (dark grey) and Nordic Walking (light grey).

4. Conclusion

In this study it was found that higher metabolic load of Nordic Walking compared to normal walking cannot be explained by differences in walking speed. In addition, we showed that this extra metabolic load can only partially be explained by the enhanced arm swing motion in Nordic Walking. Hence, instructing people to walk with exaggerated arm swing during their exercise will not replace the extra metabolic demand as found in Nordic Walking.

Apparently, significant arm muscle activity is devoted to the push off in Nordic Walking. However, because of the increased metabolic energy cost and the limited relief of the leg muscles as found in this and other studies [4], it can be wondered whether the push off work of the arms really replaces the push off work (and hence mechanical burden) of the leg muscles. The mechanical power generated during push off with the arms and legs during Nordic Walking needs to be the topic of further study

Acknowledgement
V. van Schijndel, H. Vos, S. Algera, J. van der Heeden, E. Leffelaar, R. Galiart, F. Koppenol, T. Schoots and J. Verlaan are acknowledged for their assistance in data acquisition and analyses.

References

[1]   Church T.S., C.P. Earnest, G.M. Morss. Field testing of physiological responses associated with Nordic Walking. Research Quarterly for Exercise and Sport, 73(3), 296-300, 2002
[2]   Porcari J.P., T.L. Hendrickson, P.R. Walter, L. Terry, G. Walsko. The physiological responses to walking with and without Power Poles on dtreadmill exercise. Research Quarterly for Exercise and Sport, 68(2), 161-166, 1997
[3]   Willson J., M.R. Torry, M.J. Decker, T. Kernozek, J.R. Steadman. Effects of walking poles on lower extremity gait mechanics. Medicine and Science in Sports and exercise, 33(1), 142-147, 2001
[4]   Stief F. F.I. Kleindienst, J. Wiemeyer, F. Wedel, S. Campe, B. Krabbe. Inverse dynamics analysis of the lower extremities during nordic walking, walking and running. Journal of Applied Biomechanics, 24, 351-359, 2008.

Chapter 8

FES

8.1

Oral Presentations

Rehabilitation: Mobility, Exercise and Sports
L.H.V. van der Woude et al. (Eds.)
IOS Press, 2010

311

doi:10.3233/978-1-60750-080-3-311

Effect of functional electrostimulation on impaired skin vasodilator responses to local heating in spinal cord injury

D.H.J. THIJSSEN[a,b], N.T.L. VAN DUIJNHOVEN[b], T.W.J. JANSSEN[c,d], D.J. GREEN[a,e], C.T. MINSON[f], M.T.E. HOPMAN[b]

[a]*Research Institute for Sport and Exercise Science, Liverpool John Moores University, Liverpool, United Kingdom;* [b]*Department of Physiology, Radboud University Nijmegen Medical Centre, The Netherlands;* [c]*Faculty of Human Movement Sciences, VU University, Amsterdam, The Netherlands;* [d]*Duyvensz-Nagel Research Laboratory, Rehabilitation Center, Amsterdam, The Netherlands;* [e]*School of Sport Science, Exercise and Health, The University of Western Australia, Crawley, Western Australia;* [f]*Department of Human Physiology, University of Oregon, Eugene, United States*

Abstract. Spinal cord injury (SCI) induces vascular adaptations below the level of the lesion, such as impaired cutaneous vasodilation. However, the mechanisms underlying these differences are unclear. The aim of this study is to examine arm and leg cutaneous vascular conductance (CVC)-responses to local heating in 17 able-bodied controls (39±13 years) and 18 SCI subjects (42±8 years). SCI subjects were counterbalanced for functional electro-stimulation(FES)-cycling exercise (SCI-EX, n=9) or control (SCI-C, n=9) and re-analyzed after 8 weeks. Arm and leg SkBF was measured by laser-Doppler flowmetry during local heating (42°C), resulting in an axon-reflex mediated first peak, nadir and a primarily NO-dependent plateau-phase. Data were expressed as a percentage of maximal CVC (%CVC$_{max}$; 44°C). CVC-responses to local heating in the paralyzed leg, but also in the forearm of SCI subjects, were lower than in able-bodied controls (P<0.05 and 0.01, respectively). The 8-week intervention did not change forearm and leg CVC-responses to local heating in SCI-C and SCI-EX, but increased femoral artery diameter in SCI-EX (P<0.05). Interestingly, findings in skin microvessels contrast with conduit arteries, where physical (in)activity contributes to adaptations in SCI. The lower CVC-responses in the paralyzed legs might suggest a role for inactivity in SCI, but the presence of impaired CVC-responses in the normally active forearm suggests other mechanisms. This is supported by a lack of adaptation in skin microcirculation after FES-cycle training. This might relate to the less frequent and smaller magnitude of skin blood flow responses to heat stimuli compared with controls, than physical inactivity *per se*.

Keywords. spinal cord injury, microcirculation, nitric oxide, inactivity, functional electrical stimulation.

1. Introduction

A spinal cord injury (SCI) leads to dramatic central and peripheral cardiovascular adaptations. For example, an impaired skin microcirculation below the level of the lesion has been reported [1,2], which likely contributes to frequently reported pathologies in individual with SCI such as skin breakdown lesions [3] and poor wound healing. Apart from reports of impaired axon-reflex mediated vasodilation in SCI in the leg [2,4], little is known about the mechanisms that may underlie the impaired skin microcirculation in SCI. In addition, no studies have examined the impact of FES-cycle training on microcirculatory function in SCI subjects.

The aim of the present study was to examine skin microcirculation in the upper and lower limbs of able-bodied controls and SCI individuals, while the SCI subjects were examined again after an 8-week intervention (FES-cycling or control). We utilized a local heating protocol to examine the axon-reflex mediated and NO-dependent vasodilation [5].

2. Methods

Subjects. Seventeen healthy recreationally active men (38.6 ± 13.8 years) and 18 individuals with SCI (41.5 ± 8.4 years) were recruited from the community. The group SCI subjects were allocated to a group that participated in an 8-week FES-exercise training group (SCI-EX, n=9, 38.8 ± 7.2 years) or a control group (SCI-C, n=9, 44.2 ± 9.0 years). All SCI subjects, except one (C6, SCI-EX, excluded for analysis of forearm skin microvascular function) had a complete thoracic spinal cord lesion, varying between T1 and T12, which existed for at least 4 years.

Experimental Design. Under standardized conditions, forearm and thigh skin microvascular function was examined in control subjects and SCI individuals, using laser-Doppler flowmetry. Subsequently, the SCI subjects were divided to a group that embarked upon an 8 week FES-cycling training program of the paralyzed legs to assess whether skin microvascular function can be altered by training. The other SCI subjects continued their normal daily activities during the same time frame. After 8 weeks, SCI subjects were tested at the same time of day as during the first measurement to avoid diurnal variation.

Laser-Doppler flowmetry. After an acclimatization period of 30 minutes, microvascular function was examined via recording of local skin blood flow (SkBF) responses. To obtain an index of SkBF, cutaneous red blood cell (RBC) flux (in mV) was measured in the forearm and thigh using a Moor laser-Doppler flowmetry (LDF) system (DRT-4). After instrumentation, RBC flux of both sites was monitored to examine baseline SkBF, while blood pressure was measured to eventually calculate cutaneous vascular conductance (CVC). Data were expressed as a percentage of maximal CVC obtained during maximal heating ($\%CVC_{max}$). See previous studies for more information [5].

3. Results

An extensive description of the data can be found in Van Duijnhoven *et al.* J Applied Physiology (2009;106(4):1065-71)

Controls vs SCI. Forearm baseline $\%CVC_{max}$ was not different between controls and SCI. Responses to local heating were significantly higher in able-bodied controls compared to SCI subjects. Baseline leg $\%CVC_{max}$ was not different between both groups, while leg responses to local heating in SCI subjects were significantly lower compared to able-bodied controls.

Pre vs Post-training. In the SCI subjects that performed FES-cycling as well as the control groups, no change forearm baseline $\%CVC_{max}$ or during the local heating protocol was observed. Also in the leg, %CVC$_{max}$ at baseline or during the local heating protocol was not changed in both groups.

4. Discussion

This is the first study that comprehensively examined skin blood flow responses to local heating below (leg) and above (arm) a spinal cord lesion, and whether possible differences between SCI subjects and able-bodied controls can be altered by 8 weeks of FES-cycling training. SCI subjects demonstrated impaired CVC in the paralyzed legs during local heating compared with able-bodied controls. Interestingly, the forearm CVC responses (*above* the spinal cord lesion) were also impaired in SCI subjects compared with able-bodied controls. These unexpected findings suggest that a chronic spinal cord lesion results in a systemic adaptation of the skin microcirculation to local heating, rather than changes in the paralysed region only. This hypothesis is supported by the lack of limb differences regarding skin microcirculatory responses to local heating in SCI subjects, despite the marked difference in activity level between the upper and lower limb in SCI subjects. Whilst physical inactivity is the key factor for vascular adaptations in conduit and resistance vessels in the paralysed legs of SCI subjects [6-10], our findings suggest that physical activity itself is not the key factor that affects skin microcirculation but most likely it is the exercise induced thermoregulation. This conclusion is supported by the finding that 8 weeks of FES-cycling in SCI subjects, which increases physical activity in the legs, did not alter the SkBF and CVC responses to local heating below (leg) nor above (forearm) the spinal cord lesion, despite an increase in the femoral artery. These latter findings reinforce the evolving hypothesis that a change in physical activity level has a different effect on large and small arteries and that physical activity alone may not explain the impaired skin microcirculatory responses to local heating in SCI subjects.

References

[1]   Nicotra A, Asahina M, Mathias CJ. Skin vasodilator response to local heating in human chronic spinal cord injury. *Eur J Neurol.* 2004;11:835-837.
[2]   Nicotra A, Young TM, Asahina M, Mathias CJ. The effect of different physiological stimuli on skin vasomotor reflexes above and below the lesion in human chronic spinal cord injury. *Neurorehabil Neural Repair.* 2005;19:325-331.
[3]   Deitrick G, Charalel J, Bauman W, Tuckman J. Reduced arterial circulation to the legs in spinal cord injury as a cause of skin breakdown lesions. *Angiology.* 2007;58:175-184.
[4]   Kuesgen B, Frankel HL, Anand P. Decreased cutaneous sensory axon-reflex vasodilatation below the lesion in patients with complete spinal cord injury. *Somatosens Mot Res.* 2002;19:149-152.
[5]   Minson CT, Berry LT, Joyner MJ. Nitric oxide and neurally mediated regulation of skin blood flow during local heating. *J Appl Physiol.* 2001;91:1619-1626.
[6]   de Groot PC, Bleeker MW, Hopman MT. Magnitude and time course of arterial vascular adaptations to inactivity in humans. *Exerc Sport Sci Rev.* 2006;34:65-71.
[7]   Thijssen DH, Ellenkamp R, Kooijman M, Pickkers P, Rongen GA, Hopman MT, Smits P. A causal role for endothelin-1 in the vascular adaptation to skeletal muscle deconditioning in spinal cord injury. *Arterioscler Thromb Vasc Biol.* 2007;27:325-331.
[8]   Thijssen DH, Ellenkamp R, Smits P, Hopman MT. Rapid vascular adaptations to training and detraining in persons with spinal cord injury. *Arch Phys Med Rehabil.* 2006;87:474-481.
[9]   Thijssen DH, Heesterbeek P, van Kuppevelt DJ, Duysens J, Hopman MT. Local vascular adaptations after hybrid training in spinal cord-injured subjects. *Med Sci Sports Exerc.* 2005;37:1112-1118.
[10] Hopman MT, Groothuis JT, Flendrie M, Gerrits KH, Houtman S. Increased vascular resistance in paralyzed legs after spinal cord injury is reversible by training. *J Appl Physiol.* 2002;93:1966-1972.

Rehabilitation: Mobility, Exercise and Sports
L.H.V. van der Woude et al. (Eds.)
IOS Press, 2010
© 2010 The authors and IOS Press. All rights reserved.
doi:10.3233/978-1-60750-080-3-314

Evoked EMG and muscle fatigue during isokinetic FES cycling in individuals with SCI

E.H. ESTIGONI[a, b,1], C. FORNUSEK[a, b], T. SONG[a, b], R.A. TANHOFFER[a, b],
R. SMITH[b], G.M. DAVIS[a, b]

[a]*Rehabilitation Research Centre, Faculty of Health Sciences*
[b]*Exercise Health and Performance FRG, The University of Sydney*

Abstract. Purpose – To determine if FES-evoked electromyographic signals (eEMG), collected from paralysed quadriceps muscles, could be used as a proxy of fatigue during FES-induced cycling. Methods – Five subjects with SCI performed one FES-cycling session over 30 min, with the quadriceps muscles being electrically stimulated as the prime agonist. The pedal torques and surface eEMG signals were synchronously recorded for offline analysis. Results – Eight parameters were extracted from eEMG m-waves and processed using Matlab. While pedal torque decayed exponentially over 30-min for all individuals, none of the eEMG parameters followed the same characteristic pattern. A clear change in most of the eEMG curves was detected around the 7th minute of exercise. After analysing data from the onset of exercise until the 7th minute, time variables from the m-waves seem to inversely reflect the decay of torque. From the 7th minute onwards, amplitude and frequency variables showed a moderate correlation with pedal torque. Conclusion – eEMG parameters reflected muscle fatigue only to a limited extent. A high instability period for most of the parameters was observed during the first 7 minutes of exercise.

Keywords. evoked EMG, m-waves, muscle fatigue, FES cycling.

1. Introduction

Functional electrical stimulation (FES) cycling exercise can increase muscle strength and bring substantial improvements to the health of paralysed people [1]. However, there are many physiological considerations that must be taken into account when this population undertakes FES-evoked leg exercise. One of them, and perhaps the most important one, is leg muscle fatigue. Muscle fatigue occurs considerably more quickly in paralysed muscles. Especially under FES, when the muscle fibres are being activated in a synchronized manner [2].

Recent developments in signal processing have allowed surface EMG data acquisition to be used as a method for analysing the muscle condition in real time. When muscle activity is electrically monitored during FES-exercise, the signal collected from the muscles is known as *evoked electromyography (eEMG)*.

From this signal, can be derived relative changes within the muscle regarding the intensity of contractions [3]. In the specific case of FES-evoked leg exercise, eEMG changes represent changes in muscle responses when they are artificially recruited, and

---

[1] Corresponding Author: Eduardo Estigoni; Rehabilitation Research Centre - The University of Sydney; East Street, Lidcombe, 2141; NSW - Australia. E-mail: e.estigoni@student.usyd.edu.au

during which there is an inevitable progress of muscle fatigue. The purpose of this study was to investigate eEMG changes during this exercise modality in SCI subjects, seeking relationships with the direct measurement of pedal torque during cycling via FES quadriceps neurostimulation.

2. Methods

The equipment employed on the experiment comprised an isokinetic leg cycle ergometer (iFES-LCE) [4] and a four channel portable eEMG acquisition system (e2MG), designed and constructed specifically for this study.

Five subjects with SCI performed one iFES-LCE session at a pedal cadence of 15 rev•min^{-1} over 30 minutes. The quadriceps muscles from both legs were electrically stimulated between cycling crank angles of -50° and +50° (0°=TDC). Stimulation parameters were set to 30Hz biphasic pulses of 300μs delivered at up to 100mA, according to subjects' sensation and condition. The gains of the e2MG system were adjusted as the stimulation current went up from 0 to 100mA during the first minute of exercise. From the second minute onwards, eEMG data and pedal torque (τ) were synchronously recorded for offline analysis.

3. Results

Eight variables were extracted from the averaged eEMG m-wave trains during every revolution of the pedal (see Table 1). None of them resembled the exponential decay of pedal torque observed during 30-min of iFES-LCE exercise. However, the eEMG data displayed a characteristic change of pattern around the 7th minute from the onset of exercise. A new analysis was then performed on 2 time-periods, before and after minute 7 of exercise (*P1* and *P2*) comparing the normalized τ to the 8 normalized eEMG variables.

We considered the relationship between τ and eEMG curves as simple linear regression relationships for the independent periods *P1* and *P2*. The cross-correlation index (*r*; lag=0*)* suggested "how predictive" each of the 8 eEMG curves represented τ curves for each subject-leg. The results (mean ± std) are shown in Table 1. **TNP** and **TPtP** displayed high negative *r* coefficients in *P1*, indicating that higher than average eEMG values represented lower than average τ values.

Table 1. Torque × eEMG cross-correlation coefficients (*r*) and coefficients of determination (R^2). Amplitude eEMG variables: peak-to-peak amplitude (*APtP*); positive peak amplitude (*APP*); negative peak amplitude (*ANP*); Temporal variables: time delay between stimulus artifact and positive peak (*TPP*), time delay from the artifact to the negative peak (*TNP*) and time delay between peaks (*TPtP*); Mixed variable: total area under both peaks (*RUP*); Frequency variable: total area under the power spectrum (*RPS*).

	APtP	APP	ANP	TPP	TNP	TPtP	RUP	RPS
r (*P1*)	0.40 ± 0.46	0.09 ± 0.67	0.50 ± 0.51	-0.26 ± 0.69	-0.78 ± 0.19	-0.74 ± 0.21	0.01 ± 0.57	0.10 ± 0.48
R^2 (*P1*)	0.36 ± 0.37	0.41 ± 0.29	0.49 ± 0.29	0.49 ± 0.30	0.64 ± 0.24	0.59 ± 0.23	0.29 ± 0.37	0.22 ± 0.32
r (*P2*)	0.83 ± 0.09	0.61 ± 0.33	0.85 ± 0.08	-0.11 ± 0.64	0.41 ± 0.40	0.59 ± 0.24	0.84 ± 0.09	0.80 ± 0.11
R^2 (*P2*)	0.69 ± 0.15	0.47 ± 0.34	0.72 ± 0.13	0.38 ± 0.33	0.32 ± 0.23	0.40 ± 0.26	0.71 ± 0.15	0.65 ± 0.17

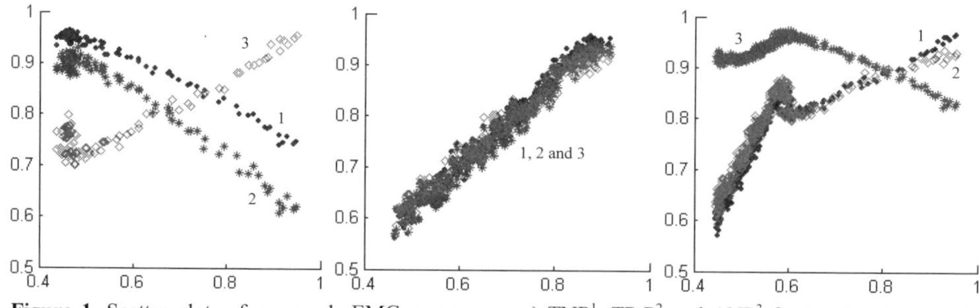

Figure 1. Scatter plots of averaged eEMG × τ curves: **a)** TNP[1], TPtP[2] and ANP[3] for t = 0 to 7min (P1); **b)** ANP[1], RUP[2] and APtP[3] for t = 7 to 30min (P2); **c)** ANP[1], TPP[2] and APtP[3] × torque for t = 0 to 30min.

For *P2*, APtP, ANP, RUP and RPS revealed correlations ≥0.80, suggesting these were good pedal torque predictors. Mean coefficients of determination (R^2) of ANP and RUP were ≥0.70, which supported the cross-correlation findings during P2. However, during P1, the R^2 of TNP and TPtP were ≤0.65, suggesting only low-moderate linear fit. Figure 1 portrays the relationships between eEMG variables and pedal torque in the first 7-min (left panel), from the 7th min to 30th min (centre panel) and over the 30-min FES-exercise period (right panel).

4. Discussion and Conclusion

Isolated m-wave parameters did not seem to be useful indicators of fatigue over 30-min of iFES-LCE. Amplitude, area and frequency curves demonstrated oscillatory patterns during the first 7 minutes, and only after that was the relationship with τ significant. Temporal variables revealed an inverse relationship to τ during P1 and no relationship during P2. The separation of curves into 2 phases around the 7th minute provided new baselines for the dataset normalization, improving the relationship between the eEMG variables and τ (Figure 1). However, it is still unclear whether this time threshold separating P1 from P2 is constant or is likely to change under different experimental conditions (cycling speeds, FES parameters, etc.).

In conclusion, evoked EMG signals represent the onset and progress of muscle fatigue during FES cycling only to a limited degree. Further research with a larger number of subjects is needed for a better understanding of the evoked EMG patterns during fatiguing leg exercise in SCI individuals.

References

[1] G.M. Davis, N.A. Hamzaid, C. Fornusek, Cardiorespiratory, metabolic and biomechanical responses during FES leg exercise: Health and fitness benefits, *Artif Organs* **32** (2008), 625-629.

[2] B. Bigland-Ritchie et al, Excitation Frequency and Muscle Fatigue - Electrical Responses During Human Voluntary and Stimulated Contractions, *Experimental Neurology* **64** (1979), 414-427.

[3] R. Merletti, M. Knaflitz, C. J. DeLuca, Electrically evoked myoelectric signals, *Crit Rev Biomed Eng* **19**, (1992), 293-340.

[4] C. Fornusek et al, Development of an Isokinetic Functional Electrical Stimulation Cycle Ergometer, *Neuromodulation* **7** (2004), 56-64.

Rehabilitation: Mobility, Exercise and Sports
L.H.V. van der Woude et al. (Eds.)
IOS Press, 2010

doi:10.3233/978-1-60750-080-3-317

Influence of FES cycling on spasticity in subjects with incomplete spastic paraplegia

W. REICHENFELSER[a], H. HACKL[a], J. WIEDNER[b], J. HUFGARD[b],
K. GSTALTNER[b], S. MINA[c], S. HANKE[c], M. GFOEHLER[a]
[a] *Dept of Engineering Design & Logistics Engineering, Vienna University of
Technology, Austria*
[b] *AUVA Rehabilitation Centre Weißer Hof, Austria*
[c] *Austrian Research Centers ARC, Austria*

Abstract. Commonly used methods for quantification of spasticity have shown
controversial reliability. In this study we propose a method for quick determination
of spasticity in spinal cord injured subjects on a cycling and measurement system.
Measurements with test persons with incomplete spastic paraplegia have shown
that spasticity is decreased after a 30 min cycling training with functional electrical
stimulation (FES).

Keywords. spasticity, paraplegia, spinal cord injury, functional electrical
stimulation.

1. Introduction

Spasticity is a common problem among paraplegic subjects that can cause pain, lead to
unwanted movements or prevent intended movements. Lance [1] defined spasticity as a
motor disorder that is characterized by a velocity dependent increase in the tonic stretch
reflex with exaggerated tendon reflexes. For quantification of spasticity manual scales,
biomechanical techniques, or neurophysiological methods have been applied. Manual
scales as the Ashworth Scale/Modified Ashworth Scale (MAS) are most commonly
used but have shown a controversial reliability [2]. Krause et al [3] found that FES
cycling training reduced spasticity (determined by MAS and pendulum test) in spinal
cord injured (SCI) subjects.
The aim of this study was the assessment of spasticity in the lower extremities using
the pedaling mechanism of a cycling system for paraplegics [4] and to quantify the
influence of cycling training with FES on spasticity in SCI subjects.

2. Methods

The cycling and measurement system

The cycling and measurement system is based on a tricycle that was especially adapted
for the FES training of paraplegic subjects (Fig.1). A motor that is mounted underneath
the crank beam can move the cranks at a given angular velocity or hold the cranks at a
defined position. Orthoses support the legs and fix the ankle joints. A 10 channel
current controlled stimulator stimulates three muscles/muscle groups of each leg (m.

quadriceps femoris, mm. hamstrings, and m. gluteus maximus) via attached surface electrodes. The motor current and the forces (Fr, Ft) applied to the cranks are continuously monitored during the therapy sessions.

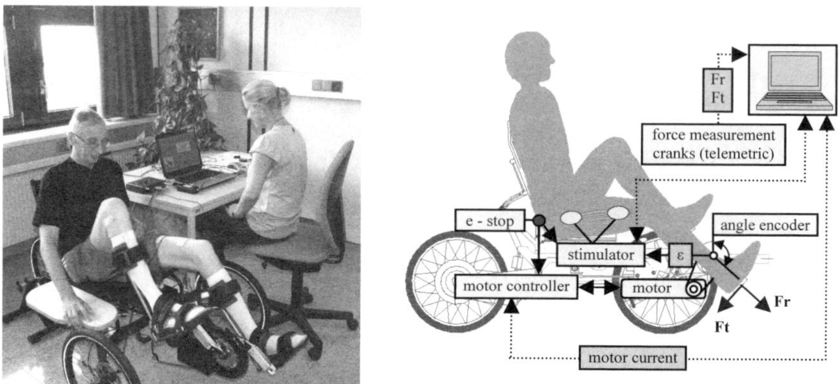

Figure 1. The cycling and measurement system during measurements and schematic of control

Measurements

Nine subjects with incomplete spastic paraplegia (age 38/ SD 16, time since injury 6.1 month/ SD 3.2, motoric lesion at L1-C6, ASIA A-C) volunteered for the study and gave informed consent. The training sessions in a period of 2 month were started with a short passive warm-up followed by the assessment of the patients' spasticity status. After a 30 min pedaling training with FES the spasticity test routine was repeated.

For the spasticity test routine the cranks were moved by the motor with constant angular velocity at 10/20/30/40/50/60 rpm, for 15 full rotations at each cadence. Therefore the patient was asked to relax to minimize his force inputs by active muscle recruitment. The subjects' geometrical position was adjusted to allow a maximum knee angle of 160°. The maximum angular velocities of knee and hip joints were about 230°/s and 160°/s, respectively.

The applied motor current is corresponding to the resistance of the legs against the movement. For evaluation the current values were averaged over 10 full rotations at each cadence.

3. Results

The results of 7 to 14 training sessions were averaged for each patient. Figure 2 shows a comparison of the results of a non-spastic test person (MAS 0) and a test person with an averaged MAS of 1.5 that dropped to 1.2 after the FES training. For non-spastic subjects resistance was usually slightly decreased after the FES training over the whole range of velocities, the curves run in parallel (Fig. 2, left side). Basically, the increase due to inertia is the same before and after the FES training. Consequently, if the difference between the two curves increases at higher velocities as in the right sided graph in Fig. 2, it can be assumed that this effect originates from the spasticity.

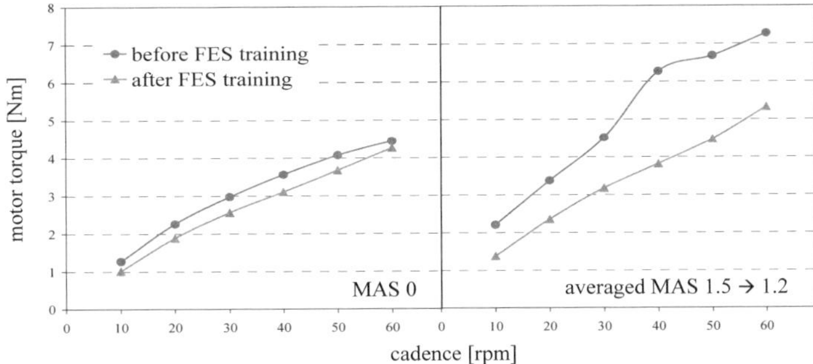

Figure 2: Comparison of averaged results of a non-spastic test person P1 (left) and test person P3 with MAS 1.5 on average before the FES training (right).

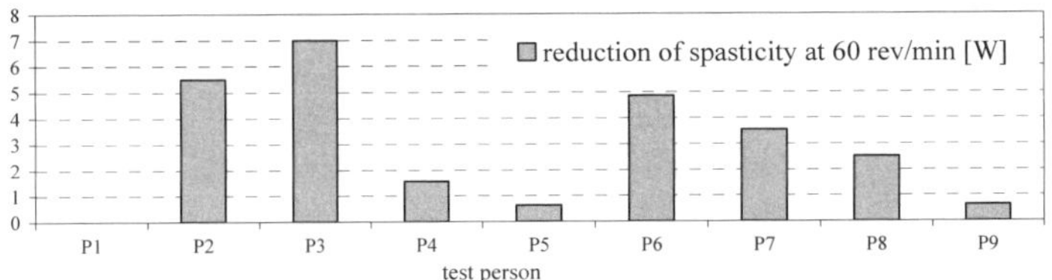

Figure 3: Reduction of spasticity in Watts at 60 rpm after the FES cycling training

Figure 3 shows the reduction of spasticity for all nine test persons, calculated as the diverence of necessary drive power before and after the FES cycling training. The general relaxation of the passive structures is taken into account by subtracting the difference in motor torque at 10 rpm. Test person P3 reaches the highest value of reduction, 7 W at 60 rpm, for the non-spastic test person P1 the value is 0.

4. Discussion and Conclusion

The proposed method of spasticity assessment has the advantage, that the spasticity of both hip and knee joints is included in one test routine. The results show that spasticity is decreased after the cycling training with FES. This is in line with the subjective feelings of the patients after the training. A permanent decline of spasticity can not be reported.

Acknowledgment: This study was sponsored by the FFG and the AUVA.

References

[1]   J W Lance, Symposium synopsis, in Spasticity: Disordered Motor Control, R G Feldman, R R Young, and W P Koella, Eds. Miami: Symposia Specialist, (1980), 485-495.

[2]   A D Pandyan, G R Johnson, C I M Price, R H Curless, M P Barnes and H Rodgers, "A review of the properties and limitations of the Ashworth and modified Ashworth Scales as measures of spasticity," Clinical Rehabilitation, 13 (1999), 373-383.

[3]   P Krause, J Szecsi, A Straube, Changes in spastic muscle tone increase in patients with spinal cord injury using functional electrical stimulation and passive leg movements Clin Rehabil 22 (2008), 627-34.

[4]   W Reichenfelser, H Hackl, S Mina, S Hanke, P Lugner, M Gföhler, Trainings- and Measurement-System for FES- Cycling, Proc 13th Ann Conf of the IFESS, Freiburg, Germany, September 2008.

Rehabilitation: Mobility, Exercise and Sports
L.H.V. van der Woude et al. (Eds.)
IOS Press, 2010

doi:10.3233/978-1-60750-080-3-320

The impact of exercise training on oxidative stress in spinal cord injured individuals

N.T.L. VAN DUIJNHOVEN[a,1], E.O. HESSE[b], T.W.J. JANSSEN[c,d],
M. KNIPPENBERG[e], P. SCHEFFER[f], M.T.E. HOPMAN[a]

[a]*Department of Physiology, Radboud University Nijmegen Medical Centre,
Nijmegen, The Netherlands,* [b]*Institute of Human Movement Sciences and
Sport, ETH Zurich, Switzerland,* [c]*Research Institute MOVE, Faculty of Human
Movement Sciences, VU University, Amsterdam, The Netherlands,* [d]*Rehabilitation
Centre Amsterdam, The Netherlands,* [e]*Department of Clinical Chemistry, Maastricht
University Medical Centre, Maastricht, The Netherlands,* [f]*Department of Clinical
Chemistry, VU University Medical Centre, Amsterdam, The Netherlands*

Abstract. Spinal cord-injured (SCI) individuals have a high risk for cardiovascular diseases. An imbalance in (anti)oxidative status would be associated with an increased cardiovascular risk. OBJECTIVE: To compare baseline levels of oxidative stress and antioxidative capacity in SCI individuals and able-bodied (AB) subjects, and to assess acute and long-term effects of functional electrical stimulation (FES) exercise on oxidative stress and antioxidative capacity in SCI. METHODS: Venous blood was taken from SCI (n=9) and age-matched AB subjects (n=9) to examine oxidative stress through malondialdehyde (MDA) levels, while superoxide dismutase (SOD) and gluthatione peroxidase (GPx) enzyme levels represented anti-oxidative capacity. Subsequently, SCI subjects performed an 8 week FES exercise training period. Blood was taken at fixed time points to examine the acute and chronic effect of FES exercise. RESULTS: Baseline levels of MDA, SOD and GPx were not different between SCI and AB subjects. Both, a single FES exercise bout and 8 weeks FES training, had no effect on MDA, SOD and GPx levels. CONCLUSION: The preserved (anti)oxidative status in SCI suggests that the increased prevalence for CVD in SCI is unlikely explained by (anti)oxidative imbalance. Furthermore, the stimulus induced by FES exercise is possibly insufficient to change (anti)oxidative status in SCI individuals.

Keywords. oxidative stress, antioxidative capacity, functional electrical stimulation, spinal cord-injury.

1. Introduction

Physical inactivity, which is an independent risk factor of CVD and a fact in SCI individuals, increases vascular oxidative stress and accelerates the atherosclerotic process [1]. Considering the extensive adaptations of the cardiovascular system to extreme deconditioning such as in SCI, an imbalance in (anti)oxidative status may contribute to the increased prevalence for CVD. The first aim of the present study was to compare baseline levels of oxidative stress and antioxidative capacity from chronic SCI individuals with levels in able-bodied subjects.

---

[1] Corresponding Author.

Physical exercise results in increased levels of oxidative stress, and elevated antioxidative enzyme activity. Functional electrical stimulation (FES) has been proven to be an efficient manner to counteract the detrimental changes in the paralyzed limbs in SCI [2]. The second aim of this study was to assess the acute and long-term effects of electrically induced exercise on oxidative stress and antioxidative capacity in chronic SCI individuals.

2. Methods

Subjects
Nine men with a SCI (41 ± 9 years, lesion C5-T11, ASIA Impermant Scale A, B, D) and nine age-matched, able-bodied (AB) controls (42 ± 10 years) participated in this study. None of the participants were familiar with CVD, diabetes or its risk factors.

Design and protocol
A cross-sectional comparison on oxidative stress and antioxidative capacity was made between SCI subjects and AB controls. Then, an intervention study was performed on the SCI participants, performing identical measurements pre and post intervention to assess the effect of training on oxidative stress and antioxidative capacity.

Oxidative stress was indirectly estimated from venous blood by malondialdehyde (MDA), while antioxidative capacity was represented by the activity of superoxide dismutase (SOD) and gluthation peroxidise (GPx). Baseline blood samples were taken before the first and last FES exercise session. Additionally, blood was drawn immediately after the first and last FES exercise session, to assess the acute effect of one bout of FES exercise. In the control group, only baseline blood samples were taken.

FES exercise training consisted of 8 wks, 2-3 times/wk, reaching 20 sessions/ person. Quadriceps, hamstrings amd gluteal muscles were stimulated for 30 minutes maximally, using surface electrodes (Stimex, Pierenkemper GmbH, Germany) and a computer-controlled leg cycle ergometer (Ergys 2, Therapeutic Alliances Inc, USA). Electrical stimulation (duration monophasic square wave pulses, 450 µs, frequency 30 Hz) was applied in coordinated sequence permitting cyclic patterns of muscle contractions resulting in leg cycling.

To assess differences between SCI and AB in subject characteristics and blood parameters, an unpaired Student's t-test was used (SPSS 16.0, Chicago, USA). The effect of FES training on blood parameters was tested with a paired Student's t-test.

3. Results

Subject characteristics were not different between SCI and AB individuals (Table I). Baseline levels of MDA, SOD and GPx were not different between SCI and AB subjects (P=0.55, 0.70 and 0.73, respectively; Table 1).

All SCI individuals successfully completed the training period. Workload during FES exercise increased significantly after training (median[25%-75%]: pre 0.0[0.0-2.2] kJ, post 11.0[5.5-19.7] kJ, Wilcoxon: P=0.008). Baseline levels of MDA, SOD and GPx were unaltered after FES exercise training, compared to before training (P=0.44, 0.39 and 0.98, respectively; Table 1). Responses of MDA, SOD and GPx levels to one bout of exercise were not different after training, compared to before (P=0.92, 0.82 and 0.37, respectively).

Table 1. MDA, SOD and GPx levels of AB and SCI before and after FES training

	AB	SCI before training		SCI after training	
	Baseline	**Baseline**	**After 1x FES**	**Baseline**	**After 1x FES**
MDA µmol/l	5.4 ± 0.4	5.3 ± 0.8	5.6 ± 1.2	5.1 ± 0.6	5.4 ± 1.3
SOD, U/g Hb	1113 ± 143	1081 ± 200	1068 ± 102	1142 ± 94	1113 ± 275
GPx, U/mmol Hb	1220 ± 475	1137 ± 523	1147 ± 515	1175 ± 570	1070 ± 494

SCI spinal cord-injured; AB able-bodied; FES functional electrical stimulation; MDA malonaldehyde; SOD superoxide dismutase; GPx gluthatione peroxidased. Data are presented as mean±SD.

4. Discussion

Baseline levels of MDA, SOD and GPx were comparable between chronic SCI and AB subjects, which is in disagreement with our hypothesis of increased oxidative stress and decreased antioxidative capacity in SCI due to their paralysis. Previous studies showed increased free radical generation in cervical SCI [3], or reduced MDA levels in SCI [4]. In our study, SCI subjects performed zero to six hours of sports a week (mainly wheelchair basketball, rugby and hand biking). Furthermore, a significant inverse correlation was found between their maximal achievable workload in a hand bike test and baseline levels of oxidative stress (R=-0.763, P=0.05), indicating that a higher upper-body aerobic fitness is associated with a lower level of oxidative stress. This confirms the idea that physical inactivity increases vascular oxidative stress. Although an acute SCI provokes an enormous increase in oxidative stress levels [5], individuals with long-standing SCI appear to show normalized oxidative stress and antioxidative capacity levels.

Levels of MDA, SOD and GPx were maintained after one bout of FES exercise and 8 weeks of FES training. These findings do not correspond to our hypothesis and some other studies on (anti)oxidative parameters related to short-term exercise or long-term training in rodents, and healthy and diseased humans. We suggest that *just* exercise is not enough to provoke significant changes in (anti)oxidative balance, but that exercise intensity level is crucial to induce adaptation processes. It might be questioned if FES exercise in this study was intense enough to induce adaptations in (anti)oxidative status measured from blood. However, the idea that this FES exercise program is moderate intense, is supported by anecdotal evidence (sweating, difficulty talking, physically tired after training), and by previous unpublished data on heart rate rise during FES exercise (rest: 75±3, steady state during FES exercise: 97±4, N=9).

In conclusion, our results suggest that baseline levels of oxidative stress and antioxidative capacity in chronic SCI individuals are similar to healthy, able-bodied controls. Furthermore, we found no changes in (anti)oxidative status after acute and long-term FES exercise in SCI individuals. Possibly, the stimulus induced by FES exercise is insufficient to change (anti)oxidative status in SCI individuals.

References

[1] U. Laufs et al., *Arterioscler Thromb Vasc Biol* **25** (2005), 809-814.
[2] M.T. Hopman et al., *J Appl Physiol* **93** (2002), 1966-1972.
[3] H. Kocak et al., *Clin Biochem* **38** (2005), 1034-1037.
[4] A. Wozniak et al., *Neurol Neurochir Pol* **37** (2003), 1025-1036.
[5] D. Liu et al., *Free Radic Biol Med* **27** (1999), 478-482.

Rehabilitation: Mobility, Exercise and Sports
L.H.V. van der Woude et al. (Eds.)
IOS Press, 2010
© 2010 The authors and IOS Press. All rights reserved.
doi:10.3233/978-1-60750-080-3-323

Functional electrical stimulation assisted cycling of patients with multiple sclerosis

J. SZECSI[a], C. SCHLICK[ac], M. SCHILLER[a], W. PÖLLMANN[b], N. KOENIG[b], A. STRAUBE[a]

[a]*A Center for Sensorimotor Research, Dept. of Neurology, Ludwig-Maximillians University*
[b]*Marianne Strauss Therapy Centre for Multiple Sclerosis, Kempfenhausen, Germany*

Abstract. Objective: To determine whether functional electrical stimulation-supported ergometric training of patients with multiple sclerosis has a prosthetic or therapeutic effect on biomechanical (power, smoothness of cycling) and functional outcomes (walking capability, strength of muscle, spasticity). Design: Twelve subjects with multiple sclerosis participated in an electrical stimulation-supported ergometric training (3 sessions/week for 2 weeks). Measurements were to study prosthetic (with and without stimulation) and therapeutic effects (before and after training). Methods: Power and smoothness were calculated, spasticity; strength and walking capability were measured by the Modified Ashworth Scale, Manual Muscle Test, and 10-Meter Walk Test. Results: The power and smoothness of pedaling significantly improved prosthetically with electrical stimulation, but did not show significant improvement over the 2 weeks of training. Significant short-term reductions of spasticity (before vs. after training session; p < 0.05) were found. Isometric strength did not increase significantly during the 2-week training period and there was no improvement in walking ability. Conclusion: Patients with multiple sclerosis are able to improve their cycling power and smoothness by pedaling with stimulation. Severely affected patients benefit more from FES-cycling therapy than slightly affected patients do.

Keywords. multiple sclerosis, functional electrical stimulation, ergometer training, cycling.

1. Introduction

FES-propelled cycling has so far been successfully applied to persons with complete spinal cord injury (SCI)(2) to strengthen muscles, to stimulate the cardiovascular system, and to improve cycling mobility.

Neither the therapeutic effect of FES coupled with cycling in MS patients is known, nor have the biomechanical parameters or functional outcome that could be improved by such therapy been investigated.

Aim of the study was to assess the effects of electrical stimulation on mechanical power output and the uniformity of pedaling during a 2-week FES-supported ergometric training of MS patients with pareses of the lower limbs. Both prosthetic effects occurring during FES-supported cycling, as well as therapeutic, long-term effects (before and after the 2-week training period) were considered. Furthermore, the impact of the intervention on walking capability, spasticity, and volitional strength was investigated.

2. Materials and methods

Twelve subjects (11 M/1 F) with chronic progressive MS in a stable time course were scheduled to undergo six FES-supported cycling training sessions for 2 weeks. The patient's quadriceps and hamstring muscle groups on both sides were electrically stimulated. Crank angular position and torque were recorded during ergometer sessions; cadence, power, and smoothness of pedaling were derived. Smoothness of pedaling was defined as roughness index (RI) of angular speed(3). Functional outcome was evaluated by the walking capability (10 MWT), the knee extensor and flexor strength (MMT), and also the spasticity (MAS). To account for the prosthetic effects, mean power and smoothness were calculated for each subject over all training (and measurement) sessions with respect to the four comparison intervals. To analyze the development of power and smoothness during the 2-week training period, averages were assigned in a first step to the six training sessions and for the four comparison

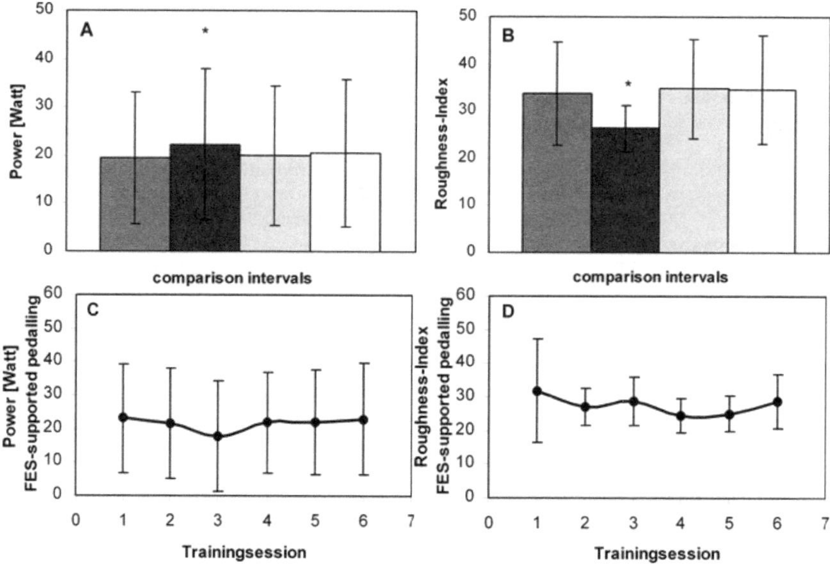

Figure 1. Upper: Course of power and smmothness in one training session before (dark grey), during (black) and after stimulation (light grey and white). Low: Power and smoothness during the 2 weeks training period.

intervals of the sessions. In a second step, a one-way ANOVA with factor session number was performed for the phase-related power and smoothness over the 2-week training time.

3. Results

Generated power significantly increased with stimulation compared to that with voluntary cycling in the pre-stimulation interval (p=0.02). Carryover of the prosthetic effect was not found in the post-stimulation intervals. No significant difference could be detected between early and late post stimulation intervals. The number of training sessions had no significant effect on the power generated with stimulation during the 2-week training period (Fig. 1; p = 0.28). This was also true for the training intervals before and after stimulation. Significantly better smoothness (Fig. 1; p=0.02) was achieved in the stimulation interval than in the voluntary cycling interval beforehand. After cessation of stimulation the smoothness worsened significantly in comparison to that during the stimulated interval (p=0.01). No significant change of smoothness was found when comparing intervals before and after stimulation, and no significant difference in smoothness could be detected between early and late stimulation intervals.

No significant changes of walking capability could be found in the short term (p >0.77) or in the long term. Both knee extensor and flexor strengths did not change significantly over the 2-week training period .MAS revealed a significant reduction of muscle spasticity in the short term (pre/post training session, p = 0.05) but no significant reduction in the long term (first/last training days, p = 0.92).

4. Discussion

Biomechanic parameters

The main finding was that subjects with MS could achieve significantly more cycling power and smoothness with FES than without it (prosthetic effect). Moreover, power in the post-stimulation phase tended to remain increased compared to that in the pre-stimulation phase. Thus a prolonged training protocol could eventually lead to a longer-lasting power increase, even after cessation of the stimulation.
The subjects who had low pain tolerance (##04 and 08), as shown by low stimulation intensities (< 40 mA supposed to be the motor threshold), could not, as expected, increase their power or improve their smoothness. In contrast, the subjects with high pain tolerance (## 01, 02 and 07, > 55 mA) improved both their power and smoothness, probably independently of the severity or asymmetry of the impairment. We recommend using the FES-cycling method in subjects with high or medium pain tolerance, depending on the severity and asymmetry of the motor impairments. It is probably inappropriate for subjects with low pain tolerance.

Functional outcome.

Walking capability did not change in the short or in the long term. The lack of therapeutic effect can perhaps be explained by the insufficiency of muscle strength and coordination improvement (as reflected by no smoothness improvement) achieved over the 2-week training period. Feedback from the participants revealed subjectively experienced outcome improvements (transfer in ## 3 and 7, more independence in activities of daily life in ## 5 and 7, and qualitative correction of foot cleaning in ## 1, 2, and 4.

References

[1]   Petrofsky JS, Phillips CA. The use of functional electrical stimulation for rehabilitation of spinal cord injured patients. Cent Nerv Syst Trauma. 1984; 1:57-74.
[2]   Chen G, Kautz SA, Zajac FE. Simulation analysis of muscle activity changes with altered body orientations during pedaling. J Biomech. 2001; 34:749-756.
[3]   Nielsen JB, Crone C, Hultborn H. The spinal pathophysiology of spasticity - from a basic science point of view. Acta Physiol (Oxf). 2007; 189:171-180.

8.2

Poster Presentations

Rehabilitation: Mobility, Exercise and Sports
L.H.V. van der Woude et al. (Eds.)
IOS Press, 2010

doi:10.3233/978-1-60750-080-3-329

Development of a tricycle for spinal cord injured

R. BERKELMANS[a, 1], J. DUYSENS[b], D. VAN KUPPEVELT[c]
[a]*BerkelBike BV, 's-Hertogenbosch, the Netherlands*
[b]*Department of Biomedical Kinesiology, KU Leuven, Belgium*
[c]*Sint Maartenskliniek Research, Development & Education, Nijmegen, the Netherlands*

Abstract. Purpose: To develop a tricycle with Functional Electrical Stimulation (FES) for the leg muscles of spinal cord injured. It has to give the therapeutical benefits of FES, but also be practical in speed, range and reliability. Methods: We combined voluntary arm cranking with FES leg cycling. Three different models are made. One model is just a front part with one wheel, which can be attached and detached to a wheelchair. Two models can also be used outdoor tricycles and all models can be used as a stationary bike. Results: Compared with FES leg cycling only, the power output and the stamina improved. The combined exercise from arms and legs gives a higher oxygen uptake then separate exercises. Conclusion: A practical outdoor tricycle for people with SCI is developed. The different models are suitable for complete spinal cord injured ranging from C5 to T12.

Keywords. FES cycling, hybrid exercise, spinal cord injury, tricycle

1.   Introduction

Since the early 80's, a lot of research has been conducted about the effects of Functional Electrical Stimulation (FES) with people who suffer from a Spinal Cord Injury (SCI). Especially riding a stationary bike seemed a very good method to obtain physiological effects. Local effects of riding this bike provides better blood circulation [1, 2] hypertrophy [1, 3-5] of stimulated muscles and alteration of muscle fiber types [4]. Cardiac output [6, 7] maximum oxygen intake [7-9] hormone metabolism [10, 11] and psychological effects [11] are the more general benefits. It has been determined that combining FES biking with voluntary arm cranking has a greater impact on the general benefits [12]. Considering the life expectancy of SCI patients still being remarkably lower than non-patients [13], it is understandable that there have been multiple attempts to make FES cycling more attractive by developing an outdoor bike [14-16].

Our goal was to develop a FES tricycle that is suitable for the largest part of the SCI population, including the spinal cord injured with an incomplete lesion. For this purpose, it has to be practical in speed, range, reliability and physiological response as well.

---

[1] Helftheuvelweg 11, 5222AV 's-Hertogenbosch, +31 (0)73-7851184, www@berkelbike.com

2. Methods

We combined voluntary arm and (FES) leg cycling. Three different models are made: a complete tricycle, a model, which the user can attach or detach to their own wheelchair and a Home trainer, which is designed for SCI in an electrical wheelchair. The first two types are developed to ride outdoors but can be used as a stationary bike as well. The Home version however can only be used as a stationary bike.

All the bikes can be equipped with a FES 8 channel stimulator. For cycling we normally used maximum 150 mA, 150 V, 20 Hz, 0.8 mS biphasic pulse. In each stimulator we preprogrammed 5 different stimulation programs. Most of the times, they only differ in timing of the muscle stimulation. The subjects can chose their own favorable program and adjust the stimulation intensity with a plus and minus button.

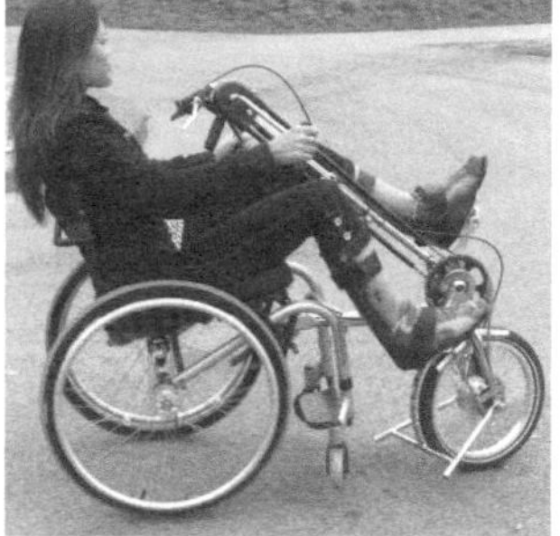

Figure 1. Front part is attached to wheelchair

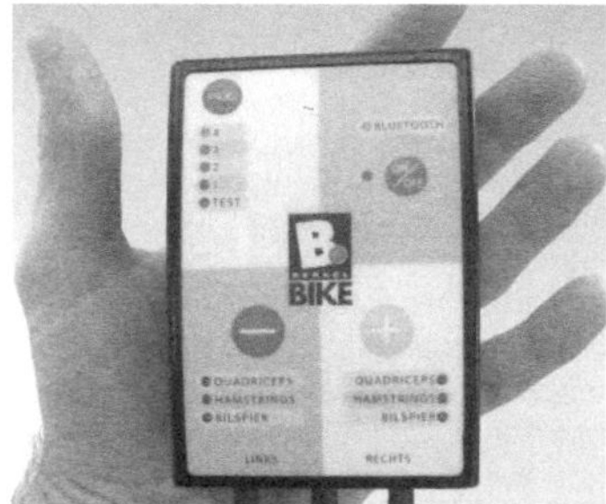

Figure 2. 8 channel FES stimulator for cycling.

3. Results

Compared with FES leg cycling only, the power output and the stamina improved. The average speed went up from 5 km/h to 15 km/h. Even when the legs where fatigued it was still possible to ride home. The combined exercise from arms and legs gives a higher oxygen uptake then separate exercises.

The Classic and the Pro are favored for SCI with lesions from C7-T12 because of the fact that they allow the possibility to ride outdoors. The home version is most suitable for C4, C5 & C6.

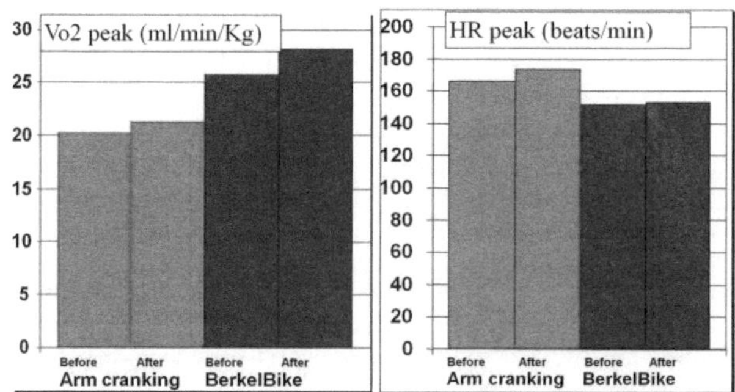

Figure 3. Results armcranking vs Hybrid cycling before and after 4 weeks training.

Almost half of the current 70 owners use it without FES. These are mostly incomplete SCI, MS and stroke patients, who still have some power left in their legs but not enough for riding on leg power alone.

The only defined problem so far occurred with injuries of joints due to rapid increase of training load. We now have a more moderate training protocol.

4. Conclusion

Adding arm cranking to the FES tricycle has practical as well as physiological advantages. We were able to develop a well functioning outdoor bike with or without the use of FES. The device can be beneficial for a large patient population. Attaching and detaching to and from one's own wheelchair is experienced as a great advantage by most SCI patients.

References

[1]   Chilibeck PD, Jeon J, Weiss C, Bell G, et al. Histochemical changes in muscle of individuals with spinal cord injury following functional electrical stimulated exercise training. Spinal Cord, 37:264-268, 1999.

[2]   Thijssen DH, Ellenkamp R, Smits P, et al. Rapid vascular adaptations to training and detraining in persons with spinal cord injury. Arch Phys Med Rehabil, 87:474-481, 2006.

[3]   Baldi JC, Jackson RD, Moraille R, et a. Muscle atrophy is prevented in patients with acute spinal cord injury using functional electrical stimulation. Spinal Cord, 36:463-469, 1998.

[4]   Crameri RM, Weston A, Climstein M, et al. Effects of electrical stimulation-induced leg training on skeletal muscle adaptability in spinal cord injury. Scand J Med Sci Sports, 12:316-322, 2002.

[5]   Scremin AM, Kurta L, Gentili A, et al. Increasing muscle mass in spinal cord injured persons with a functional electrical stimulation exercise program. Arch Phys Med Rehabil, 80:1531-1536, 1999.

[6]   Faghri PD, Glaser RM, Figoni SF: Functional electrical stimulation leg cycle ergometer exercise: Training effects on cardiorespiratory responses of spinal cord injured subjects at rest and during submaximal exercise. Arch Phys Med Rehabil, 73:1085-1093, 1992.

[7]   Hooker SP, Figoni SF, Rodgers MM, et al. Physiologic effects of electrical stimulation leg cycle exercise training in spinal cord injured persons. Arch Phys Med Rehabil, 73:470-476, 1992.

[8]   Barstow TJ, Scremin AM, Mutton DL, et al. Changes in gas exchange kinetics with training in patients with spinal cord injury. Med Sci Sports Exerc, 28:1221-1228, 1996.

[9]   Hooker SP, Scremin AM, Mutton DL, et al. Peak and submaximal physiologic responses following electrical stimulation leg cycle ergometer training. J Rehabil Res Dev, 32:361-366, 1995.

[10] Hjeltnes N, Galuska D, Bjornholm M, et al. Exercise-induced overexpression of key regulatory proteins involved in glucose uptake and metabolism in tetraplegic persons: Molecular mechanism for improved glucose homeostasis. FASEB J, 12:1701-1712, 1998.

[11] Twist DJ, Culpepper-Morgan JA, Ragnarsson KT, et al. Neuroendocrine changes during functional electrical stimulation. Am J Phys Med Rehabil, 71:156-163, 1992.

[12] Mutton DL, Scremin AM, Barstow TJ, et al. Physiologic responses during functional electrical stimulation leg cycling and hybrid exercise in spinal cord injured subjects. Arch Phys Med Rehabil, 78:712-718, 1997.

[13] National spinal cord injury statistical center, The 2006 Annual Statistical Report for the Model Spinal Cord Injury Care System. 1-121; 2006.

[14] Hunt KJ, Stone B, Negard NO, et al. Control strategies for integration of electric motor assist and functional electrical stimulation in paraplegic cycling: Utility for exercise testing and mobile cycling. IEEE Trans Neural Syst Rehabil Eng, 12:89-101, 2004.

[15] Pons DJ, Vaughan CL, Jaros GG: Cycling device powered by the electrically stimulated muscles of paraplegics. Med Biol Eng Comput, 27:1-7, 1989.

[16] Szecsi J, Fiegel M, Krafczyk S, et al. The electrical stimulation bicycle: A neuroprosthesis for the everyday use of paraplegic patients. MMW Fortschr Med, 146:37-8, 40-1, 2004.

Rehabilitation: Mobility, Exercise and Sports
L.H.V. van der Woude et al. (Eds.)
IOS Press, 2010
© 2010 The authors and IOS Press. All rights reserved.
doi:10.3233/978-1-60750-080-3-332

Electrical stimulation-induced Gluteal and Hamstring muscle activation can reduce sitting pressure in individuals with a spinal cord injury

T.W.J. JANSSEN[a,b], A. DE KONING[a,b], K.J.A. LEGEMATE[a,b], C.A.J. SMIT[a]

[a]*Duyvensz-Nagel Research Laboratory, Rehabilitation Centre Amsterdam*
[b]*Research Institute MOVE, Faculty of Human Movement Sciences,*
VU University Amsterdam, The Netherlands

Abstract. Individuals with spinal cord injury (SCI) are at high risk of developing pressure sores, in part due to high sitting pressures under the buttocks. PURPOSE: To evaluate the effect of ES-induced activation of the gluteal and hamstring muscles on the sitting pressure in individuals with SCI. METHODS: Five men with SCI received ES in their own daily-use wheelchair while sitting pressure under the buttocks was measured. The subjects wore a Bioshort (Bioflex Inc.) with built-in electrodes. Two 3-hr protocols were randomly applied, both consisting of 3 min of stimulation (all muscles simultaneously activated) followed by 17 min rest. Prot. A had a 1s:1s and prot. B a 1s:4s on-off duty cycle. Peak pressure under the buttocks and pressure gradient were calculated. RESULTS: For both protocols, peak pressure decreased (p<0.05) from 183±13 (A) and 179±14 (B) during rest to 168±17 (A) and 147±24 (B) mmHg during the 3-hr stimulation periods. The pressure gradient tended (p<0.1) to decrease for both protocols indicating an improved pressure distribution. Prot. B showed in general superior effects. CONCLUSIONS: ES-induced activation of the gluteal and hamstring muscles in sitting individuals with SCI causes a temporary decrease in peak sitting pressure under the buttocks and an improved pressure distribution.

Keywords. spinal cord injury, electrical stimulation, pressures sores.

1. Introduction

Individuals with spinal cord injury (SCI) are at high risk of developing pressure sores, partly due to high sitting pressures under the ischial tuberosities. Methods to prevent pressure sores include the use of special cushions and protective behavior (lifting, weight shifting). Although these methods may help reduce the risk, pressure sores are still common, indicating that these methods are not adequate.

A method that may accomplish both an improvement in interface pressure distribution, a reduction of muscle atrophy, and improved circulation is activation of the gluteal muscles using electrical stimulation (ES), temporarily changing the shape of the buttocks. In a recent pilot-study,[1] we showed that ES of the gluteal muscles using surface electrodes indeed acutely reduced peak sitting pressure. However, placing electrodes under the buttocks is not desirable and we did not study effects outside the lab during longer periods or different protocols. In this study we therefore used custom-made shorts with built-in electrodes to simultaneously activate gluteal ánd hamstring muscles during 3 hours in a more daily-life situation using 2 different protocols. To evaluate the effect of ES-induced activation of the gluteal and hamstring muscles on the sitting pressure distribution in individuals with SCI.

2. Method

Subjects

Five men with an (in-)complete SCI (41±13 yrs; 83±15 kg, lesion C5-T11; TSI 162±99 months) participated in this IRB-approved study after signing an informed consent form. Individuals with a flaccid paralysis, a history of severe autonomic dysreflexia, current pressure ulcers under the tuber areas, and intolerance for ES were excluded.

Protocol

Subjects received ES (50 Hz, 70-80 mA, 2-ch NeuroPro stimulator; Fig.1) in their own daily-use wheelchair while sitting pressure was measured using a 32x32-sensor pressure mapping system (FSA, Vista Medical). The subjects wore a custom Bioshort (Bioflex Inc., Columbus, USA) with built-in electrodes one over the gluteus and one over the hamstrings. During 2 days, two 3-hr protocols were randomly applied, both consisting of 3 min of stimulation (all muscles simultaneously activated) followed by a 17-min rest. Prot. A had a 1s:1s and prot. B a 1s:4s on-off duty cycle.

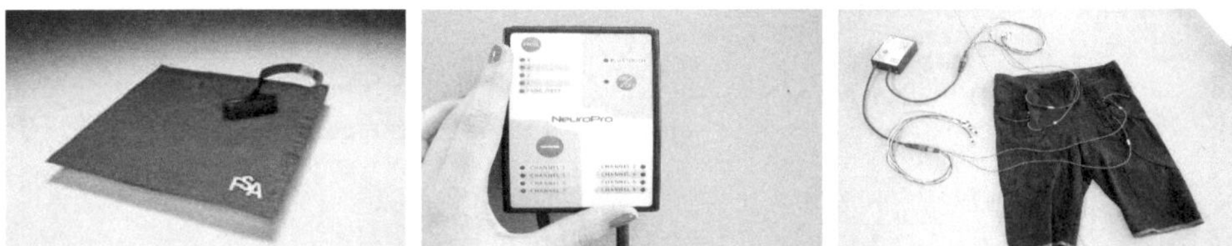

Figure 1. From L to R: pressure mapping system, stimulator, and Bioshorts with ES system

Data collection and statistics

Pressure values were recorded (10 Hz) at start (t0), after 1 (t1), 2 (t2), and 3 (t3) hrs during the 3 min stimulation and the last min before the stimulation. Peak and mean (9-sensor) pressure under the tuber areas and pressure gradient (difference between mean pressure and surrounding sensors) were calculated (see Fig. 2). A 2-way repeated measures ANOVA was used to compare pressure values of the 2 protocols ($\alpha=0.05$).

3. Results

For both protocols, peak pressure decreased ($p<0.05$) from 183±13 (A) and 179±14 (B) during rest to 168±17 (A) and 147±24 (B) mmHg during the 3-hr stimulation periods. The pressure gradient tended ($p<0.1$) to decrease for both protocols indicating an improved pressure distribution. Protocol B showed in general superior effects.

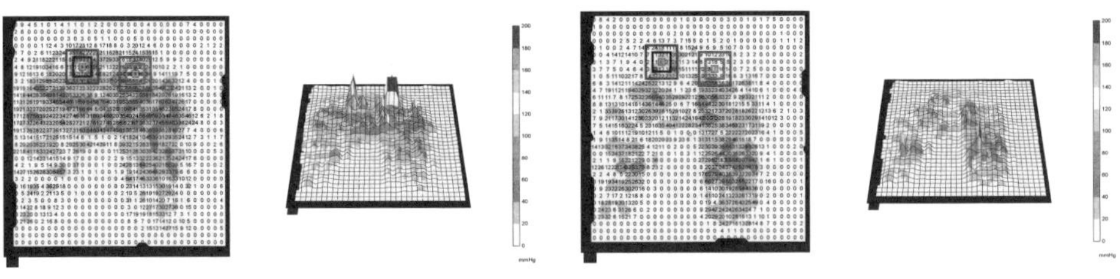

Figure 2. Example of the pressure profile during rest (left panels) and during Protocol B stimulation (right panels). Squares indicate areas used for analysis.

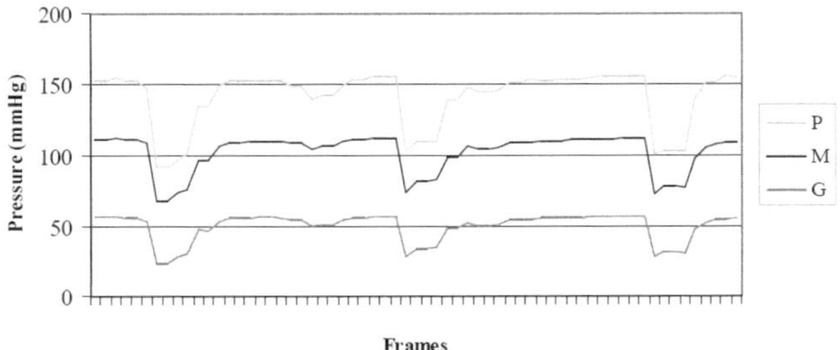

Figure 3.. Example of ES-induced reductions for peak (P) and mean (M) pressure and pressure gradient (G) during the first 14s of Protocol B (1:4).

Within the 3 min stimulation, muscle fatigue apparently occurred during Prot. A, but not in Prot. B, because pressure reductions disappeared. No differences in maximal pressure reductions were found between t1, t2, and t3 for both protocols, indicating that the 17-min rest was sufficient and no significant fatigue occurred during the 3 hours.

4.   Conclusion

ES-induced activation of the gluteal and hamstring muscles in sitting individuals with SCI causes a temporary decrease in peak sitting pressure under the tuber areas and an improved pressure distribution during a 3-hr daily life situation. A protocol with longer rest periods (1:4) results in larger pressure reductions and less fatigue. This method appears practical in daily life and well tolerated by the individuals. Since ES not only reduces sitting pressure but also increases circulation and muscle mass, this technique seems very promising.

References

[1]   A. van Londen, M. Herwegh, C.H. van der Zee, A. Daffertshofer, C.A. Smit, A. Niezen, T.W. Janssen. The effect of surface electric stimulation of the gluteal muscles on the interface pressure in seated people with spinal cord injury. *Arch Phys Med Rehabil* 89:1724-32, 2008.

Rehabilitation: Mobility, Exercise and Sports
L.H.V. van der Woude et al. (Eds.)
IOS Press, 2010
© 2010 The authors and IOS Press. All rights reserved.
doi:10.3233/978-1-60750-080-3-335

A comparison of low and high frequency functional electrical stimulation during standing in spinal cord injury

A.I.P. TANHOFFER [a,1], J. CROSBIE [a], G.M. DAVIS [a], J.W. MIDDLETON [b],
J.E. BUTLER [c]
*[a] Faculty of Health Sciences, [b] Faculty of Medicine, The University of Sydney,
[c] Prince of Wales Medical Research Institute, Australia*

Abstract. Functional electrical stimulation (FES) using a low frequency [LF] of 35 – 50 Hz can assist people with spinal cord injury (SCI) to stand, however recent work suggests that a higher frequency [HF] (100Hz) might be preferable, eliciting longer duration muscle contractions at lower current intensities. We compared the two FES paradigms in people with incomplete SCI, with respect to the duration and stability of their upright standing. Subjects stood unassisted, and with LF and HF FES. Stimulation was applied to quadriceps and gluteus muscles, intensity being increased according to the tolerance and requirement of the individual. Postural sway characteristics were measured using a force platform to capture the variance of the horizontal shear forces plus the AP and lateral motion of the Centre of Pressure. Preliminary findings indicate that duration and stability parameters are significantly and substantially improved by both forms of FES compared to no stimulation. There is some indication that HF stimulation evokes a more stable response than LF.

Keywords. incomplete spinal cord injury, functional electrical stimulation, low frequency, high frequency, standing.

1. Introduction

Following spinal cord injury (SCI), patients are often left with significant motor deficits in the lower limbs. The most obvious functional limitation of these impairments is the inability to walk unaided. For many, however, their ability to stand with minimum support is of short duration. The use of strategically applied functional electrical stimulation (FES) to the extensor muscles of the lower limbs (quadriceps femoris and gluteus maximus) may extend this duration and hence allow functionally relevant independent standing. Conventional stimulation patterns utilize low frequency (LF) stimuli trains of between 35 and 50 Hz. Some current opinion has suggested that higher frequency (HF) stimulation paradigms using 100Hz may elicit longer duration muscle contractions without rapid onset of fatigue, through the evocation of "plateau potential" phenomena [1]. The purpose of this study was to test the ability of SCI

---

[1] Corresponding Author: Aldre I.P. Tanhoffer, Clinical and Rehabilitation Sciences, Discipline of Physiotherapy, Faculty of Health Sciences, The University of Sydney, NSW, Australia, E-mail: a.tanhoffer@usyd.edu.au

subjects with incomplete motor lesions to stand continuously with minimum support under conditions of voluntary muscle recruitment, LF stimulation and HF stimulation and to compare the results obtained from each condition. At this stage, only preliminary data from three subjects will be reported.

2. Methods

Three individuals with motor-incomplete SCI (Table 1) were tested on their standing ability using two different FES paradigms (LF 35Hz and HF 100Hz) and via voluntary muscle recruitment. Testing occurred on different days but at the same time of day and in random order.

The subject was lifted to an upright posture by an overhead support harness and was positioned to stand on a floor-mounted (AMTI) force platform. Stimulation was then applied (when the LF or HF were tested) to quadriceps femoris and gluteus maximus muscles. Stimulation intensity was increased incrementally according to the tolerance and requirement of the individual. Continuous collection of force platform data was carried out until the subject was unable to continue the test due to muscle fatigue beyond the capacity of FES stimulation. The variance (standard deviation) of the horizontal shear forces provide a reliable and valid measure of postural sway [2] as do the amplitudes of anteroposterior (AP) and medio-lateral (ML) motion of the Centre of Pressure.

3. Results

The duration of standing under the three conditions is detailed on (Table 1). Subjects 1 and 2 demonstrated substantial improvements in their standing duration with FES stimulation. Subject 3 demonstrated no real difference in this aspect of standing with or without FES.

Table 1. Participant characteristics and standing durations

Subjects	Gender	Age (years)	Time since injury	Level of injury	ASIA	Type of standing	*Duration*
1	Male	59	23 years	T 8	C	Free (No stim)	*7min 14s*
						LF	*37min*
						HF	*39min*
2	Male	53	6 years	T 12	C	Free (No stim)	*2min 07s*
						LF	*7min*
						HF	*6min 12s*
3	Female	22	6 years	T 12	C	Free (No stim)	*22min*
						LF	*23min*
						HF	*23min*

The Standard Deviation of the horizontal shear forces during sustained quiet standing [Figure 1]. In subjects 1 and 2 there are clear improvements in the stability measured by this variable when stimulation is applied. It is not clear from these values, however, whether HF or LF is more effective. Subject 3 demonstrated low variance even under free-standing conditions and stimulation does not seem to make much difference.

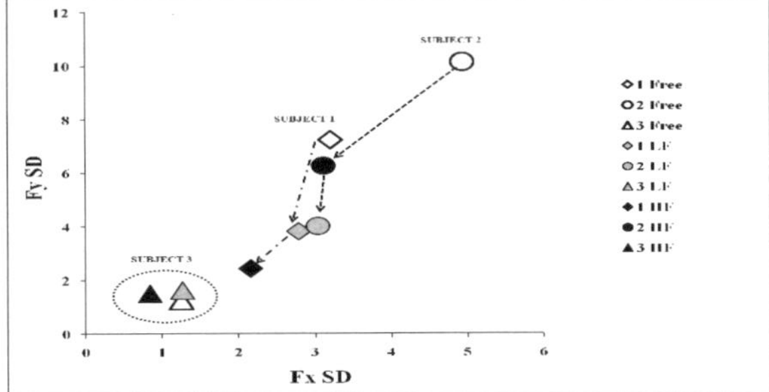

Figure 1. The Standard Deviation of the horizontal shear forces during sustained quiet standing.

The total amount of "sway" [Figure 2] as shown by the amplitude of centre of pressure (CoP) movement in the antero-posterior (Y direction) direction and the mediolateral direction (X direction) is, in each case, improved by HF stimulation. Mediolateral sway seems to be particularly improved with FES, antero-posterior sway (Y direction) is more variable.

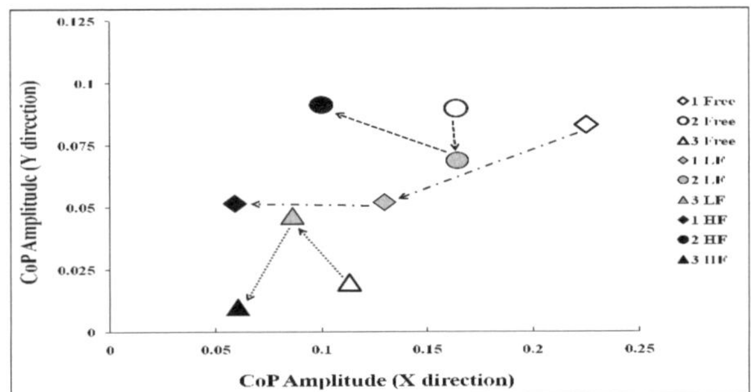

Figure 2. The total amount of "sway" as shown by the amplitude of centre of pressure movement in the antero-posterior (Y) direction and the mediolateral direction (X).

4.   Conclusion

There is some indication that HF stimulation evokes a greater stability during sustained standing than conventional LF FES, indicating that it could be related to the development of *'plateau potentials'* what can provide an on-going motoneuron 'after discharge' and thereby continued force output.

References

[1]   D.F. Collins et al., Sustained contraction produced by plateau-like behavior in human motoneurons. *J. Physiology*, **538** (2002), 289-301.
[2]   P. A. Goldie, Postural control in standing following stroke: test-retest reliability of some quantitative clinical tests. *Physical Therapy*, **70**(1990), 234-243.

Rehabilitation: Mobility, Exercise and Sports
L.H.V. van der Woude et al. (Eds.)
IOS Press, 2010
© *2010 The authors and IOS Press. All rights reserved.*
doi:10.3233/978-1-60750-080-3-338

No significant muscle atrophy occurs in first dorsal interosseus muscle after incomplete cervical spinal cord injury

A. TEUNISSEN[a], R. BAKELS[a], C.K. THOMAS[b], D. MULDER[c], I. ZIJDEWIND[a]

[a] *Department of Neurosciences, Medical Physiology, UMCG, Groningen, The Netherlands*
[b] *The Miami Project to Cure Paralysis, University of Miami Miller School of Medicine, Miami, Florida, USA*
[c] *UMCG-Center for Rehabilitation Beatrixoord, Groningen, The Netherlands*

Abstract. Purpose: Following spinal cord injury (SCI), atrophy is often observed in muscles innervated from spinal segments below the lesion. We used the twitch interpolation technique to estimate the total force capacity of the first dorsal interosseus muscle (FDI, index finger abductor) and compared these data to the maximal voluntary contraction (MVC) actually produced by the subject. Methods: Four SCI subjects who had partial voluntary control over their hand muscles, 7 control SCI subjects with intact hand function and 10 able-bodied subjects (AB) performed 3 MVCs and 3 voluntary contractions at 10, 30, 50 and 70% MVC with the right FDI muscle. During the contractions the ulnar nerve was electrically activated (two pulses, interval 10 ms). Muscle force evoked by the stimulation was expressed as a percentage of the potentiated rest twitch and plotted against the background force. Results: MVCs were smaller in the incomplete SCI-group (19.1±3.5N, p<0.005) compared to the control SCI group (40.8±9.1N) and AB-controls (38.1±10.2N). However, the total force capacity as estimated on the basis of regression analysis between the superimposed twitch and background forces resulted in similar forces for all groups (incomplete SCI: 28.5±7.3N, control SCI: 36.4±16.0N, AB-controls: 30.3±6.2N). Conclusion: Comparable total force capacity for all groups suggests that muscle atrophy was insignificant in the SCI-subjects with incomplete injuries.

Keywords. incomplete spinal cord injury, muscle atrophy, twitch interpolation technique, total muscle force, first dorsal interosseus.

1. Introduction

Following spinal cord injury (SCI), muscle atrophy is often observed in muscles innervated from spinal segments below the lesion. Incomplete SCI is characterized by a deterioration of function and deficits in force production in some muscles, but these muscles can still be activated voluntarily to some extent. Force reductions (muscle weakness) after incomplete injury are expected to be largely due to decreased drive from the central nervous system. However, if muscle fibers are denervated chronically or not used that much then muscle atrophy likely also contributes to the force loss. In the present study we used the twitch interpolation technique [1] to approximate the total force capacity of the first dorsal interosseus muscle. Since muscle force is proportional to the cross-sectional area of a muscle [2], the predicted total force capacity can be used as an indicator of possible muscle atrophy [3]. We compared data obtained from subjects with incomplete spinal cord injury with able bodied control subjects and with spinal cord injured subjects who had thoracic lesions and so uncompromised hand function. The latter control group was added to compensate for possible differences in hand use after spinal cord injury (e.g. due to wheelchair use).

2. Methods

Subjects

Four chronic SCI-subjects with impaired hand function (incomplete SCI group; 3 males, lesion level: C4-C6), 7 control SCI-subjects with unimpaired hand function (control SCI-group; 5 males, lesion level: T3-T10) and 10 able-bodied, age-matched control subjects (AB-controls; 7 males) were included in this study.

Protocol

We assessed the maximal voluntary abduction force of the right index finger. Subjects gripped an isometric force transducer [4] and looked at a computer screen that showed the force and a command line. When the command line went up subjects were instructed to perform a maximal voluntary contraction (MVC) with the first dorsal interosseus (FDI, index finger abductor) muscle. After determining the maximal voluntary force, 3 voluntary contractions were performed at several submaximal forces (10, 30, 50 and 70% MVC). During the submaximal and maximal contractions the ulnar nerve was electrically activated (two pulses, interval 10 ms) at 150% of the intensity that produced a maximal EMG response (M-wave) at rest. The stimulation resulted in a twitch superimposed on the voluntary contraction (twitch interpolation technique). Twitches were evoked at rest after the maximal contractions.

Data analysis

Additional muscle force evoked by the stimulation was expressed as a percentage of the rest twitch and plotted against the background force (voluntary force at the time of stimulation). Regression analysis was used to predict the total force capacity of the FDI.

3. Results

The MVC force were significantly lower in the incomplete SCI-group (19.1 ± 3.5N) compared to both the control SCI group (40.8 ± 9.1N, $p<0.005$) and AB-controls (38.1 ± 10.2N, $p<0.005$). The superimposed twitches recorded during the MVCs were significantly larger in the incomplete SCI-subjects (incomplete SCI: $37.6\pm29.2\%$ of rest twitch, SCI-control: $2.1\pm2.5\%$ of rest twitch, AB-controls: $5.6\pm8.8\%$, $p=0.001$) suggesting that the lower voluntary force of the incomplete SCI-subjects was partly due to insufficient drive to the motoneurons. The total force capacity however, estimated on the basis of regression analysis between the twitch amplitude and background forces was not significantly different between the groups (incomplete SCI: 28.5 ± 7.3N, control SCI: 36.4 ± 16.0N, AB-controls: 30.3 ± 6.2N).

4. Discussion

The fact that the estimated total force capacity of the incomplete SCI group was similar to the two control groups indicates there was no evident muscle atrophy. The decrease in voluntary force without muscle atrophy can be explained: 1) by inadequate drive to the motoneuron pool without significant changes in the number of innervated muscle fibers (and therefore no muscle atrophy) [5]; or 2) by innervation of fewer muscle fibers from higher brain centers without changes in muscle fiber integrity (possibly due to passive movements imposed on the paralyzed muscle fibers by the remaining functional muscle fibers [6]). Both theories have interesting and important implications. If all motor units are still under voluntary control but are more difficult to activate because of impaired drive, it implies that techniques that enhance the corticospinal excitability could be an important tool in rehabilitation. However, if passive exercise is capable of maintaining muscle fibers properties, more attention is needed to include this therapy in rehabilitation programs.

Acknowledgement

Funded by USPHS grant NS-3-2351, NS-30226, The Miami Project to Cure Paralysis, and the University of Groningen.

References

[1]   Shield and S. Zhou, Assessing voluntary muscle activation with the twitch interpolation technique, *Sports medicine* **34** (2004), 253-267.
[2]   S.A. Bruce, S.K. Philips and R.C. Woledge, Interpreting the relation between force and cross-sectional area in human muscle, *Medicine and science in sports and exercise* **29** (1997), 677-683.
[3]   C.K.Thomas, E.Y. Zaidner, B. Calancie, J.G. Broton. and B.R. Bigland-Ritchie. Muscle weakness, paralysis and atrophy after human cervical spinal cord injury. *Exp Neurol* **148** (1997), 414-423.
[4]   H. van Duinen , M. Post, K. Vaartjes, H. Hoogduin , I. Zijdewind. MR compatible strain gauge based force transducer. J Neurosci Methods. **164** (2007), 247-54.
[5]   I. Zijdewind and C.K. Thomas, Motor unit firing during and after voluntary contractions of human thenar muscles weakened by spinal cord injury, *Journal of neurophysiologogy* **89** (2003), 2065-2071.
[6]   T. Sasa, K. Sairyo, N. Yoshida, M. Fukunaga, K. Koga, M. Ishikawa and N. Yasui, Continuous muscle stretch prevents disuse muscle atrophy and deterioration of its oxidative capacity in rat tail–suspension models, *American journal of physical medicine & rehabilitation* **83** (2004), 851-856.

Chapter 9

Sports Performance

9.1

Keynote

Rehabilitation: Mobility, Exercise and Sports
L.H.V. van der Woude et al. (Eds.)
IOS Press, 2010
doi:10.3233/978-1-60750-080-3-343

Research in sport performance and rehabilitation

Y.C. VANLANDEWIJCK[a], Y. BHAMBHANI[b], J. MACTAVISH[c], S. WARREN[b],
P. VAN DE VLIET[c,d], S.M. TWEEDY[e]
[a]*Faculty of Kinesiology and Rehabilitation Sciences, Katholieke Universiteit
Leuven, Belgium*
[b]*Faculty of Rehabilitation Medicine, University of Alberta, Canada*
[c]*Faculty of Physical Education & Recreation, University of Manitoba, Canada*
[d]*International Paralympic Committee, Bonn, Germany*
[e]*School of Human Movement Studies, University of Queensland, Brisbane,
Australia*

1. Introduction

The research agenda of the Sport Science Committee (SSC) of the International Paralympic Committee (IPC) is driven by questions of interest in the Paralympic Movement. While many of these questions concern elite athletes at the summit of their careers, the research outcomes have implications for novice athletes and, in some situations, people in rehabilitation. From the research agenda of the SSC, 'boosting' (deliberate induced autonomic dysreflexia to improve performance) is selected for discussion, with conclusions drawn in relation to rehabilitation and grassroots' sport.

2. Boosting in Athletes with High Level Spinal Cord Injury: Incidence, Knowledge and Attitudes of Athletes in Paralympic Sport

People with spinal injuries at or above the 6th thoracic segment can experience from an abnormal sympathetic reflex called Autonomic Dysreflexia (AD). This reflex is caused by any noxious stimulus below the level of the lesion, such as distension or irritation of the urinary bladder or musculoskeletal trauma. The symptoms of AD include a rapid rise in blood pressure, headache, sweating, skin blotchiness and goose bumps. This reflex may happen spontaneously or may be deliberately self-induced to improve performance, a practice known among athletes and coaches as "Boosting". However significant health risk are associated with AD - in serious cases, confusion, cerebral haemorrhage and even death can occur – and consequently the IPC forbids athletes to deliberately induce AD or to compete when under the influence of AD.

Currently, there is no research that has systematically examined the incidence of boosting, or which has investigated the knowledge and attitudes of competitive athletes pertaining to boosting. The objectives of this WADA approved and funded research study were to: (1) examine the incidence of boosting in competitive high level spinal cord injured athletes, (2) evaluate their knowledge and beliefs with respect to the effects of boosting on sport performance and overall health, and (3) document their attitudes towards boosting and other performance enhancement strategies in competitive sport.

3.   Methods

The target population was athletes with a spinal cord injury at or above T6 who were currently competing in Paralympic sport at state / provincial level or above. Data was collected via a questionnaire designed by the IPC SSC which was piloted for content validity and readability prior to circulation. Data were collected via three main avenues: Members of the International Network for the Advancement of Paralympic Sports through Science (INAPSS) distributed the questionnaire to eligible athletes in their home countries; eligible athletes competing at the 2008 Paralympic Games in Beijing; and via an on-line version on the IPC website. Data were statistically analyzed using Chi square test of frequency and the Fisher Exact test.

4.   Results

A total of 99 (84♂, 11♀, 4 not identified) participants completed the questionnaire. The majority of the participants were aged 22 to 45 years (86.8%) and were more than 5 years post-injury (89%). Lesion levels were predominantly at the cervical spine (C5-C7: 70.7%, T1-T3: 3.0%, T4-T6: 14.1%). A large majority of the participants (54.2%) competed in wheelchair rugby, followed by wheelchair sprint events (10.4%), wheelchair basketball and middle distance events (9.4% each), long distance events including marathon racing (12.6%) and throwing events (6.3%).

Awareness and Incidence of Boosting

Of the 99 participants who completed the survey, 54.5% had heard of boosting prior to reading about it in the questionnaire, while 39.4% had not heard of boosting previously and 6% did not respond?. Sixty participants responded the question: *"Have you ever intentionally induced autonomic dysreflexia to boost your performance in training or competition?"*, 10 (16.7%) in the affirmative and 50 (83.3%) in the negative. All the positive responses were obtained from the males who played wheelchair rugby (55.5%) or competed in long distance wheelchair racing (44.4%). Of the 10 respondents who used boosting, a small proportion (6% to 14%) used it during training or national competition. Only one participant indicated that he used boosting all the time during national and international competitions to improve performance.

Knowledge and Beliefs about Boosting

The participants identified the following variables that they felt benefited from boosting during competition: *increased arm strength and endurance, less arm stiffness, less difficulty breathing, improved circulation, less overall fatigue, increased aggression, and increased alertness.* However, a small number of participants also reported *increased anxiety and greater frustration* as possible effects of boosting during competition.

   Beliefs about how dangerous boosting is were evenly divided: On a 5 point scale, 52.9% of participants believed that boosting was not dangerous or somewhat dangerous, and 46.8% believed boosting was dangerous or very dangerous to
   health.

The main source of knowledge regarding the symptoms of boosting was their personal experience (61.7%) and reports from other athletes (50%). The participants gained some information by reading about boosting (22.9%) and only 2.1% had received information from their coaches.

Attitude towards Boosting

Almost 100% of the participants believed it was unacceptable to use banned drugs to improve training capacity or maximize performance. Although the majority of the respondents (61.3%) indicated that boosting was *"completely unacceptable"* for improving training capacity or maximizing performance in competition (64.5%), their opinion was split when queried whether *"boosting should not be banned because it can happen unintentionally"* (25% thought this is unacceptable while 37% were in agreement with the statement). Similarly, the participants expressed opposing views in responding to the statement *"boosting should not be banned because any athlete with T6 or higher spinal cord injury can decide to induce autonomic dysreflexia."*

5. Conclusion

Although this study has some drawbacks such as geographical and sport representation of respondents, clear recommendations for stakeholders are nevertheless evident. There is an important role for the physiotherapist/physician during rehabilitation to educate every SCI patient, vulnerable for AD, about boosting. National and International Federations should start educational programmes about AD for all athletes from novice to elite level, as well as coaches and support staff. Testing for AD during National and International competition should be improved and should be implemented more frequently.

Acknowledgement

The authors want to acknowledge the International Network for the Advancement of Paralympic Sport through Science (INAPSS) for their contribution in the boosting survey (Dr. L. Malone, Dr. E. Colantonio, Dr. M. Tulio de Mello, Dr. E. Bressan, Dr. B. Burkett, Mr. K. Frojd, Dr. Yves Vanlandewijck, Dr. S. Tweedy). Furthermore, the authors want to thank the World Anti-Doping Association (WADA) for their financial support.

9.2

Oral Presentations

Rehabilitation: Mobility, Exercise and Sports
L.H.V. van der Woude et al. (Eds.)
IOS Press, 2010
© *2010 The authors and IOS Press. All rights reserved.*
doi:10.3233/978-1-60750-080-3-349

The influence of glove type on mobility performance for wheelchair rugby players

B.S. MASON[a], L.H.V. VAN DER WOUDE[b], V.L. GOOSEY-TOLFREY[a]
[a]*School of Sport and Exercise Sciences, Loughborough University, U.K.*
[b]*Centre for Human Movement Sciences, University Medical Centre Groningen, RUG, Groningen, The Netherlands*

Abstract. The purpose of this study was to determine the effectiveness of different glove types on mobility performance specific to wheelchair rugby. Ten international wheelchair rugby players performed three field drills in four glove conditions: i) players' current glove selection (CON), ii) American football glove (NFL), iii) building glove (BLD) and iv) new prototype glove (HYB). Performance was assessed by times taken, peak velocities and accelerations within each drill through the use of a velocometer sampling at 100Hz and a short likert scale questionnaire. A Two-way analysis of variance with repeated measures revealed that participants' performed significantly better for measures of acceleration and sprinting when wearing CON in comparison to HYB ($p < 0.05$). Subjective data identified that players also favoured CON ahead of other gloves. It may be concluded that gloves which have been modified to cater for the specific demands of wheelchair rugby players are more effective for aspects of mobility performance.

Keywords. wheelchair propulsion, wheelchair athletes, sports performance.

1. Introduction

The majority of wheelchair rugby (WCR) players use some form of gloves and/or taping on the hands in order to improve coupling with the hand rim and to provide hand protection. Players currently wear a variety of gloves designed for other purposes and often modify these in order to accommodate the demands of their sport, as a glove designed specifically for WCR does not exist.

Research into the use of gloves and its effect on wheelchair sports performance is extremely limited. It has been revealed that a glove/splint combination can reduce wrist extension, which may contribute to decreased injury incidence, without negatively affecting maximal wheeling speed [1]. Only Lutgendorf et al. [2] have investigated the effects of glove type on aspects of mobility performance specific to WCR. This study revealed that American football gloves and building gloves performed consistently better than multipurpose gloves and no gloves at all during field tests with able-bodied participants.

The aim of the current investigation was to determine the effectiveness of four different glove types upon aspects of mobility performance specific in WCR.

2. Method

Ten international WCR players (30 ± 5 years, 66.2 ± 6.9 kg) participated in the study. Each participant performed three sport specific field tests in their own sports wheelchair in four different glove conditions: i) participants' current glove modified for competition (CON) ii) American football glove (NFL) iii) building glove (BLD) iv) a new glove developed specifically for WCR (HYB).

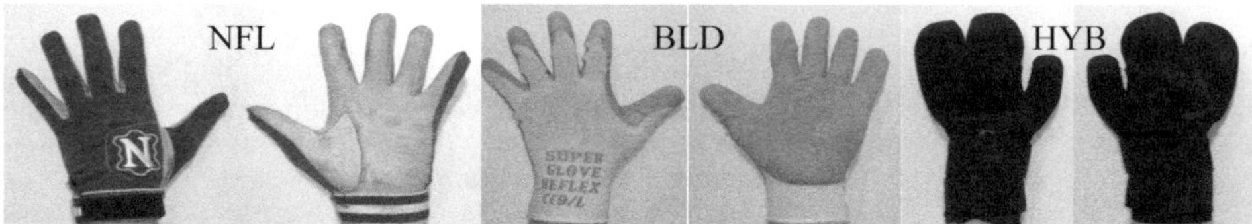

Figure 1. Illustration of three glove types sampled

Glove performance was assessed using the times taken to complete drills in conjunction with velocity, acceleration and deceleration data derived from a velocometer sampling at 100Hz. The velocometer as documented by Moss et al. [3] was attached to each participants chair and produced velocity traces with respect to each push. Measures of glove performance were grouped into three categories based on the aspects of performance they assessed: i) Acceleration, ii) Braking, iii) Sprinting. Participants were also required to complete a short likert scale questionnaire to ascertain their subjective ratings of each gloves performance. A series of two-way ANOVA's with repeated measures were conducted on all measures of performance.

3. Results

Objective Measures

Glove type had no significant effect on braking performance. However, the peak velocities reached within 2.5m and 5m revealed that CON was significantly more proficient for accelerating in comparison to all other glove types. Measures of sprinting performance also revealed that participants performed a linear 15m sprint significantly quicker in CON than HYB and completed an agility drill significantly quicker than all glove types.

Subjective Measures

The results of the questionnaire revealed that participants subjectively valued CON ahead of all other gloves for the comfort and the grip they offered. HYB were shown to be least favourable for the preparation time they required, although along with CON, this glove rated highly for its protection properties than other glove types.

4. Discussion

The results of the current investigation revealed that participants mobility was improved when wearing gloves which had been modified specifically to each individual (CON). The superior performance of CON may be attributed to the improved familiarity that participants had with these gloves. It may also be possible that the condition of CON may be better associated with improved mobility performance, as all other gloves were either brand new or worn once, whereas the condition of CON was not controlled. Therefore, a breaking in period may exist for gloves in order to perform optimally. Although beyond the scope of this study, it is possible that CON induced improved coupling at the wheelchair-user interface, as was subjectively reinforced by participants in the questionnaire.

The only area that HYB performed well in was participants subjective ratings of hand protection. These gloves may have been bulky and rigid enough in design to provide protection, yet too bulky to allow for optimal mobility performance. The materials used for HYB were similar to those that participants strategically located to modify CON. Therefore, these materials seem to provide sufficient protection, yet the more strategic location in CON does not impinge upon hand dexterity and wheelchair handling skills.

Future Recommendations

In order to develop a greater understanding of the topic area, further investigations under more controlled laboratory conditions would be desirable. A force application investigation would provide more detailed information as to how gloves of different materials and configurations interact directly at the wheelchair-user interface. More also needs to be known about the exact location of pressure distributed on the hands during wheelchair propulsion so that gloves can be reinforced in areas that are specific to users' individual techniques. Finally a kinematic and electromyographic investigation of the joint and muscular activity of the lower arm would provide a better assessment of gloves protection properties.

References

[1]　L.A. Malone, P.L. Gervais, R.S. Burnham, M. Chan, L. Miller & R.S. Steadward, An assessment of wrist splint and glove use on wheeling kinematics, *Clinical Biomechanics* **13** (1998), 234-236.

[2]　M. Lutgendorf, B.S. Mason, L.H.V. van der Woude & V.L. Goosey-Tolfrey, The effect of glove type on wheelchair rugby skill performance, *British Paralympic Association 6th Annual Sports Science and Medicine Conference* (2008).

[3]　A.D. Moss, N.E. Fowler & V.L. Goosey-Tolfrey, A telemetry based velocometer to measure wheelchair velocity, *Journal of Biomechanics* **36** (2003), 253-257.

352

Rehabilitation: Mobility, Exercise and Sports
L.H.V. van der Woude et al. (Eds.)
IOS Press, 2010
© 2010 The authors and IOS Press. All rights reserved.
doi:10.3233/978-1-60750-080-3-352

Sports participation in adolescents and young adults with Myelomeningocele

L.M. BUFFART[a,1], H.P. VAN DER PLOEG[b], A.E. BAUMAN[b], F.W. VAN ASBECK[c], H.J. STAM[a], M.E. ROEBROECK[a], H.J.G. VAN DEN BERG EMONS[a]
[a]*Department of Rehabilitation Medicine, Erasmus MC Rotterdam, The Netherlands*
[b]*Centre for Physical Activity and Health, Sydney, Australia*
[c]*Department of Rehabilitation Medicine, University Medical Center Utrecht, The Netherlands*

Abstract. To assess sports participation in young adults with spina bifida and its association with personal, condition-related and psychosocial factors, physical activity and fitness. Fifty-one persons (26 males) participated, mean age 21.1 (standard deviation 4.5) years. We assessed self-reported sports participation, ambulatory status, presence of hydrocephalus, functional independence, social support, perceived competence, exercise enjoyment, self-reported physical activity, peak oxygen uptake and muscle strength. Associations were studied using regression analyses. Thirty-five persons (69%) participated in sports. Sports participation was not associated with condition-related characteristics, but was associated with social support from family, perceived athletic competence and physical appearance ($p \leq 0.05$) and tended to be associated with global self-worth. Sports participants had higher self-reported physical activity levels than non-participants ($p \leq 0.05$). Furthermore, sports participated tended to be less likely to have subnormal muscle strength (odds ratio= 0.26; p= 0.08) and their peak oxygen uptake was 0.19 l/min higher, but not statistically significant (p= 0.13). In conclusion, sports participation seems to be due to personal preferences rather than physical ability; it could benefit from improving social support and perceived competence, and is associated with higher self-reported physical activity.

Keywords. spina bifida, exercise behaviour.

1. Introduction

Physical inactivity has negative consequences for health. It may lead to reduced physical fitness, an increased risk of secondary conditions such as overweight or obesity, diabetes mellitus type 2, and cardiovascular diseases, and to reduced social participation and lower quality of life.

Almost half of the Dutch population is insufficiently active. Due to mobility limitations, people with physical disabilities are at increased risk to develop inactive lifestyles. In a previous study, we showed that adolescents and young adults with spina bifida are less active compared to able-bodied people of the same age [1], and that they have low physical fitness [2]. Persons with spina bifida nowadays survive into adulthood [3] which raises the importance of a healthy lifestyle.

Sports and exercise can be seen as a subcategory of physical activity, which is planned, structured and repetitive [4]. Sports-related physical activities can easily be

---

[1] Corresponding Author.

provided through rehabilitation services and could increase physical activity behaviour and fitness in persons with spina bifida.

Due to the lack of knowledge about sports participation in people with spina bifida is scarce, the present study aimed to investigate sports participation and its association with personal, disease-related and psychosocial factors, physical activity and fitness.

2. Methods

Fifty-one persons (26 males) diagnosed with myelomeningocele (most open and severe form of spina bifida) participated. Mean age was 21.1 (SD 4.5) years and 55% was wheelchair-bound.

The main outcome measure was self-reported current sports participation ($\geq$ 1 hour per week, yes/no). The following personal and condition-related factors were registered: age, gender, educational level, ambulatory status, the presence of shunted hydrocephalus, and functional independence using the total motor score and total cognitive score of the functional independence measure and functional assessment measure (FIM+FAM).

We assessed the following psychosocial factors using questionnaires: social support from family and friend using the Dutch version of the scales for measuring Social Support for Diet and Exercise Behaviours; perceived athletic competence and global self worth using the Dutch version of the Harter's Social Perception Profile for Adolescents scale; and enjoyment in exercise using the Groningen Enjoyment Questionnaire.

The total self-reported physical activity pattern was assessed using the Physical Activity Scale for Individuals with Physical Disabilities (PASIPD). Aerobic fitness was measured during a progressive maximal exercise test. Depending on whether the main mode of ambulation was walking or wheelchair driving, participants performed the test on an electronically braked cycle ergometer or an arm ergometer, respectively. The mean oxygen uptake during the last 30 sec of exercise (peakVO$_2$, expressed in l/min) was used as indicator of aerobic fitness. Muscle strength of upper or lower extremity was determined by hand-held dynamometry and normalised to Z-scores using reference values of able-bodied males and females. A person's lowest Z-score of upper or lower extremity was used as an indicator of muscle strength, dichotomizing it into normal (Z-score > -2) or subnormal (Z-score $\leq$ -2) muscle strength.

Linear and logistic regression analyses were performed to study associations with sports participation. Gender and ambulatory status were potential confounders adjusted for in al multivariable analyses.

3. Results

Thirty-five (69%) adolescents and young adults participated in sports. No relationships were found between sports participation and personal- and condition related factors, except for gender; females tended to be less likely to participate in sports than males (odds ratio= 0.30, p= 0.06).

Sports participation was related to psychosocial factors. People who received more social support from family were more likely to participate in sports (odds ratio =1.12 – 2.12, p< 0.05). In addition, those who received social support from friends (odds ratio=0.17, p= 0.09) and those who reported higher perceived enjoyment of exercise (odds ratio= 1.05, p= 0.10) tended be more likely to participate in sports. Furthermore, sports participation was associated with athletic competence (odds ratio= 1.47, p= 0.001) and physical appearance (odds ratio= 1.24, p= 0.03), and appeared to have some association with global self-worth (odds ratio = 1.20, p= 0.10).

Results of the PASIPD showed that persons who engaged in sports were more physically active during the day (p< 0.05). Besides, they also reported 56 min more on non-exercise related walking or wheelchair driving (p= 0.04). In sports participants, the contribution of sports and exercise to total physical activity was 16%. Time spent on household and occupational activities did not differ between persons who participated in sports and those who did not.

Average peakVO$_2$ was 0.19 l/min higher in persons who participated in sports compared to those who did not; however, this difference was not significant (p= 0.13). The percentage of participants with subnormal muscle strength tended to be lower in those who participated in sports (52%) compared to those who did not (81%; odds ratio= 0.26, p= 0.08).

4. Conclusion

Sports participation seems to be due to personal preferences rather than physical ability. It could benefit from social support (particularly from a person's family) and perceived competence, and is associated with higher self-reported physical activity. Conclusive evidence is needed on whether sports participation improves physical fitness. Improving physical activity behaviour and fitness in persons with spina bifida is important for health, and increasing sports participation may contribute.

References

[1]   L.M. Buffart et al. Triad of physical activity, aerobic fitness, and obesity in adolescents and young adults with myelomeningocele. *J Rehabil Med* **40** (2008), 70-75.
[2]   L.M. Buffart et al. Health-related physical fitness of adolescents and young adults with myelomeningocele. *Eur J Appl Physiol* **103** (2008), 181-188.
[3]   R.M. Bowman et al. Spina bifida outcome: a 25-year prospective. *Pediatr Neurosurg* **34** (2001), 114-120.
[4]   C.J. Caspersen et al. Physical activity, exercise and physical fitness: definitions and distinctions for health-related research. *Public Health Rep* **100** (1985), 126-131.

Rehabilitation: Mobility, Exercise and Sports
L.H.V. van der Woude et al. (Eds.)
IOS Press, 2010
© 2010 The authors and IOS Press. All rights reserved.
doi:10.3233/978-1-60750-080-3-355

Essential wheeled mobility skills for daily life – an international survey among elite wheelchair athletes with SCI

O. FLIESS-DOUER[a], Y.C. VANLANDEWIJCK[a], L.H.V. VAN DER WOUDE[b]

[a] *Faculty of Physical Education and Physiotherapy, Department of Rehabilitation Sciences, K.U. Leuven, Belgium*
[b] *Centre for human Movement Sciences, University Medical Centre Groningen, University of Groningen, The Netherlands*

Abstract. To develop a universal wheelchair skill test battery, a survey among wheelchair athletes was initiated. Opinions of athletes with a spinal cord injury (SCI) regarding the most essential skills for everyday life were collected. Where and by whom they learned to perform these skills, were also asked. A survey with 24-skills was presented to wheelchair athletes with SCI during the Beijing Paralympics. Respondents were asked to state the essentiality of each skill (1-5; Not essential - extremely essential), and to inform where and by whom they learned to perform each skill. Three visual analog scales (VAS 1-10) were used to examine 1) how SCI perceived their level of wheeled mobility (WM) gained during rehabilitation, 2) to determine the amount of time that was dedicated for teaching WM skills during rehabilitation; and 3) to express their level of WM at present. The study sample (M/F: 49/30, Para/Tetra 64/15) represents 18 countries and 14 sports disciplines. Results revealed that the most essential skill for daily life is "transfer in/out a car" (4.67±0.69). Judged as less essential is a "one-handed wheelie" (1.96±1.36). Of the respondents 57% learned the most essential skills in clinical rehabilitation, while 40% claimed to have learned those skills afterwards in a community setting. Mean ±SD of 'WM skills gained in rehabilitation' was 5.4±2.5 and of 'WM at present' 8.5±1.5. This revealed a significant increase in WM skill level perceptions over time. The Swedish rehabilitation system received the highest (7.6), and Spanish hospitals the lowest (2.8) scores. It is of greatest importance to incorporate skills that were graded "Very-extremely essential" in inpatient rehabilitation and in post hospital WM workshops. It is recommended to conduct a comparative study of rehabilitation programs in different countries in order to improve WM teaching methods.

Keywords. hand rim wheelchair, mobility, spinal cord injury, skill survey.

1. Introduction

Wheeled mobility skills (WM) are essential to daily functioning of people with spinal cord injury (SCI), and assumed to contribute to their participation and quality of life. According to the International Classification of Functioning Disability and Health (ICF), the most appropriate definition to wheeled mobility is "**Moving around using equipment**: moving the whole body from place to place, on any surface or space, by using specific devices designed to facilitate moving or create other ways of moving around, such as with skates, skis, or scuba equipment, or moving down the street in a wheelchair or a walker"[1]. For individuals with SCI this definition relates to their ability to move around, using a wheelchair, in different and changing environments.

To develop a universal wheelchair skill test battery, a survey among wheelchair athletes was initiated during the Paralympic games in Beijing 2008, in order to collect SCI athletes' opinions regarding the most essential skills for everyday life and to find out where and by whom the participants learned to perform these skills.

2.   Method

Design

Survey with 24-skills was presented among wheelchair athletes with SCI during the games. Decisions about survey content were gathered from a literature review of WM skill tests that were published between 1970 and 2007 [2], the researchers' own experiences working with individuals with SCI, and the British Spinal Injuries Association "Turning the Corner" video cassette (2003 © all rights reserved). The participants were asked to:

- State the essentiality of each skill (1-5; Not essential - extremely essential);

- State where and by whom they learned to perform each skill;

- Answer three questions using a VAS scale from poor to excellent[3]:

    o   "How would you describe the level of your wheeled mobility skills gained during the rehabilitation period?"

    o   "How would you describe the amount of time dedicated for teaching wheeled mobility skills during your inpatient stay at the hospital?"

    o   "How would you describe your level of wheeled mobility skills performance today?"

Sample

The study sample (N=79, M/F: 49/30, Para/Tetra 64/15) represented 18 countries and 14 sports disciplines. Age Range 14-53 (M= 33±8.18), Time since Injury varied between 3 and 31 years (M= 15.5±6.63). Three categories for athlete's subgroups were determined: Gender, Lesion level/completeness and type of sport (static wheelchair sport, dynamic - team and/ or individual - wheelchair sport, and non wheelchair sport).

3.   Results

Survey analysis results

The most essential skills were: "Transferring into a car / out of a car" (4.7±0.7), "50 meter forward" (4.5±1) and "Going up a ramp and opening a door (4.35±1). The less essential skills were: One handed wheelie (1.96±1.6), Going up & down a flight of 5 stairs with a handrail (2.3±1.4) and 5 minutes on a treadmill (2.8±1.4). 57% of the respondents learned to perform the most essential skills during rehab, 33% claimed to have learned to perform those skills after rehab elsewhere, 7% of the respondents learned to perform the most essential skills in sport activity after rehab while 3% never learned to perform those skills. 42% of the respondents stated that they learned to perform the most essential skills by themselves, the same percentages were learned these skills by a professional instructor, 13% by a peer and 3% never learned them. The Swedish athletes learned WM skills during inpatient by peers who came to the hospital on a regular base for that purpose.

Athlete's subgroups investigation results

Two significant differences in perception of WM at present were found: persons with tetraplegia perceive lower WM levels than those with paraplegia, and athletes who participate in team wheelchair sports perceived the highest level of WM, while athletes competing in static wheelchair sports perceived the lowest WM levels.

4.　Discussion and conclusions

There is a great importance to incorporate the skills that were graded "Very and extremely essential" during inpatient rehabilitation and in post rehabilitation WM workshops. It is recommended to conduct a comparative study of WM rehabilitation programs in spinal cord units in different countries, in order to improve WM teaching methods. Future studies should also focus on the peer learning process and its potential influence on enhancing WM skills performances for SCI. Encouraging wheelchair users to join dynamic wheelchair sports in order to improve WM performances is a rational conclusion based on this study's findings.

References

[1]　ICF: International Classification of functioning, disability and health; Geneva: *World Health Organization*, 2001; p.138, 146

[2]　O. Fliess-Douer, L.H.V. van der Woude, G. Lubel, Y.C. Vanlandewijck (2009). Towards a standardized wheelchair skill assessment tool – A critical review. in preparation

[3]　D.D. Price, P.A. McGrath, A. Rafii, B. Buckingham, The validation of visual analogue scales as ratio scale measures for chronic and experimental pain. *Pain* **17** (1983), 45—56

Rehabilitation: Mobility, Exercise and Sports
L.H.V. van der Woude et al. (Eds.)
IOS Press, 2010
© 2010 The authors and IOS Press. All rights reserved.
doi:10.3233/978-1-60750-080-3-358

Spirometric assessment of wheelchair athletes at home and during the Paralympics in Beijing 2008

C. PERRET[a,1], J. LEUPPI[b], F. MICHEL[c], M. STRUPLER[a]
[a]*Institute of Sports Medicine and* [c]*Swiss Paraplegic Centre, Nottwil, Switzerland*
[b]*Department for Internal Medicine, University Hospital Basel, Switzerland*

Abstract. The aim of the present study was to assess possible effects of expected air pollution on lung function of Swiss wheelchair athletes at the Paralympic Games 2008 in Beijing. For this purpose forced vital capacity, forced expiratory volume in 1s and peak expiratory flow was determined during the medical examination of the Swiss wheelchair athletes (n=13, whereof 4 asthmatics) at home (pre-test) as well as between day 2-7 (post-test 1) and 15-20 (post-test 2) after the arrival at the Paralympic Village in Beijing. Concomitantly concentration of particulate matters (PM10) was measured. Post-test lung function measurements where performed 4.1 ± 1.6 days and 16.7 ± 0.5 days after arrival at the Paralympic Village. Analysis of variance revealed no differences concerning pre- and post-test lung function measurements. Average daily concentration of PM10 ranged between 22 and 119 µg/m^3. No significant correlations were found between PM10 concentrations and lung function measurements. In conclusion, although quite high at some days, air pollution was less than suspected in advance of the Paralympic Games 2008 presumably due to restrictive sanctions (reduced traffic, closing down of factories) of the organising committee. The measured PM10 concentrations seemed to have no effect on lung function as none of the athletes showed any respiratory complications or decreased lung function during the stay at the Paralympic Village.

Keywords. respiration, exercise, spinal cord injury, wheelchair racing, air pollution.

1. Introduction

Beijing is among the most air polluted megacities in the world. Based on this fact, many experts warned of decreased athletic performance and serious health problems in view of the Olympic and Paralympic Games 2008 [1]. Amongst other health problems, difficulties in breathing, respiratory discomfort, airway irritation, asthma like symptoms and a reduced forced expiratory volume in one second were expected to appear due to bad air quality [2]. The aim of the present investigation was to assess possible effects of the expected air pollution on lung function of Swiss wheelchair athletes participating at the Paralympic Games 2008 in Beijing.

---
[1] Corresponding Author: Claudio Perret, Institute of Sports Medicine, Swiss Paraplegic Centre, CH-6207 Nottwil, Switzerland; E-mail: claudio.perret@paranet.ch.

2. Methods

In order to detect possible changes in lung function parameters forced vital capacity, forced expiratory volume in one second and peak expiratory flow were determined by means of a hand-held spirometer in 13 wheelchair athletes (4f/9m) during the medical examination at home (pre-test) as well as between day 2-7 (post-test 1) and day 15-20 (post-test 2) after arrival at the Paralympic Village in Beijing. Four of the athletes were known asthmatics and were adequately treated before as well as during the Paralympic Games.

Concentration of particulate matters (PM10) was measured during the whole duration of the stay in the Paralympic Village by a commercially available analyser (Aerosol Spektrometer 1.107, Eco Analytics, Pratteln, Switzerland).

To compare pre- and post-test lung function data a one way analysis of variance (ANOVA) was performed. Spearman correlation coefficients were calculated for delta and absolute values to test the relationship between lung function measurements and PM10 concentrations. Statistical significance was set at $p<0.05$.

3. Results

Post-test measurements where performed after 4.1 ± 1.6 days and 16.7 ± 0.5 days after arrival at the Paralympic Village. No significant differences concerning pre- and post-test lung function measurements were found (Table 1) and none of the athletes complained about respiratory problems.

Table 1. Mean ($\pm$ standard deviation) forced vital capacity (FVC), forced expiratory volume in one second (FEV1) and peak expiratory flow (PEF) of 13 wheelchair athletes at home (pre-test) and during the first (post-test 1) and the third week (post-test 2) at the Paralympic Village

Parameter	pre-test	post-test 1	post-test 2
FVC [L]	4.24 ± 1.05	4.10 ± 1.05	4.03 ± 1.04
FEV1 [L]	3.64 ± 0.91	3.48 ± 0.88	3.44 ± 0.85
PEF [L/s]	8.61 ± 3.04	8.13 ± 2.38	8.25 ± 2.64

Average daily concentration of PM10 ranged between 22 and 119 $\mu g/m^3$ (Figure 1). No significant correlations were found between PM10 concentrations and lung function measurements.

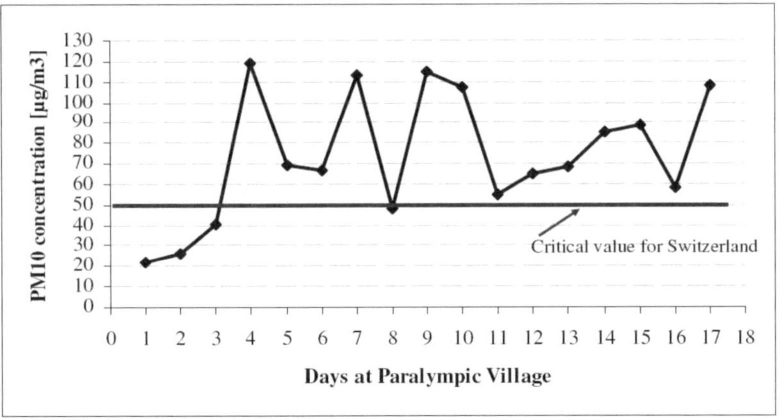

Figure 1. Average daily PM10 concentrations during the stay at the Paralympic Village. Note that the critical value for Switzerland of 50µg/m^3 was exceeded on most days.

4. Discussion

Between 2000 and 2004 average annual PM10 concentrations in the urban areas of Beijing were reported to range between 141 and 166 µg/m^3 [3]. Although during some days quite high (PM10 concentration up to 120 µg/m^3), air quality at the Paralympic Games was much better (Figure 1) compared to the above reported data, presumably due to the restrictive sanctions (reduced traffic, closing down of factories) of the organising committee. However, one has to be aware that the critical value (50µg/m^3) specified for Switzerland was clearly exceeded on most days (Figure 1).

Surprisingly, neither the four treated asthmatic nor the non-asthmatic athletes were complaining about respiratory problems during the three week stay in the Paralympic Village and it can be concluded that neither lung function (Table 1) nor athletic performance seems to be negatively influenced due to PM10 concentrations of up to 120 µg/m^3 in spinal cord injured athletes.

References

[1] G. Lippi, G.C. Guidi, N. Maffulli: Air pollution and sports performance in Beijing. *Int J Sports Med.* **29** (2008), 696-698.

[2] G. Florida-James, K. Donaldson, V. Stone: Athens 2004: the pollution climate and athletic performance. *J Sporst Sci.* **22** (2004), 967-980.

[3] M. Zhang, Y. Song, X. Cai: A health-based assessment of particulate air pollution in urban areas of Beijing in 2000-2004. *Sci Total Environ* **376** (2007), 100-108.

9.3

Poster Presentations

Rehabilitation: Mobility, Exercise and Sports
L.H.V. van der Woude et al. (Eds.)
IOS Press, 2010
© 2010 The authors and IOS Press. All rights reserved.
doi:10.3233/978-1-60750-080-3-363

363

The effect of glove type on wheelchair rugby sports performance

M. LUTGENDORF[a], B.S. MASON[b], L.H.V. VAN DER WOUDE[c],
V.L. GOOSEY-TOLFREY[b]

[a]*Faculty of Human Movement Sciences, Free University, Amsterdam, The Netherlands*
[b]*School of Sport and Exercise Sciences, Loughborough University, U.K.*
[c]*Centre for Human Movement Sciences, University Medical Centre Groningen, RUG, Groningen, The Netherlands*

Abstract. The purpose of this study was to determine the influence of glove type upon skill performance in wheelchair rugby. Eleven able-bodied males performed three sport specific field tests in four glove conditions: building gloves (BLD), multipurpose gloves (MLP), American football gloves (NFL) and no gloves(NO). Timing gates and a velocometer sampling at 100Hz were used to objectively assess aspects of mobility performance. One-way ANOVA's with repeated measures revealed that acceleration performance was significantly quicker in NFL and BLD than MLP ($p<0.01$), as were the times taken to perform an agility drill ($p<0.05$). Subjectively, participants also valued the performance of NFL over MLP. To conclude, glove type had a significant bearing upon wheelchair handling skills in able bodied participants, with NFL and BLD shown to perform the best. Future testing would be advised using disabled participants from wheelchair rugby.

Keywords. wheelchair rugby skills, wheelchair-user interface, able-bodied.

1. Introduction

Gloves are an important part of the equipment for wheelchair rugby players, as they directly influence the wheelchair-user interface. Besides protection of the hands, gloves are predominantly used to obtain extra grip and aid with chair mobility and ball handling. Since gloves, specifically developed for wheelchair rugby, are not yet available, athletes currently select a variety of gloves originally used for other purposes.

To the author's knowledge, the interaction between the gloves and hand rim on wheelchair sports performance have not been studied before. Instead, studies focusing on the wheelchair-user interface have manipulated the wheelchair handrim tube diameter, profile and texture. Although focused on daily-life purposes, Koontz et al. [1] demonstrated that a hand rim with added high friction coating and an ergonomic design had a significantly favourable effect on grip moments and force application. Van der Woude et al. [2] observed no physical differences from using hand rims of different size and texture at steady state conditions, but a foam coated rim was subjectively favoured by subjects.

The aim of the current study was to evaluate the effect of different glove conditions – currently used among level GB wheelchair rugby players - on standardised wheelchair rugby skills performance in able-bodied subjects and in comparison to not using gloves at all.

2. Method

Eleven able-bodied physically active males (age = 24.3±5 years; mass = 79.9 ± 8.4kg), unfamiliar with wheelchair propulsion, volunteered to participate in the study. Each participant performed three sport specific field tests in a standard offensive rugby wheelchair. All trials, held in two identical sessions a week apart, were performed in randomised order without gloves (NO) and in three different glove conditions: building gloves (BLD), multipurpose gloves (MLP) and American football gloves (NFL). Prior to commencing the first testing session, a 30-min familiarisation period of wheelchair propulsion was completed.

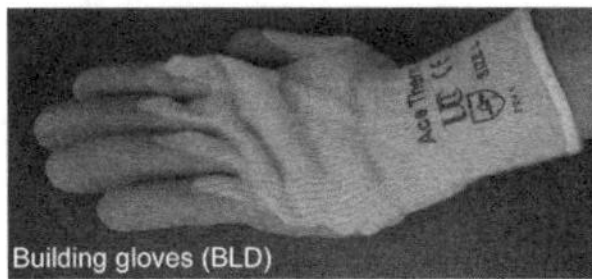

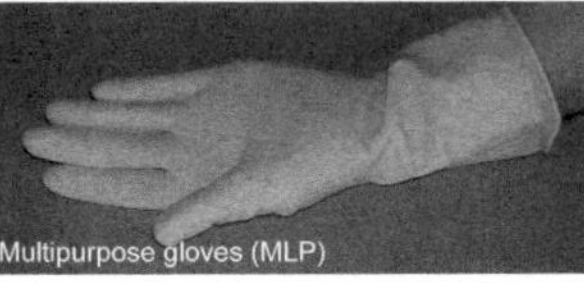

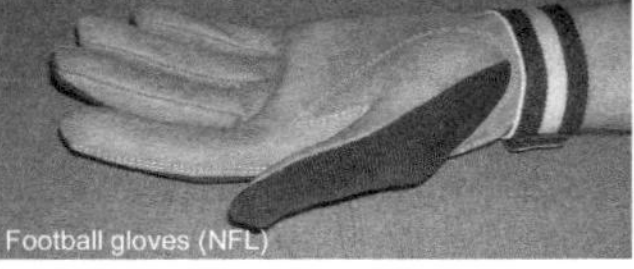

Figure 1. Illustration of three glove types sampled.

Glove performance was assessed by the overall time taken to complete the drill, using timing gates. Furthermore, a velocometer [3] mounted to the wheelchair produced velocity traces with respect to each push. Data derived from this velocometer sampling at 100Hz was used to assess peak velocities reached, obtain an acceleration profile over the 1st three pushes and measure deceleration (braking). After the first session participants completed a short likert-scale questionnaire to ascertain their subjective ratings of each gloves performance. A one-way ANOVA's with repeated measures was conducted on all performance measurements.

3. Results

Due to a learning effect visible in the data between both sessions, although results seemed to be consistent, only data from session 2 was used for further analysis.

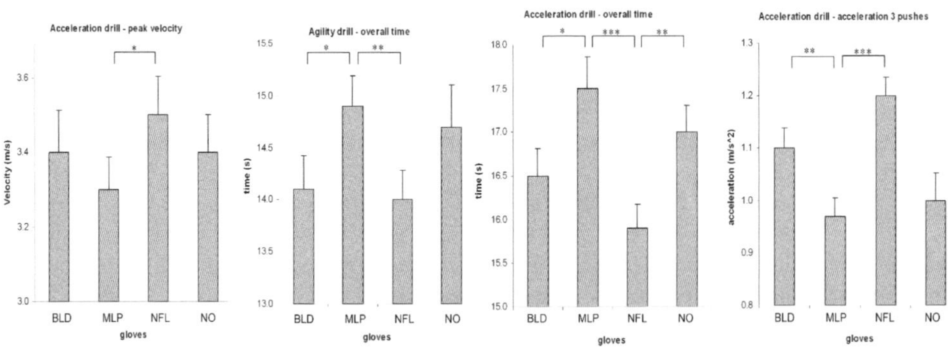

Figure 2. Results of glove performance in session 2 (Means ±SD), * p<0.05, ** p<0.01, *** P<0.001

Glove type had no significant effect on accuracy of ball handling. NFL And BLD produced significantly quicker overall times and acceleration profiles compared to other glove conditions. Significantly higher peak velocities were observed for NFL compared to MLP (p<0.05). BLD were significantly more effective at braking (decelerating) than MLP (p< 0.05). Main results are given in figure 1.

Subjective data identified that NFL were favoured over MLP. Participants particularly valued the comfort, grip and fit of the NFL over other gloves.

4. Discussion

The results suggest that NFL produced the most favourable performance in this group of able-bodied participants, with BLD also shown to perform positively. The positive performance of NFL may have been due to the improved grip provided by the tackified material on the palm of the hand. The good fit of NFL, which subjects felt allowed for superior comfort of pushing, was likely to be due to the fact that only NFL were remotely designed with sporting performance as its primary purpose. It would appear that BLD also provided an adequate grip, having scored highly in the questionnaire.

Although some trends seemed to appear in favour of NO in comparison to MLP, this is not to suggest that NO would be more suitable for wheelchair rugby, as obviously able-bodied subjects have full control of their hands to aid with gripping the wheels, as opposed to athletes with tetraplegia. NO obviously would not be suitable, as gloves are predominantly worn to protect and it was frequently commented that this was a drawback of the NO condition. The results do suggest that MLP are not likely to be effective for wheelchair rugby. As well as scoring poorly in all the objective measures of performance, MLP also scored poorly amongst subjects for the questionnaire outcomes. They were deemed to be ineffective for sports performance, as the material was very thin and provided little protection, as well as being elasticated.

Hand rim configuration is an area that would be strongly recommended for future testing. It would be interesting to establish how gloves of different materials interact with the push rims of differing materials and design. The sport specific drills used for the current study seemed to be a success and would be recommended for future testing, as although there had been a significant improvement in performances in session 2, the results of glove performance were found to be consistent. Further recommendations testing the effectiveness of gloves for wheelchair rugby would also involve the inclusion of wheelchair rugby players with tetraplegia.

Even though NFL performed the best, subjective issues still arose concerning the gloves durability and protection. Therefore, the development of a glove suitable for the specific demands of wheelchair rugby should be considered.

References

[1]   L.H.V. van der Woude, M. Formanoy, S. de Groot, Hand rim configuration: effects on physical strain and technique in unimpaired subjects, *Medical Engineering and Physics* **25** (2003),765-774.

[2]   A.M. Koontz, Y. Yang, D.S. Boninger, J. Kanaly, R.A. Cooper, M.L. Boninger, K. Dieruf, L. Ewer, Investigation of the performance of an ergonomics handrim as a pain relieving intervention for manual wheelchair users, *Assistive Technology* 18 (2006), 123-143.

[3]   A.D. Moss, N.E. Fowler & V.L. Goosey-Tolfrey, A telemetry based velocometer to measure wheelchair velocity, *Journal of Biomechanics* **36** (2003), 253-257.

Chapter 10
Running
10.1
Oral Presentations

Rehabilitation: Mobility, Exercise and Sports
L.H.V. van der Woude et al. (Eds.)
IOS Press, 2010

doi:10.3233/978-1-60750-080-3-369

Wheel-assisted running training in children with cerebral palsy: a controlled clinical trial

Y. HUTZLER [a,1] R. LEVIN [b], E. CARMELI [b], Z. YIZHAR [b]

[a] *Zinman College for Physical Education and Sports Sciences @ Wingate Institute*
[b] *Faculty of Medicin, School of Physiotherapy, Tel Aviv University*

Abstract. The purpose was to evaluate the effects of adding a wheel assisted running training (WART) to conventional mixed physical activity training (CT) program on function, and walking in children with cerebral palsy (CP). Method: Thirty children with CP, GMFCS 2–4 were assigned to either WART or CT groups (15 in each group). Energy Expenditure Index (EEI), the Gross Motor Function Measure 66 (GMFM), and walking velocity using the 10-meter test were administered by a trained physical therapist. The intervention period was six months, with tone to two sessions per week. Results: No significant group and time differences were found, except for cadence, which was lower in the CT group Post test. Conclusion: Both types of intervention appear to conserve and buffer the trend of decreased motor performance and efficiency often observed in children with CP without training intervention.

Keywords. cerebral palsy, walking, wheel-assisted running.

1. Introduction

Community exercise and physical fitness programs are recommended to increase the walking ability of children with CP.[1] In addition to strength training, intensive and motivational training modalities have been strongly encouraged for this purpose.[2] Treadmill training has become a common practice in children with CP, since as an externally paced exercise modality it requires continuous activity.[1] In order to assist participants with severe limitations in keeping an upright position during walking, the partial body weight supported treadmill training (PBWSTT) modality was introduced and proved to improve function. Recent research studies have investigated the impact of PBWSTT on walking performance and gross motor function in participants with CP. And have demonstrated significant improvements in energy expenditure index (EEI), velocity, step length, heart rate and blood pressure,[3]

The principle of body weight support is central to another movement-enhancing system that has been utilized in participants with CP, named the "Race-Runner" also called "Petra".[4] This is an athletic device where the athlete is running with his or her feet on the ground while using a running frame equipped with three large bicycle wheels supporting the athlete's body. Support is provided by a regular cycle saddle, a frontal body support plate, and the steering handle bars. We hypothesized that the

---

[1] Corresponding Author.

wheel assisted running training (WART) may increase duration of exercising and reduce the onset of fatigue, thus contributing to participants' physical performance, particularly in children with moderate to severe locomotor dysfunction.

The purpose of this study was to compare the effects of a training program that includes body weight supported WART to a conventional mixed training program (CT) on walking efficiency and activity criteria, including gross motor function (GMFM), walking velocity, step length and cadence.

2. Method

A controlled group design was applied with a convenience group allocation (n=15 each group). GMFCS, age and previous exposure to physical activity were similar in both groups.

Participants

Thirty children (15 in each group; 16 females and 14 males)) with CP, ages 6-18 were assigned to the study, after screening for medical procedures involving the lower limbs. Pre-test participation in physical activity training varied among participants with a range of up to 10 years. Participation rate also varied from nearly full participation to 30% of the training sessions.

Instruments

- Functional level was assessed by means of the *Gross Motor Function Classification System* (GMFCS) and used to classify severity of participants' activity limitation.
- Walking performance was assessed by means of the *10-meter test*. Outcomes were normalized, and included self-selected velocity (SSV), fast velocity (FV), cadence and step length in the SSV.
- Predicted energy cost of locomotion was calculated by *Energy expenditure index (EEI),* calculated by extracting the steady state resting HR from the steady state walking HR (measured with a Polar Electro [Kempele, Finland] S610), divided by walking velocity.
- The 66 item-version of the *Gross Motor Function Measure (GMFM)* was administered by a physiotherapist.

Procedure

Participants in both groups attended a community-based training program for children with disabilities in a specialized center, including two to three consecutive classes including swimming, table-tennis, fitness, and / or judo, provided twice a week for a period of six months. One of the classes attended by participants in the WART group consisted of the running bike intervention. Participants in the CT did not attend this class during the intervention period.

Statistical analysis

Repeated measures analyses of variance (ANOVA), using the confidence interval adjustment by Bonferroni for post hoc comparison tests, were employed for each dependent variable, comparing between groups. Percent gains between pre and post tests were calculated for each group.

3. Results

The statistic analysis did not reveal any significant differences in EEI, Velocity indices and GMFM between the groups prior to the intervention, and no significant time or group by time interaction effects. However, a considerable reduction in EEI (Figure 1) was observed in the CT (-21.71% gain), with a moderate effect size (ES= 0.5), while no change occurred in the WART (2.38%; ES= -.0.04). Significant changes in the CT group were observed only in cadence (Table 1).

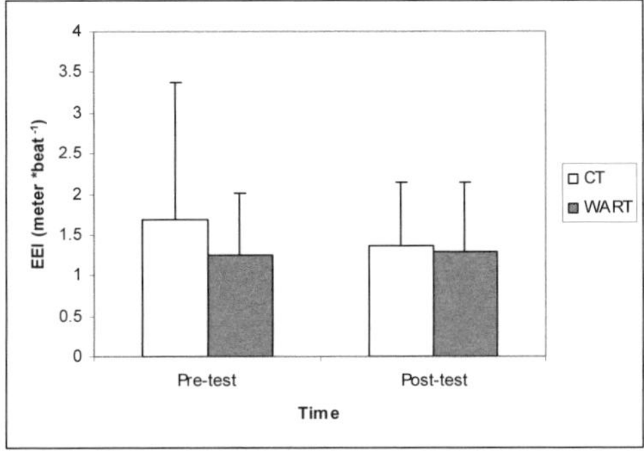

Figure 1. EEI across groups and test times

Table 1. Descriptive values of cadence outcomes

Variable	CT Pre-test	CT Post-test	WART Pre-test	Wart Post-test	Group effect P
Cadence Steps*min^{-1}	121.58 (30.77)	115.22 (28.00)	93.90 (35.67)	92.31 (28.06)	.025*
Normalized Cadence	0.53 (.13)	0.51 (.13)	0.42 (.16)	0.42 (.13)	.040*

4. Summary

Based on the findings in our sample of mainly trained participants, both WART and CT appear mainly to maintain walking performance and conserve efficiency, thus buffering the trend of decreased motor performance and efficiency typically observed in children with CP without training intervention. Contrary to our hypothesis, the WART training did not prove to be more efficient than CT. Future research is warranted to investigate larger groups of untrained participants.

References

[1] Fowler EG,, Kolobe THA, Damiano DL, et al. Promotion of physical fitness and prevention of secondary conditions for children with cerebral palsy: Section on pediatric research summit proceedings. *Phys Ther* **87** (2007), 1-15.
[2] Leonard C. Motor behavior and neural changes following perinatal and adult-onset brain damage: Implications for therapeutic interventions. *Phys Ther* **74** (1994), 753-67.
[3] Dodd KJ, Foley S. Partial body-weight supported treadmill training can improve walking in children with cerebral palsy: a clinical controlled trial. *Dev Med Child Neurol* **49** (2007), 101-05.
[4] Beginners race running compendium. www.petrabike.com.

Rehabilitation: Mobility, Exercise and Sports
L.H.V. van der Woude et al. (Eds.)
IOS Press, 2010

doi:10.3233/978-1-60750-080-3-372

Motion control shoe affects the lower leg muscle activities in runners with over-pronation

G.Y.F. NG[a], R.T.H. CHEUNG[b]

[a,b] *Department of Rehabilitation Sciences, Hong Kong Polytechnic University, China HKSAR*

Abstract. Motion control shoe is a well developed technology in running shoe design for controlling excessive rearfoot pronation and plantar force distribution. There is, however, little evidence on the lower leg muscle activation response to different shoes. This study examined the shank muscles EMG activity with different footwear. Methods: Twenty female recreational runners with excessive rearfoot pronation were tested with running for 10km on a treadmill on 2 days. Subjects wore either motion control running shoe or neutral running shoe during each day. Activities of their right tibialis anterior (TA) and peroneus longus (PL) were recorded with surface EMG. Their normalized root mean square (RMS) EMG and median frequency (MF) were compared between the two shoe conditions. Results: Significant positive correlations were found between the RMS EMG and running mileage in both TA and PL in the neutral shoe condition (p<0.001). There was MF drop in both shoe conditions with mileage but paired t-tests revealed significantly larger drop in the neutral shoe (p<0.001 for PL, p=0.074 for TA). Conclusions: Motion control shoe may facilitate a more stable activation pattern and higher fatigue resistance of TA and PL in people with excessive rearfoot pronation during running.

Keywords: running, footwear, leg, electromyography.

1. Introduction

Excessive rearfoot pronation may cause various overuse injuries in runners such as posterior tibial syndrome (shin splints), plantar fasciitis and Achilles tendinopathy [1]. Footwear is essential in running and the motion control shoe technology was developed to prevent lower leg muscles overuse in runners. A recent study found that motion control shoe could reduce rearfoot pronation by an average of 6.5° [2] and balance the uneven plantar load distribution [3]; and the effect was maintained even after fatigue of the leg muscles.

Most running injuries are associated with imbalanced activities of the leg muscles [4]. Hitherto, the effects of motion control shoe on lower leg muscle activations have not been well examined. Therefore, this study aimed to investigate the lower leg muscle activations between different shoe conditions and to compare motion control shoe with cushioned shoe on the activation of lower leg musculature in subjects who had excessive foot pronation.

2. Methods

Twenty female runners with mean age of 25.8 years and 4.6 years of running experience were tested. All subjects had excessive rearfoot pronation of $> 6°$.

Two shoe models were tested, namely, "Adidas Supernova control" which is a motion control shoe model and "Adidas Supernova cushion" which is a neutral shoe model. Both shoe models are comparable in design except for the midsole that the "Supernova control" was composed of two materials with different hardness, whereas the "Supernova cushion" only has a single midsole material that reduces the impact loading rate but not controlling foot pronation.

Treadmill running at a speed of 8 km/hr without inclination was used in this study. All the subjects ran for 10 km in two sessions with 1 week apart. In each session, the subjects wore either test shoe models in a randomized sequence.

The right tibialis anterior (TA) and peroneus longus (PL) were tested in this study in light of their roles as the major stabilizing muscles of the subtalar joints [5,6]. The EMG activities of these muscles were recorded using the DelSys (DelSys Inc., Boston, U.S.A.) double differential Ag-AgCl surface electrodes.

In order to compare different stages of running, the total 10 km running distance was equally divided into 10 recording sessions. To reduce the data acquisition and storage problem, the EMG data was only collected during the last minute of each recording session and all the recording sessions were included for analysis. The root mean squared (RMS) EMG from all the running steps were averaged and normalized against the EMG value of the respective muscles' MVC taken in the beginning of each running bout.

Repeated measures ANOVA was used to test the effects of footwear and mileage on the normalized RMS EMG values of both muscles with α adjusted to 0.0025. The relationships between mileage and EMG were examined with Pearson's correlation. For the fatigue profile, the corresponding median frequency (MF) difference between session 1 and 10 was analyzed with paired t-tests with α maintained at 0.05.

3. Results

The normalized RMS EMG of TA and PL revealed significant difference with different footwear and mileage ($p<0.001$). When comparing to the baseline value at the 1st check point, the TA and PL activities increased since the 5th and 2nd check-point respectively.

Significant correlations are found between the change in TA activities of both shoe conditions with mileage, whereas for the PL muscle, such a correlation is only revealed in the neutral shoe condition. As a whole, the correlations are more evident in the neutral shoe than the motion control shoe condition.

There is a significant downward shift ($p < 0.001$) in MF after the 10-km running bout. Comparing the two shoe conditions, significantly larger shift in MF was found in PL during the neutral shoe testing condition ($p < 0.001$). For the TA however, the difference between shoe conditions was insignificant ($p = 0.074$).

4. Discussion

The subject pool of this study was homogeneous in terms of gender, running skill level and foot type. Recruitment of subjects from a single gender would minimize the variance due to gender difference despite the limitation on the generalisability of this study to both genders.

The RSM EMG findings revealed an increased activation in TA and PL in the neutral shoe condition and there are also significant correlations between the change in RMS EMG of both muscles and mileage of running with neutral shoe. For the motion control shoe however, the activation levels of both muscles were more stable throughout the running bout.

Different from foot orthosis, the design feature of motion control footwear allows more time for loading response during landing, thus a longer duration for the foot stabilizers to work which results in an overall lesser muscle activities. In contrast to foot orthosis which provides extra support to foot arch so that the muscles can contract in a more efficient position, muscle activation is therefore expected to be lower in motion control shoe whereas orthosis might increase muscle activation.

The present findings revealed that MF had dropped in both muscles after running with motion control or neutral shoe conditions, but the drop was significantly more in the neutral shoe condition than the motion control shoe condition for PL ($p<0.001$) and a similar trend was also observed for TA ($p=0.074$). These suggest that PL and possibly, TA, had developed more fatigue in the neutral shoe testing condition throughout the 10 km running. As both TA and PL are important dynamic stabilizers [5,6] that control rearfoot pronation, fatigue of these muscles might lead to further increase in pronation with running mileage [2]. Therefore, motion control shoe which helps delay muscle fatigue in PL and TA would be beneficial for long distance running in maintain stability of the foot.

5. Conclusions

We conclude that motion control shoe could enhance more stable activation and fatigue endurance of TA and PL than neutral shoe during a 10 km running distance in recreational runners who have rearfoot over-pronation problem.

References

[1]   Cook SD, Brinker MR, Poche M. Running shoes: their relationship to running injuries. Sports Med 1990;10:1-8.
[2]   Cheung RTH, Ng GYF. Efficacy of motion control shoes for reducing excessive rearfoot motion in fatigued runners. Phy Ther Sport 2007(8):75-81.
[3]   Cheung RTH, Ng GYF. Influence of different footwear on force of landing during running. Phy Ther 2008;88:620-8.
[4]   Nigg BM. The role of impact forces and foot pronation – a new paradigm. Clin Sports Med 2001;11:2-9.
[5]   Kirby KA. Rotational equilibrium across the subtalar joint axis. J Am Podia Med Assoc 1989;79:1-14.
[6]   Payne C, Danaberg H. Sagittal plane facilitation of the foot. Aust J Podia Med 1997; 31:7-11.

Rehabilitation: Mobility, Exercise and Sports
L.H.V. van der Woude et al. (Eds.)
IOS Press, 2010
© 2010 The authors and IOS Press. All rights reserved.
doi:10.3233/978-1-60750-080-3-375

Amputees and sports: a systematic review

M. BRAGARU[a,b], R. DEKKER[a], J.H.B. GEERTZEN[a,b], P.U. DIJKSTRA[a,b,c]
[a]Centre for Rehabilitation, University Medical Centre Groningen, University of Groningen, P.O. Box 30.001, 9700 RB Groningen, The Netherlands
[b]Graduate School for Health Research SHARE, A. Deusinglaan 1, PO box 196, 9700 AD Groningen, The Netherlands
[c]Dept of Oral and Maxillofacial Surgery, University Medical Centre Groningen, University of Groningen, P.O. Box 30.001, 9700 RB Groningen, The Netherlands

1. Introduction

Sport participation by the general population has a positive effect on the quality of life. [1] It is assumed that sports participation of disabled individuals also has a positive effect on their quality of life.

In the Netherlands more than 2000 major amputations are performed each year. [2] It is claimed that amputees have specific needs, problems and gains, different from other physically disabled individuals when performing sports. [3,4] Screening literature, it appeared that little scientific evidence is available concerning the specific needs, problems and gains of amputees when performing sports. Aim of this study was to systematically search the literature regarding amputees performing sports and scientific evidence for their specific needs, problems and gains.

2. Methods

Three databases were searched (Medline, Embase and Cinahl), using database specific MESH terms and search strategies. Taking into account the fact that energy expenditure and oxygen uptake are higher in amputees compared to able bodied individuals [5, 6], the following definition of sport and physical activity was used for this review: *"physical activity (PA) is any bodily movement produced by skeletal muscles that requires energy expenditure (WHO). Additionally, sports were defined as: an activity involving physical exertion, with or without game or competition elements, with a minimal duration of half an hour, where skills and physical endurance are either required or aim to be improved."* [7]

Included in this systematic review were studies concerning major limb amputation and sport and physical activity. Excluded were papers concerning minor amputations (e.g. toe, finger), letters to the editor, notes, narrative reviews and case studies. Of the studies identified in the search, the title was assessed by two independent observers. Studies on doubt concerning their topic were kept for further assessment. Thereafter, abstracts and full text were assessed. Additionally, the reference lists of studies relevant for this review were checked. All the selected studies were assessed according to a list of qualitative criteria. Additionally, the main outcome of the studies was assessed.

3. Results

The search identified more than 1800 papers. After title and abstract assessment and reference list check, 25 studies were selected for qualitative assessment of the full text. Main outcomes in these studies concerned sport injuries, psychological aspects and quality of life, prosthetic devices, biomechanics, cardio-pulmonary function, rehabilitation and functional outcome. The results of this review will be communicated during the oral presentation.

Keywords: amputee, sport, physical activity, systematic review.

References

[1]   W.L. Mosterd, et al., *Measures in motion*. Utrecht: Rijksuniversiteit Utrecht, 1996.
[2]   G.M. Rommers, *The elderly amputee*, 2000, Ponsen & Looyen BV, Wageningen, The Netherlands.
[3]   K. Naugle, C. Stopka, Medical Conditions of athlete with amputations, *Athletic Therapy Today*, (2006 July).
[4]   S.J. Hanraharn, Practical considerations for working with athletes with disabilities, *The Sport Psychologist* **12** (1998), 346-357.
[5]   F. Nowroozi, M.L. Salvanelli, L.H. Gerber, Energy expenditure in hip disarticulation and hemipelvectomy amputees, *Arch Phys Med Rehabil.* **64(7)** (1983 Jul), 300-3.
[6]   C.T. Huang, J.R. Jackson, N.B. Moore, P.R. Fine, K.V. Kuhlemeier, G.H. Traugh, P.T. Saunders, Amputation: energy cost of ambulation, *Arch Phys Med Rehabil.* **60(1)** (1979 Jan), 18-24.
[7]   H.G.C. Kemper, W.T.M. Ooijendijk, Consensus over de Nederlandse Norm voor Gezond Bewegen. *Tijdschrift Sociale Gezondheidszorg* **78** (2000), 180-183.

10.2

Poster Presentations

Rehabilitation: Mobility, Exercise and Sports
L.H.V. van der Woude et al. (Eds.)
IOS Press, 2010
© 2010 The authors and IOS Press. All rights reserved.
doi:10.3233/978-1-60750-080-3-379

Combining a dynamic balance protocol and statistical parametric mapping to better understand floor pedobarography in shod dynamic sports activities

J. VANRENTERGHEM [a,1], S. CHAMBERS [a], R. GARCIA [b], M. HAWKEN [a],
M. LAKE [a], T. PATAKY [c]

[a] *Research Institute for Sport and Exercise Sciences, Faculty of Science, Liverpool John Moores University, Liverpool, UK*
[b] *Fontys University of Applied Sciences, Eindhoven, The Netherlands*
[c] *School of Biomedical Sciences, University of Liverpool, Liverpool, UK*

Abstract. The purpose of this study was to evaluate the scientific potential of floor pedobarography to understand balance control mechanisms in dynamic sport activities. One participant underwent single-footed balance conditions of static standing, standing on medio-lateral sinewave perturbed surface (6 degrees roll, 0.5 Hz) and standing on medio-lateral suddenly perturbed surface (3 degrees roll either side), each in barefoot, standing on shoe sole and shod footwear conditions. The effects of balance and footwear conditions were evaluated from floor pedobarographic recordings (RSScan International, 100 Hz) using statistical parametric mapping, a label-free technique. Statistical significance was assessed using random field theory. Despite being smaller than expected, shifts in peak pressure patterns between footwear conditions indicated across balance conditions an increased balance control through heel motion in the shod condition; peak medial (p=0.014) and lateral (p<0.001) heel pressures were greater in shod than non-shod tasks. Loading and unloading rates were greater during dynamic balancing in all footwear conditions, especially along the medial (p<0.001) and lateral mid-/forefoot (p<0.001). Effects of footwear and balance conditions demonstrated strategic differences in balance control. Such findings indicate some potential of floor pedobarography in the growing scientific interest to understand balance control in dynamic sports activities.

Keywords. biomechanics, pressure, perturbation.

1. Introduction

Rapid developments over the past few decades have caused a shift in studies of balance and posture from traditionally static paradigms to more dynamic methods (e.g. [1]). This offers the possibility of designing comprehensive studies linking knowledge from

---

[1] Corresponding Author: Jos Vanrenterghem, Research Institute for Sport and Exercise Sciences, Liverpool John Moores University, Henry Cotton Campus, 15-21 Webster Street, Liverpool L3 2ET, E-mail: j.vanrenterghem@ljmu.ac.uk

investigations on balance, perturbed balance, proprioception, footwear, sports skills, etc. to provide a more sophisticated view of balance aspects of dynamic activities in sports.

One particular area with opportunities for both technological and scientific development is the role of foot-floor interaction in dynamic balance. Technological developments have made available 6-degree-of-freedom moving platforms [2], and pixel-based pedobarography analyses [3]. Scientific development has improved the design of test protocols which allow standardized balance perturbations to simulate the dynamics of sport activity [4], and the linking of detailed foot functions with whole body actions used in maintaining balance [5].

Our study was an exploration of the feasibility of using contemporary methods of pedobarography analysis in conjunction with a novel dynamic balance protocol. By using a multi-task protocol, we intend to highlight opportunities for future work in this emerging area, and any potential pitfalls.

2. Methods

Floor pedobarography data (RSScan International, Belgium) was recorded for a single subject standing on a 6-degree-of-freedom moving platform (CAREN, Motek, The Netherlands).The dynamic balance protocol was designed to perturb medio-lateral balance by rotation around the anterior-posterior center line of the sole of the foot (= roll) minimizing shear forces caused by the perturbation (Figure 1). Rotations were either a continuous sinewave (3°, 0.5 Hz) or a single ramp lifting the medial/lateral side (3°). The participant was asked to balance on one foot, either barefoot, shod, or standing on the cut-off sole of an identical shoe, which was not attached to the foot. Comparison of peak pressure, loading, and unloading images from 5 s recordings was carried out on a pixel-based basis using linear registration techniques [3].

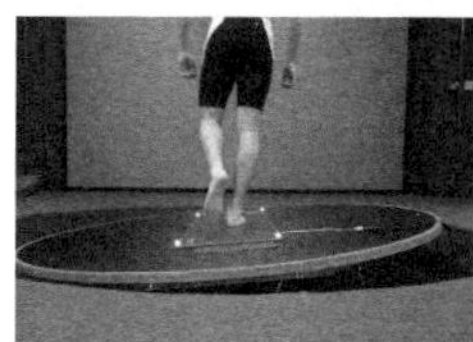

Figure 1. Indication of magnitude of perturbations.

3. Results

In the barefoot and shod condition peak pressure profiles showed that pressures were higher under lateral areas than in the loose sole condition (Figure 2). Loading rates were greater during dynamic balancing in all footwear conditions, especially along the medial and lateral mid-/forefoot (Figure 3).

4. Discussion

The subject clearly noted least stability in the 'sole' condition. This suggests reduced stability compared to 'barefoot' due to the cushioning effect, and compared to 'shod' arising from lack of attachment of the shoe to the foot. This hypothesis was supported by the presence of increased balance control through heel motion and/or sensory information in the shod condition compared to barefoot and sole conditions, indicating the importance of attachment of the shoe to the foot in dynamic balancing activities.

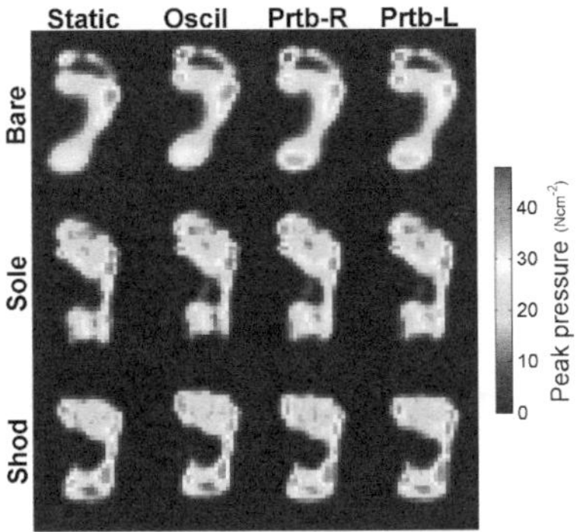

Figure 2. Peak pressure images.

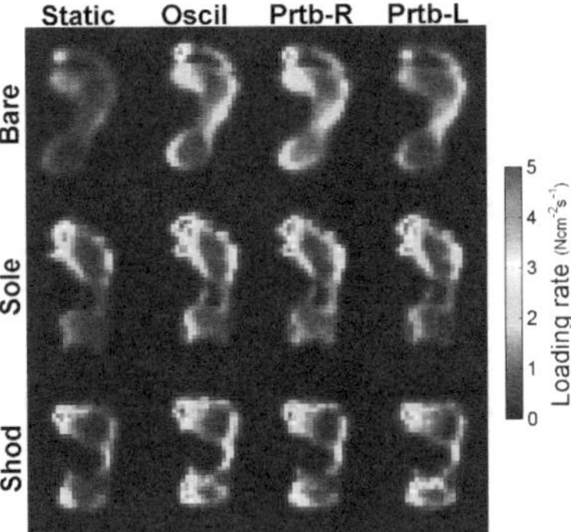

Figure 3. Loading rate images.

The sine wave motion appeared to be most effective in highlighting differences between barefoot, sole and shod conditions, because of the repetitive loading and symmetrical nature of the perturbation.

In conclusion, the use of floor pedobarography in dynamic balance protocols appears feasible. It offers an opportunity to understand more clearly the nature of foot-shoe-floor interactions during dynamic balance activities. Future challenges are in statistical analysis techniques that relate temporal characteristics of the movement to pedobarography data, and in analyzing diagnostic merit of these methods in clinical populations.

Acknowledgments

This project was co-funded by RSScan International (www.rsscan.com) and the Institute for Health Research of Liverpool John Moores University (www.ljmu.ac.uk/ihr).

References

[1] A.L. Hof, M.G.J. Gazendam, W.E. Sinke. The condition for dynamic stability, *Journal of Biomechanics* **38** (2005), 1-8.

[2] Lees, J. Vanrenterghem, G. Barton, M. Lake. Kinematic response characteristics of the CAREN moving platform system for use in posture and balance research, *Medical Engineering and Physics* **29** (2007), 629-635.

[3] T. Pataky, J.Y. Goulermas. Pedobarographic statistical parametric mapping (pSPM): A pixel-level approach to foot pressure image analysis, *Journal of Biomechanics* **41** (2008), 2136-2143.

[4] D.A.C.M. Commissaris, P.H.J.A. Nieuwenhuijzen, S. Overeem, A. De Vos, J.E.J. Duysens, B.R. Bloem. Dynamic posturography using a new movable multidirectional platform driven by gravity, *Journal of Neuroscience Methods* **113** (2002), 73-84.

[5] P.-I. Wong K.Chamari, D. Wei Mao, U. Wisloff, Y. Hong. Higher plantar pressure on the medial side in four soccer related movements, *British Journal of Sports Medicine* **41** (2007), 93-100.

Chapter 11

Wheeled Sports

11.1

Keynote

Rehabilitation: Mobility, Exercise and Sports
L.H.V. van der Woude et al. (Eds.)
IOS Press, 2010

doi:10.3233/978-1-60750-080-3-385

Supporting the Paralympic Athlete: focus on wheeled sports

V. L. GOOSEY-TOLFREY
*The Peter Harrison Centre for Disability Sport, School of Sport and Exercise
Sciences, Loughborough University, U.K*

Abstract. The complexity of wheelchair sports provide the scientist with a unique challenge. There are two major components that contribute towards 'wheeled sports' performance, these are the athlete and the chair. It is the interaction of these two that enable wheelchair propulsion and the sporting movements required within a given sport. This presentation will provide an insight into the applied sport science research that has been provided to the Great Britain wheelchair athletes over the last decade. It will focus on four sports; wheelchair racing, wheelchair basketball, wheelchair tennis and wheelchair rugby. This session will discuss how sport scientists have worked with coaches and practitioners to help optimise training leading to a major competition through evidence base practise. As changes in different mechanical variables have been shown to affect the energy requirements of wheelchair propulsion then the first topic will discuss the concept of pushing economy and mechanical efficiency of wheelchair propulsion. The second topic will illustrate the concept of sports classification, and show how training volume 'in terms of basketball shooting' may need to be individually assigned. The third topic will show how technology assists the coaching process and finally future research within wheelchair team sports and chair configurations will be examined.

Keywords. wheelchair propulsion, mechanical efficiency, wheelchair basketball, racing, tennis and rugby.

1. Introduction

The British Wheelchair Racing Association were the first disabled sports organisation in the UK to be granted sport science support project, under the scheme run by the National Coaching Foundation for the Sports Council in 1994. The aim of this project was to provide appropriate sport science support to the Wheelchair Racing squad in preparation for the 1996 Paralympics. Following this successful programme, the Great Britain men's Wheelchair Basketball Association were successfully granted support through the UK lottery to assist their preparations for the 2000 Paralympics and Wheelchair Tennis bought into a University support package leading to both the 2004 and 2008 Paralympics. This paper will highlight key areas of these support programmes and in doing so, will demonstrate the scientific study of 'wheeled sports' covering racing, basketball, tennis and rugby.

Wheelchair propulsion: Pushing economy and efficiency: From a sports perspective, both biomechanical and physiological techniques have been employed to investigate wheelchair propulsion performance related issues. It has been proposed, that three basic qualities of the wheelchair-user combination are crucial in determining the final performance in hand-rim wheelchair use. First, there is the athlete, who produces the energy and power for propulsion; second, the mechanics and technical status of the wheelchair; finally the interaction of the athlete and wheelchair which essentially will determine the efficiency of the power transfer from the athlete to the wheelchair [1]. Hand-rim propulsion is a guided movement that is regulated highly by the rim curvature and its speed and direction of movement. Within these constraints athletes are free to adopt different arm frequencies, propulsion modes or both in such a way that suits their requirements at a given wheelchair propulsion velocity or task. Interventions to improve pushing economy and mechanical efficiency are constantly sought after by athletes, coaches and sport scientists. One intervention that has received attention is manipulations of push strategy in the form of 'push frequency' and 'pushing style (synchronous vs. asynchronous arm movements)' [1,2,3]. We know from this previous work that operating at the freely chosen frequency (FCF) is the most optimal with respect to pushing economy (Figure 1). Yet regardless of achieving an optimal push strategy (in terms of oxygen cost), this form of locomotion still remains relatively inefficient (12% has been reported for trained wheelchair racing athletes [4]) and sport scientists are still looking at ways to improve these reported values.

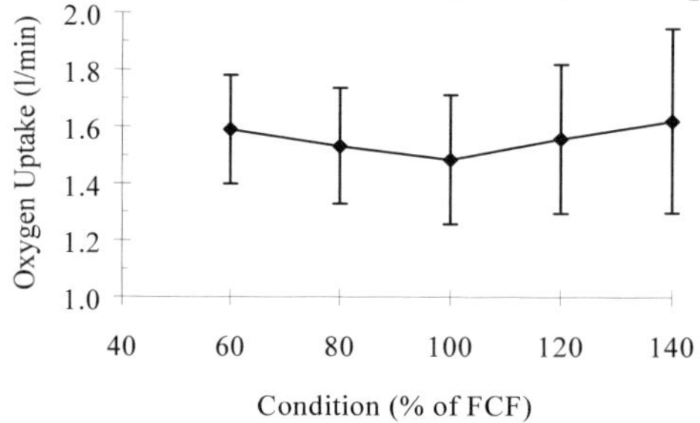

Figure 1: Pushing Economy at each push frequency (percentage of FCF) for 8 wheelchair athletes [2].

Sports classification: Implications on technical training volume (basketball shooting): Sports classification is a key topic of interest within the International Paralympic movement. Wheelchair basketball is a good example of a disability sport where athletes with varying degrees and levels of disabilities participate together based on an individual player classification system. Researchers have tended to focus their interest on the functional capacity of wheelchair users and the physiological adaptations to training of persons with a spinal cord injury. Consequently, the sports practitioner can refer to the literature for guidance about exercise tolerance, normative values based upon classification and understand the key physiological differences in relation to lesion level [5]. However, as the knowledge of basketball technical shooting programmes remains unclear, understanding the differences across classes is paramount to coaches so that the appropriate coaching models can be developed. This paper highlights which differences in technique during the completion of a successful free throw exist by players of different functional classifications [6].

Technology and coaching: A velocity meter is a device that measures the instantaneous speed of a person or object. It does this continuously and in real time. Velocity meters are not a new concept although the technology has advanced significantly in recent years. Technicians and Sport Scientists at Manchester Metropolitan University in the UK, have developed a velocity meter which can be mounted on a wheelchair to measure the intra-push profiles of over-ground wheelchair propulsion [7]. A case study within the sport of wheelchair tennis will be illustrated and the paper will explain how the coaches have used this innovative tool to aid and assist with their coaching.

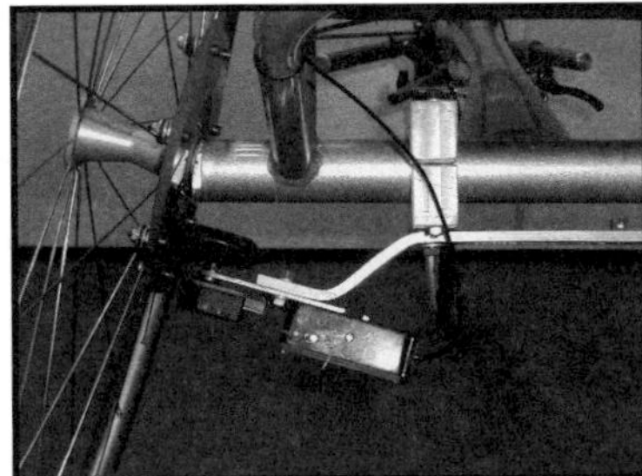 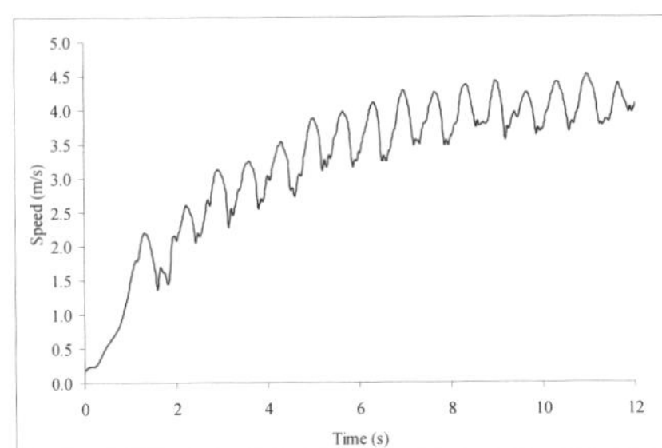

Figure 2: The velocometer mounted on a wheelchair (left) and a typical trace obtained from velocometer during a 20m sprint in a games sports wheelchair (right).

Chair configurations and wheeled sports performance: Wheelchairs used within the court sports of basketball, rugby and tennis have undergone major developments over recent years in terms of their design. Very little is known about the contribution that specific areas of wheelchair configuration has towards performance improvements, due to the limited amount of quantitative research that exists in this field. The final aspect of this paper is to highlight a current research programme that is designed to examine selected physiological and propulsion technique parameters associated to chair-set up for the execution of on-court wheelchair propulsion skills.

2. Conclusion

It is difficult to appreciate the extent to which this work has had on overall performance, although we feel that the sport science knowledge and its application to coaching within each sport has improved. Despite the coaching staff being satisfied with the support to date, further developments are warranted.

References

[1] L.H.V. van der Woude, H.E.J. Veeger & R.H. Rozendal, Ergonomics of Wheelchair Design: A Prerequisite for Optimum Wheeling Conditions. *Adapted Physical Activity Quarterly* **6** (1989), 109-132.

[2] V.L. Goosey, I.G. Campbell & N.E. Fowler, Effect of push frequency on the economy of wheelchair racers. *Medicine Science in Sports and Exercise* **32** (2000), 174-181.

[3] J.P. Lenton, N.E. Fowler, L.H.V. van der Woude & V.L. Goosey-Tolfrey, Wheelchair propulsion: effects of experience and propulsion strategy on efficiency and perceived exertion. *Applied Physiology, Nutrition and Metabolism* **33** (2008), 870-879.

[4] V.L. Goosey & I.G. Campbell, Pushing economy and wheelchair propulsion technique at three speeds. *Adapted Physical Activity Quarterly* **15** (1998), 36-50.

[5] T.W. Janssen & M.E. Hopman, The physiology of spinal cord injury. In J.S. Skinner (ed) *Exercise Testing and Exercise Prescription for Special Cases: Theoretical Basis and Clinical Applications.* Lippincott Williams and Wilkins, Baltimore, 2005.

[6] V.L. Goosey-Tolfrey, C. Morriss & D. Butterworth, A biomechanical analysis of the free throw in Paralympic wheelchair basketball players of varying classifications. *Adapted Physical Activity Quarterly* **19** (2002), 238-250.

[7] A.D. Moss, N.E. Fowler & V.L. Tolfrey, A telemetry-based velocometer to measure wheelchair velocity. *Journal of Biomechanics* **36** (2003), 253-257.

Rehabilitation: Mobility, Exercise and Sports
L.H.V. van der Woude et al. (Eds.)
IOS Press, 2010
© 2010 The authors and IOS Press. All rights reserved.
doi:10.3233/978-1-60750-080-3-388

Sports, disability & classification: a philosophers debate?

I.M. VAN HILVOORDE[a,1]

[a] Faculty of Human Movement Sciences, Research Institute MOVE, VU University,
Amsterdam, The Netherlands

Abstract. Technological developments within elite sports for disabled athletes raise intriguing philosophical questions that challenge dominant notions of the body and of normality. The case of 'bladerunner Oscar Pistorius' in particular is used to illustrate and defend 'transhuman' ideologies, in which the use of technology is promoted to extend all human capabilities. Some argue that new technologies will undermine the sharp contrast that still dominates between the athlete as a cultural hero and icon and the disabled person that needs extra attention or care; the one incorporating the peak of normality, human functioning at its best, the other often representing the opposite. Do current ways of classification do justice to the performances of disabled athletes? The case of Oscar Pistorius will be used to further illustrate the complexities of these questions, in particular when related to notions of normality and extraordinary performances. Pistorius' wish to become part of 'normal' elite sport may be framed as a way of 'inclusion' or 'integration', but at the same time reproduces new inequalities and asymmetries between performances of able and dis-abled athletes. Accepting Pistorius to compete within the 'regular' Olympic Games paradoxically underlines the differences and reproduces the current order and hierarchy between able and disabled bodies.

Keywords. disability sports, ethics, classification, enhancement; prostheses, Oscar Pistorius.

1. Introduction

The case of South African sprinter Oscar Pistorius, also known as 'the fastest man on no legs' has attracted the attention of scholars from a variety of disciplines, including philosophers (of sport). [1,2,3] Pistorius runs with carbon-fiber legs and is world record holder in the 100, 200 and 400 meters. He can even compete with elite athletes on 'natural legs'. His wish to participate in a regular competition is surrounded by controversy and raises a variety of both empirical and (sport)philosophical questions on the concepts of dis-ability, super-ability, enhancement and a fair competition.

In daily life, there is little reason to qualify people who integrate their prostheses into their 'lived bodies' as disabled. It is clear that Pistorius challenges our understanding of disability and that his case contributes to the blurring of some traditional boundaries. New technologies such as prostheses apparently help to turn 'disabled' people into 'normal' subjects. What may be considered 'normalisation' in the context of daily life is at least ambivalent in the context of elite sport. If Pistorius'

---

[1] Corresponding Author.

label as dis-abled does not relate to his body image and way of life, what does this mean for the construction of a boundary between ability sports and disability sports? Are there valid arguments to exclude him from running against able bodied athletes? And how does this discussion relate to the general discussion on classification?

2. The ideology of the ICF versus the logic of sports

The 'International Classification of Impairments, Disabilities and Handicaps' (ICIDH) has been replaced by the International Classification of Functioning, Disability and Health (ICF) at the start of this century. Generally spoken, this change of terminology reflects a shift in focus from disabilities to abilities and capacities. Disability is not regarded a characteristic (that is present all the time) but a state that may be present in certain environments or results from specific interactions with other people. The concept of health evolved from a bio-statistical ('objective') conception to a more contextual conception. Being disabled is not something one is by definition ('by its nature'), but something one becomes in relation to specific environments. People can become disabled by the environment or by specific (lack of) technologies.

Following the ideology of the ICF (an ideology of 'inclusion' and 'sameness') there is hardly any reason to exclude Pistorius from running at the regular Olympic Games. However, Oscar Pistorius is qualified as 'super-abled'. Based on a biomechanical study, the IAAF concluded that an athlete running with prosthetic blades has a clear mechanical advantage (more than 30 per cent) when compared to 'someone' not using the blades. Pistorius responded that his prosthetics also confront him with disadvantages, such as the fact that some of his energy is more easily dispensed at the start of the race than the energy of other runners.

The fact that running with prosthetics needs less additional energy than running with natural limbs is however in itself insufficient to keep Pistorius from competing in the Olympics. There is no standard test available to judge different bionic legs and compare them with 'normal' legs.' [3] The discussion on Pistorius and classification is in the end a conceptual and philosophical question on the unity of the human body, on the definition of sport and on the question whether Pistorius can be or should be considered a normal athlete or not.

Prostheses not necessarily define Pistorius as 'dis-abled'. Based upon a definition of his abilities there is no good argument to exclude Pistorius from the Olympic Games. Prostheses are however part of the definition of the game. Whereas the ICF aims at the removal of obstacles (in order to minimalize any dis-ability) sport however is defined by a voluntary attempt to overcome *unnecessary obstacles*. [4] The question if Pistorius should be labelled as either super- or dis-abled is not so relevant for his in- or exclusion. More relevant is the question: What kind of a game is he playing? Disability sports are about showing performances within categories of similar disabilities, without making those disabilities the central element of athletic prowess. Running on prostheses may be defined as crucial for the specific talent that is tested in a competition against 'relevant others': athletes who have the ability to show a similar talent.

At first sight it seems that the inclusion of Pistorius in the Olympic Games is in accordance with the ideology behind the ICF and in accordance with the realization of his *vital goals*. [5] It could be argued that Pistorius is blurring the distinction between elite sports and the disabled sports. His 'promotion' to the elite level of sport may be considered empowering and a symbol for non-discrimination. On the other hand, one can foresee a new boundary between disabled people into two categories: on the one hand the invalid, dependent and incapable and on the other hand 'that much celebrated media persona of the disabled person who has "overcome adversity" in a heartwarming manner and not been restricted by his or her "flaws", but believes that "everything is possible" for those who work hard.' [6] It is the paradox of Oscar Pistorius that he could develop into a symbol for the 'normalization of dis-abilities', but at the same time symbolizes a neo-liberal ideology in which specific talents of the individual 'superhuman' and 'inspirational overcomer' [7] are used as an heroic example.

3.   Conclusion

On the one hand, society invests quite willingly in the super-abilities of the elite athlete whilst on the other it only does this reluctantly, and from an ethics of inclusion, with respect to the disabled. In the case of disabilities, one wants to eradicate abnormalities by equalizing on the basis of 'sameness', while in the case of super-abilities we support abnormalities. This 'selective investment in the abnormal' and the admiration for the 'genetically superior' could be seen as a token of a society that cannot meet up with the criteria for justice. On the other hand, sport is a competitive practice, whose internal logic consists of the display of an unequal distribution of abilities and talents.

There are good arguments for a radical change of the organization and classification of traditional sports and for the need of a critical rethinking of the traditional boundary between Olympic Games and Paralympic Games. Starting from a more liberal definition of categories one can also imagine the organization of competitions that are not contrasted on the basis of an opposition between able and dis-able, but rather around the equal distribution and accessibility of new technology (including prostheses).

The claim that Pistorius has the right to compete directly against non-disabled athletes in Olympic events does not appear to be a strong claim. A stronger claim can be made for a separate bionic track event to be part of the Olympics. This however needs consistent rules on technical aids as well as an equal and standardized access to new technology. The inclusion however of just one ('Paralympic') event creates new inequalities and asymmetries between performances of able and dis-abled athletes. Pistorius' wish to become part of 'normal' elite sport may be framed as a way of 'inclusion' or 'integration', but paradoxically underlines the differences and reproduces the current order and hierarchy between able and disabled bodies.

References

[1]   S.D. Edwards, Should Oscar Pistorius be Excluded from the 2008 Olympic Games. In: *Sport, Ethics & Philosophy*, **2**(2) (2008), 112-125.

[2]   I. van Hilvoorde, L. Landeweerd, Disability or extraordinary talent; Francesco Lentini (3 legs) versus Oscar Pistorius (no legs). In: *Sport, Ethics & Philosophy* **2**(2) (2008) 97-111.

[3]   G. Wolbring, Oscar Pistorius and the Future Nature of Olympic, Paralympic and Other Sports. *ScriptEd* **5** (1) (2008) pp 139-160.

[4]   B. Suits, (1978/2005). *The Grasshopper*. Toronto: University of Toronto Press.

[5]   L. Nordenfelt, On health, ability and activity: comments on some basic notions in the ICF. *Disability and rehabilitation* **28**(23) (2006) 1461-5.

[6]   L. Swartz, B. Watermeyer, Cyborg Anxiety: Oscar Pistorius and the Boundaries of what it Means to be Human. *Disability & Society* **23** (2) (2008) 187–190.

[7]   C. Sandahl, P. Auslander (eds.) (2005). *Bodies in Commotion; Disability and Performance*. Ann Arbor: The University of Michigan Press.

11.2

Oral Presentations

Rehabilitation: Mobility, Exercise and Sports
L.H.V. van der Woude et al. (Eds.)
IOS Press, 2010

doi:10.3233/978-1-60750-080-3-393

393

Validity of the international wheelchair basketball and rugby classification systems

C.R. WEST[a,1], B.J. TAYLOR[a], I.G. CAMPBELL[a], L.M. ROMER[a]

[a]*Centre for Sports Medicine and Human Performance, Brunel University, UK*

Abstract. The classification systems used in wheelchair sport are based primarily upon sensory and motor ability. We asked whether the classification systems are also related to respiratory function at baseline and during exercise. Purpose: To investigate the relationship between functional class and respiratory function in GB Paralympic wheelchair basketball and rugby players. Methods: 11 wheelchair basketball and 15 wheelchair rugby players were classified using the IWBF (2004) and IWRF (2006) systems, respectively. Pulmonary function (spirometry) and respiratory muscle strength (mouth pressures) were assessed at rest. Additionally, for 11 wheelchair rugby players, ventilation and pulmonary gas exchange were assessed during maximal incremental arm-cranking exercise. Results: For wheelchair basketball, there were significant ($P < 0.01$) correlations for functional class vs. pulmonary function (% predicted FEV_1, $r = 0.76$; % predicted FVC, $r = 0.78$). For wheelchair rugby, there were also significant ($P < 0.05$) correlations for functional class vs. pulmonary function (% predicted FEV_1, $r = 0.63$; % predicted FVC, $r = 0.64$). For the wheelchair rugby players assessed during exercise, there were significant ($P < 0.05$) correlations for functional class vs. peak exercise responses (VO_2/kg, $r = 0.66$; V_E, $r = 0.62$; V_T, $r = 0.75$). Conclusion: Based on selected measures of respiratory function, IWBF and IWRF classification systems group athletes into the appropriate functional class.

Keywords. classification, paralympics, respiratory, wheelchair basketball, wheelchair rugby.

1. Introduction

Paraplegics and tetraplegics are eligible to compete in wheelchair basketball and wheelchair rugby, respectively. Historically, classification for wheelchair basketball and rugby has been dictated clinically by the vertebral level of the spinal cord injury (SCI). Currently, classification in these sports is based upon an athlete's functional ability (trunk, lower limb, upper limb and hand) at rest and during sport specific tasks. Some authors have suggested that when evaluating wheeled sport performance, the ability to complete specific tasks in that sport should be assessed in combination with cardiorespiratory function (1).

Respiratory function is significantly reduced in persons with SCI, with the degree of respiratory insufficiency improving as the level of injury moves caudally. For example, SCI has been shown to cause respiratory muscle weakness, reduce lung volumes, decrease chest wall and lung compliance, adversely affect gas exchange and

---

[1] Corresponding Author: Christopher West, Centre for Sports Medicine and Human Performance, Brunel University, Uxbridge, UK, UB8 3PH; Email: Christopher.West@Brunel.ac.uk

alveolar ventilation, and increase dyspnoea (2). Despite the evidence for respiratory insufficiency, no study has investigated the relationship between respiratory function and wheeled-sport classification in athletes with SCI. Thus, we aimed to determine the validity of the current classification systems for wheeled-sport by investigating the relationship between functional classification and respiratory function in elite wheelchair basketball and rugby players with SCI.

2. Methods

With institutional ethics approval and written informed consent, 26 GB Paralympic wheelchair athletes with traumatic SCI (T12-C5) participated in the study. Eleven of the athletes competed in wheelchair basketball (stature: 174.8 ± 11.1 cm, body mass 64.2 ± 10.7 kg, age: 31.2 ± 6.5 y) and fifteen of the athletes competed in wheelchair rugby (stature: 177.9 ± 9.9 cm, body mass 67.7 ± 11.5 kg, age: 30.9 ± 5.5 y). Prior to the study the athletes were classified according to either the International Wheelchair Basketball Federation (IWBF, 2004) or the International Wheelchair Rugby Federation (IWRF, 2006) classification system. Resting measurements were made in the following order: static and dynamic pulmonary function (forced expiratory volume in one second, FEV_1; forced vital capacity, FVC; maximum voluntary ventilation, MVV) using spirometry (MicroLab, Micro RPM, Micro Medical Ltd, Chatham, Kent, UK); and maximal inspiratory (MIP) and expiratory (MEP) mouth pressures (Micro RPM, Micro Medical Ltd, Chatham, Kent, UK). All of the measurements were expressed in absolute units and as a percentage of able-bodied predicted values. In addition, 11 of the wheelchair rugby players performed maximal incremental arm-cranking exercise (5 W every 2 min, 60-70 rpm) on a computer-controlled electromagnetically braked arm ergometer (Lode Angio, Groningen, The Netherlands). Peak ventilatory and pulmonary gas exchange indices (minute ventilation, $\dot{V}_E$; tidal volume, V_T; oxygen uptake, $\dot{V}O_2$) were measured using an online gas analysis system (Oxycon Pro, Jaeger, Höchberg, Germany).

The relationship between functional class and each of the dependent variables was investigated for each of the groups (basketball and rugby) using Pearson product-moment correlation coefficient. An alpha level of 0.05 was selected to represent statistical significance.

3. Results

There were strong, positive correlations for functional class vs. % predicted FEV_1 and % predicted FVC for wheelchair basketball and rugby (Figure 1). For wheelchair rugby, there were also strong positive correlations for functional class vs. absolute FEV_1 ($r = 0.78$, $P = 0.001$) and absolute FVC ($r = 0.75$, $P = 0.001$). For the subgroup of wheelchair rugby players, there were strong positive correlations for functional class vs. MVV ($r = 0.87$, $P = 0.001$), peak $\dot{V}_E$ ($r = 0.62$, $P = 0.04$), peak V_T ($r = 0.75$, $P = 0.007$), peak $\dot{V}O_2$/kg ($r = 0.66$, $P = 0.027$) and peak power ($r = 0.76$, $P = 0.006$). None of the other dependent variables correlated significantly with functional class.

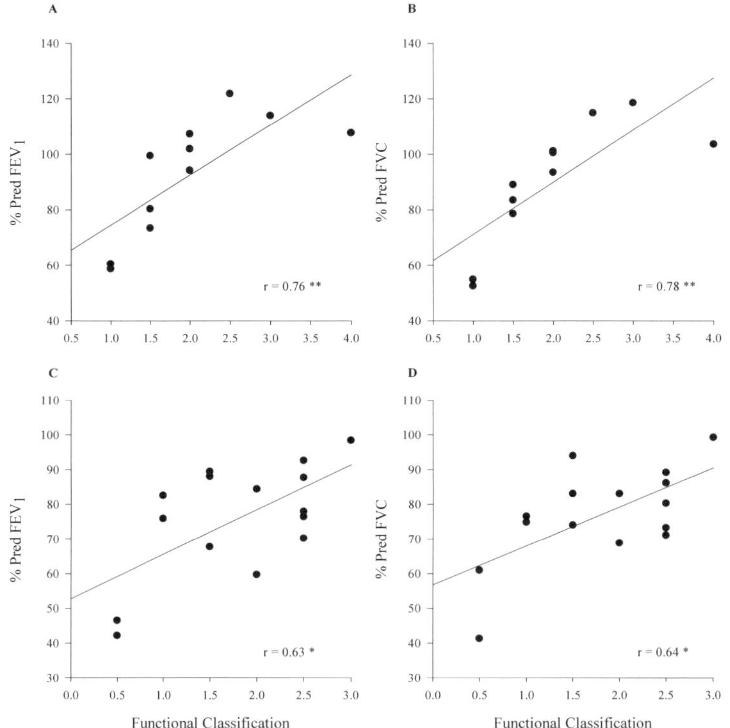

Figure 1., Pearson product-moment correlation coefficient for functional class vs. % predicted FEV$_1$ and % predicted FVC for wheelchair basketball (panels A and B) and wheelchair rugby (panels C and D). *$P < 0.05$, **$P < 0.001$

4. Conclusion

The current IWBF and IWRF classification systems are based upon a subjective, observational assessment of function. Assessment of respiratory function provides an objective measure that is easily quantifiable. Strong relationships between measures of respiratory function and functional class lend credence to the validity of the current IWBF and IWRF classification systems for use in elite athletes with SCI. Moreover, the strong positive correlations between functional class and respiratory function during exercise provide additional support to the contention that the respiratory system may be an important contributor to exercise performance in wheeled sport.

References

[1]   Y.C. Vanlandewijck, D.J. Daly, D.M. Theisen.   Field test evaluation of aerobic, anaerobic, and wheelchair basketball skill performances. *Int J Sports Med* **20** (1999), 548-554.
[2]   R Brown, A.F. DiMarco, J.D. Hoit, E. Garshick. Respiratory dysfunction and management in spinal cord injury. *Respiratory Care* **51** (2006), 853-868.

Supported by UK Sport and ParalympicsGB

396

Rehabilitation: Mobility, Exercise and Sports
L.H.V. van der Woude et al. (Eds.)
IOS Press, 2010
© 2010 The authors and IOS Press. All rights reserved.
doi:10.3233/978-1-60750-080-3-396

Practical application of the heart rate-based lactate minimum test in wheelchair racing athletes preparing for the Paralympics

C. PERRET[a,1], M. STRUPLER[a]
[a]*Institute of Sports Medicine, Swiss Paraplegic Centre, Nottwil, Switzerland*

Abstract. The aim of the present investigation was to describe the development of endurance performance between 2006 and 2008 in paraplegic wheelchair racing athletes competing at the Paralympic Games 2008 based on a heart rate-based lactate minimum test (LMT). For this purpose data of two standardised LMTs performed in 2006 and 2008 were compared in seven (4m/3f) world-class wheelchair racing athletes and correlated with individual competitive marathon racing times. Analysis included values for top speed, peak heart rate, peak lactate concentration as well as speed, heart rate and lactate concentration at lactate minimum. Significant improvements in speed at lactate minimum (9.5±3.9%, P<0.001) as a reliable predictor of maximal lactate steady-state as well as in top speed (7.3± 6.8%, P= 0.007) were found, whereas all other parameters showed no significant differences between measurements in 2006 and 2008. Seasonal best average marathon racing speed significantly correlated with speed at lactate minimum (r=0.824, P=0.004) and top speed (r=0.896, P<0.001) determined by means of the heart rate based LMT. In conclusion, even in well trained athletes impressive performance improvements can be achieved over a two year training period. The heart rate-based LMT seems to be a valuable and reliable tool to monitor such improvements in endurance performance in top-class wheelchair racing athletes and may be used for prediction of individual marathon racing times in the future.

Keywords. exercise testing, wheelchair racing, spinal cord injury, performance, maximal lactate steady state.

1. Introduction

The heart rate-based lactate minimum Test (LMT) was found to be a highly reproducible exercise test, which allows the determination of individual training intensity zones [1]. Further, it is known that there exist close relationships between heart rate as well as speed at lactate minimum compared to the corresponding values at maximal lactate steady state [2].

Based on this knowledge, the heart rate-based LMT was used for exercise testing and training prescription purposes of Swiss wheelchair racing athletes during the past few years. The present analysis aimed to determine, if the heart rate-based LMT is an adequate tool to predict competitive endurance - namely marathon - performance in well trained Paralympic wheelchair racing athletes.

---

[1] Corresponding Author: Claudio Perret, Institute of Sports Medicine, Swiss Paraplegic Centre, CH-6207 Nottwil, Switzerland; E-mail: claudio.perret@paranet.ch.

2.   Methods

In seven (4m/3f) world-class paraplegic wheelchair racing athletes data of two heart rate-based LMTs performed in 2006 and 2008 where compared and correlated (Spearman correlation) with the marathon racing performance of the corresponding year. Subjects performed LMTs in their own racing wheelchair on a treadmill at an inclination of 2% according to the protocol described in detail by Strupler and colleagues [1].

For comparison of the two LMTs data for top speed, peak heart rate, peak lactate concentration as well as speed, heart rate and lactate concentration at lactate minimum were analysed by means of a paired t-Test. The level of significance was set at p<0.05.

3.   Results

Significant improvements in speed at lactate minimum (9.5±3.9%, P<0.001) as a reliable predictor of maximal lactate steady-state and in top speed (7.3±6.8%, P= 0.007) were found, whereas all other parameters showed no significant differences between measurements in 2006 and 2008 (Table 1).

Table 1. Data (mean ± standard deviation) of the lactate minimum tests (LMT) in 2006 and 2008.

Parameter	2006	2008
Speed at lactate minimum	14.6 ± 2.9 km/h	16.0 ± 2.9 km/h*
Heart rate at lactate minimum	166 ± 3 bpm	161 ± 3 bpm
Blood lactate at lactate minimum	3.6 ± 2.1 mmol/l	4.1 ± 2.1 mmol/l
Top speed of LMT	22.9 ± 3.8 km/h	24.4 ± 3.2 km/h*
Peak heart rate of LMT	191 ± 6 bpm	189 ± 5 bpm
Peak blood lactate of LMT	9.3 ± 1.5 mmol/l	10.4 ± 2.6 mmol/l

*Significant difference between LMT of 2006 and 2008

Seasonal best average marathon racing speed significantly correlated with speed at lactate minimum (r=0.824, P=0.004) and top speed (r=0.896, P<0.001) determined by means of our LMT (Figure 1).

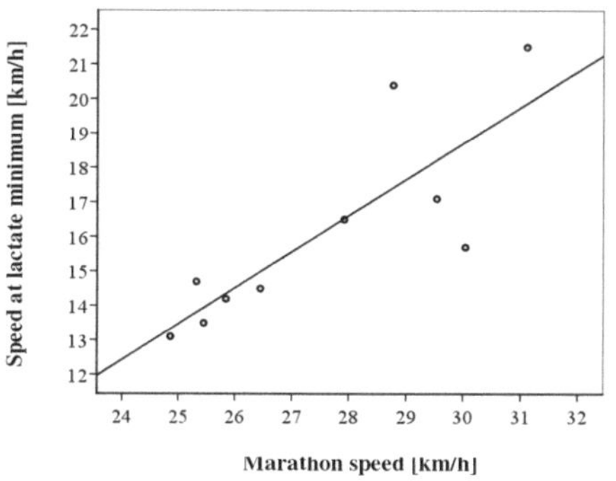
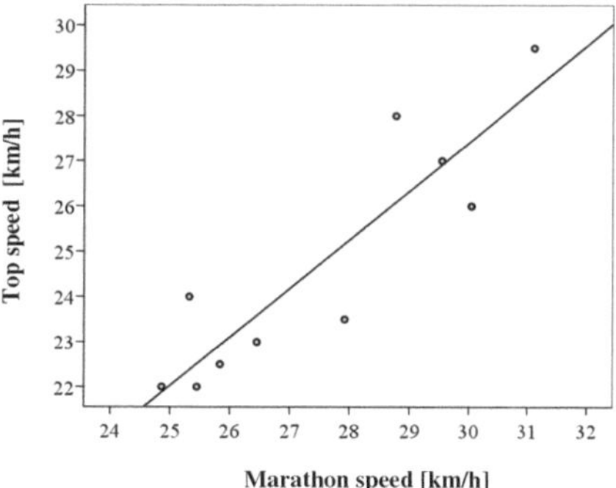

Figure 1. Correlations of marathon racing speed vs. speed at lactate minimum (left panel) and top speed (right panel).

4. Discussion

Even in well trained athletes preparing for the Paralympics impressive endurance performance improvements can be achieved. In this context, the heart rate-based LMT seems to be a valuable and reliable tool to monitor such improvements of endurance performance in top-class wheelchair racing athletes over a two year training period. Moreover, there seems to be a close relationship between results of a heart rate-based LMT and competitive marathon racing performance, which might allow an adequate prediction of marathon time in the future based on a single exercise test. In order to investigate, if such a relationship also exists between LMT data and other racing distances in wheelchair sports, further studies are needed.

References

[1]   M. Strupler, G. Mueller, C. Perret: Heart rate based lactate minimum test - a reproducible method. *Brit J Sports Med* (2008), in press.
[2]   C. Perret, R. Labruyère, G. Müller, M. Strupler: Does the lactate minimum of a heart rate based lactate minimum test correspond to the maximal lactate steady state? *Schweiz Zeitschr Sportmed Sporttraum* **55** (2007), 109.

Rehabilitation: Mobility, Exercise and Sports
L.H.V. van der Woude et al. (Eds.)
IOS Press, 2010

doi:10.3233/978-1-60750-080-3-399

Use of biomechanical analysis to classify basketball players in wheelchairs

A. GIL-AGUDO[1], A. DEL AMA-ESPINOSA, B. CRESPO-RUIZ, S. PÉREZ-NOMBELA

Biomechanical and Technical Aids Department of National Hospital for Spinal Cord Injury, Toledo (SESCAM), Spain

Abstract: The purpose was to applicate a methodology for the biomechanical analysis of wheelchair propulsion by wheelchair basketball players, which is one of the key elements for determining their functional classification. Ten basketball players of a high-performance basketball team with different functional classification scores were included in the study. A kinematic analysis system consisting of 4 camcorders (Kinescan-IBV) was used. Shoulder, elbow and wrist joint kinematics were obtained using an inverse dynamics model. A statistically significant negative correlation was found between player classification score and the time variables of push time, the ratio of the push phase/recovery phase duration, contact angle, the percentage of the cycle corresponding to hand off, and the percentage of the cycle corresponding to follow thru. The only statistically significant kinematic correlations were found between the player classification score and some carpal parameters. We propose a method for using techniques of biomechanical analysis to one of the elements used to classify wheelchairs basketball players.

Key words: wheelchair, basketball, propulsion, classification

1. Introduction

Most studies on the biomechanical analysis of manual wheelchair propulsion by athletes have been carried out for the same purposes that such studies are done in the general population, to determine the possible influence of different positional parameters on the appearance of repetitive strain injuries of the upper limbs[1,2].On the other hand, one of the most determinant elements of sports for physically challenged people are the functional classifications that allow players with a similar level of functional capacity based on residual movements to be grouped, thus avoiding competitive inequalities caused by the greater or lesser severity of the impairment of different athletes. Although the viability of these classification systems, in the case of wheelchair basketball, has been validated in earlier experiments in which field performance analysis was conducted at the national level and in elite athletes [3,4], it is interesting to examine further the biomechanical analysis of player classes.

Wheelchair basketball is one of the sports with the best developped functional classification system [5]. The system establishes a serie of player profiles that are

---

[1] Ángel M. Gil Agudo. Biomechanics and Technical Aids Department.
Hospital Nacional de Parapléjicos. Finca la Peraleda s/n. 45071 Toledo. Spain.
+34925247763 E-mail: amgila@sescam.jccm.es

determined by residual functional capacity and how specific actions are performed, such as propulsion, throwing, dribbling, or shooting the ball. The definition of the actions and categories of athletes makes it relatively easy to introduce biomechanical analysis techniques. In fact, some groups have already conducted experiments with actions like shooting [6] but, until now, manual propulsion has not been studied much in this context. The objectives established in the present experiment were the following:

- To study manual propulsion of wheelchair basketball players with kinematic analysis, taking into account the functional classification of each athlete.
- To identify possible relations between kinematic and temporal variables and the classification.

2. Methods

Ten wheelchair basketball players participated in this study. All of them had been classified by European IWBF classifiers and were considered elite players because they had participated in international events. The sample was grouped into IWBF functional classes [5]: 3 players in class 1, 3 in class 2, 2 in class 3, and 2 in class 4. A treadmill of suitable dimensions for wheelchairs was used to simulate realistic propulsion conditions (Bonte Zwolle B.V., BO Systems, GTR-2.50). Each athlete was analyzed in the usual playing situation for the player's classification with regard to the wheelchair configuration and strapping. The kinematic variables were recorded using 4 camcorders with infrared filter supported by infrared torches to observe the displacement of the reflective markers by Kinescan-IBV® at a recording rate of 150Hz. The treadmill speed was the mean reached previously in three 20-m sprints on the playing court. The test itself lasted for 1 minute. Data were collected in the middle 20-second interval. The reflective markers were positioned following I.S.B. recommendations for hand, forearm and arm [7], defining local reference systems on these segments and trunk.

Five cycles were selected from the 20-second data recording, analyzing each cycle separately and obtaining the mean value of the 5 cycles. The cycles then were normalized from 0% to 100%. They were analyzed temporal variables and the upper limb kinematics, which consisted of the maximum and minimum values of each articular movement and its range. The relation between the selected variables and the functional class was analyzed by calculating the coefficient of correlation of the Spearman rank. Correlation coefficients of $|r| \geq 0, 77$ were required to attain statistical significance at the 0, 05 levels of probability (n= 10).

3. Results

The descriptive results, expressed as the mean and standard deviation, of the temporal variables and kinematic variables for each class are listed in Table 1 and 2, respectively.

Table 1. Temporal variables by functional class (mean +/- SD)

Temporal variables	Class 1	Class 2	Class 3	Class 4
Speed (Km/h)	10.97±1.97	11.3±2.33	12.1±1.05	13.43±2.46
Cadence (strokes/s)	1.6±0.34	1.69±0.3	1.9±0.42	1.8±0.85
Duration of push phase (s)	0.21±0.03	0.15±0.05	0.14±0.02	0.09±0.02
Duration of recovery phase (s)	0.39±0.12	0.37±0.12	0.41±0.1	0.54±0.29

Push phase/Recovery phase	0.59±0.23	0.4±0.08	0.34±0.04	0.19±0.06
Contact angle (°)	119.12±2.71	107.27±14.09	101.72±0.93	81.4±6.76
Release angle (°)	19.96±15.28	13.95±4.17	7.84±4.05	20.16±14.23
Propulsion angle (°)	99.16±14.35	93.32±11.53	93.88±3.12	61.24±7.47
Top center, percentage of the cycle (%)	-20.99±52.3	5.37±3.57	3.29±0.03	-1.26±1.16
Hands off, percentage of the cycle (%)	36.33±8.63	28.41±3.83	25.44±2.43	15.6±4.57
Follow thru, percentage of the cycle (%)	39.74±9.32	31.63±2.47	27.79±3.39	22.94±6.51
Hand preparation, percentage of the cycle (%)	72.09±16.45	87.85±4.97	71.77±13.42	76.96±10.45

Table 2. Kinematic wrist variables by functional class (mean +/- SD)

Kinematic Variables	Class 1	Class 2	Class 3	Class 4
Wrist: maximum ulnar deviation	20.16±0.91	26.19±3.17	22.41±1.01	29.42±7.74
Wrist: maximum radial deviation	23.08±4.98	16.22±4.04	0.94±5.91	-7.64±11.94
Wrist: ROM ulnar-radial	4.64±2.01	9.98±3.65	21.46±4.9	37.06±19.69
Wrist: maximum flexion	29.77±13.3	12.31±14.92	5.44±12.91	-0.18±9.86
Wrist: maximum extension	17.55±9.36	34.06±6.61	32.62±4.23	25.98±6.97
Wrist: ROM flexo-extension	18.51±14.53	21.75±19.5	27.18±17.14	26.16±2.9

A statistically significant negative correlation was found between the classification score and the following variables: push time ($r=-0.81$, $p<0.05$), ratio of the duration of the push phase/recovery phase ($r=-0.88$, $p<0.05$), contact angle ($r=-0.90$, $p<0.05$), percentage of the cycle at which hand off occurs ($r=-0.87$, $p<0.05$), percentage of the cycle at which follow thru occurs ($r=-0.84$, $p<0.05$), maximum carpal radial deviation ($r=0.91$, $p<0.05$), and maximum carpal flexion ($r=-0.79$, $p<0.05$). In contrast, as the class increased from 1 to 4, the value of carpal range of movement in ulnar-radial deviation increased ($r=0.94$, $p<0.05$).

4. Discussion

It should be noted that this study was a pilot experiment to assess the possible suitability of using biomechanical analysis techniques as the methodology for comparing and defining functional classifications in wheelchair basketball. The results should be interpreted with caution due to the small number of players analyzed in each class and the many potential errors associated with the tests.

Until now, several previous experiments on the analysis of different wheelchair basketball player classes have been presented. In a very complete study, the characteristics of each class were analyzed, evaluating the generation of force, maximal aerobic power, and propulsion technique [8]. In a later study of 59 female players who participated in the World Championship for Wheelchair Basketball in Sydney 1998, high scoring players were found to perform better than low scoring players for most of the variables that determine the quality of play [9]. Biomechanics already has been used in a study to analyze shooting mechanics in relation to player classification and free throw success [6]. Interesting experiments have been made on the application of kinematic techniques to the analysis of functional classifications in other sports like shot-putting or javelin throw performed by wheelchair athletes [10, 11].

With regard to temporal variables, it was found that as the class score rose from 1 to 4, less time and a briefer hand contact angle on the pushrim were needed to propel the wheelchair, probably because the force exerted by the arms was greater when more muscular groups were available. For the same reason, hand off and follow thru took place earlier in the cycle in higher ranked players. Significant correlations with kinematic variables were found only with some carpal parameters. For instance, the maximum radial deviation and flexion were smaller in high ranked classes, whereas the range of motion in ulnar-radial deviation was greater in the highest ranked classes. This is because the classes with higher scores had more muscular groups available and could bring more force to bear to propel and increase the inertia to carry the carpus into ulnar deviation just after releasing the pushrim.

One of the most controversial aspects may be the fact that functional classifications are defined in terms of playing actions, whereas the scenario of the biomechanical analysis laboratory is experimental. We also think that it would be interesting to continue this study with a larger sample and expand the analysis to the rest of key points of the classification (shooting, dribbling, rebound, manual propulsion, etc).

References

[1] Boninger ML, Robertson RN, Wolff M, Cooper RA., Upper limb nerve entrapments in elite wheelchair racers. *Am J Phys Med Rehab* 75(1996) , 170-176.

[2] Burnham RS, Chan M, Hazlett C, Laskin J, Steadward RD., Acute median nerve dysfunction from wheelchair propulsion: the development of a model and study of the effect of hand protection, *Arch Phys Med Rehab* 75 (1994), 513-518.

[3] Vanlandewijck YC, Spaepen AJ, Lysens RJ., Relationship between the level of physical impairment and sports performance in elite wheelchair basketball players, *Adapt Phys Act Quart* 12 (1995), 139-150.

[4] Vanlandewijck YC, Evaggelinou C, Daly DD, Van Houte S, Verellen J, Aspeslagh V, Hendrickx R, Piessens T, Zwakhoven B., Proportionality in wheelchair basketball classification, *Adapt Phys Act Quart* 20 (2003), 369-380.

[5] Internacional Wheelchair Basketball Federation. IWBF. Player Classification System Wheelchair Basketball. 2002. IWBF web site. Avalaible online at: www.iwbf.org/classification/.

[6] Malone LA, Gervais Pl, Steadward RD., Shooting mechanics related to player classification and free throw success in wheelchair basketball, *J Rehabil Res Dev* 39 (2002), 701-709.

[7] Wu G, van der Helm F, Veeger H.E.J., Makhsous M, Van Roy P, Anglin C, Nagels J, Karduna A, McQuade K, Wang X, Werner F, Bucholz B., ISB recommendation on definitions of joint coordinate systems of various joints for the reporting of human joint motion- Part II: shoulder, elbow, wrist and hand, *J Biomechanics* 38 (2005), 981-992.

[8] Vanlandewijck YC, Spaepen AJ, Lysens RJ., Wheelchair propulsion: functional ability dependent factors in wheelchair basketball players. *Scand J Rehabil Med* 26 (1994), 37-48.

[9] Vanlandewijck YC, Evaggelinou C, Daly DD, Van Houte S, Verellen J, Aspeslagh V, Hendrickx R, Piessens T, Zwakhoven B., The relationship between functional potential and field performance in elite female wheelchair basketball players. *J Sports Sci* 22 (2004), 668-675.

[10] Chow JW, Chae WS, Crawford MJ., Kinematic analysis of shot-putting performed by wheelchair athletes of different medical classes. *J Sports Sci* 18 (2000), 321-330.

[11] Chow JW, Kuenster AF, Young-tae L., Kinematic analysis of javelin throw performed by wheelchair athletes of different functional classes. *J Sports Sci Med* 2 (2003), 36-46.

Rehabilitation: Mobility, Exercise and Sports
L.H.V. van der Woude et al. (Eds.)
IOS Press, 2010

doi:10.3233/978-1-60750-080-3-403

Improving classification: who is eligible for wheelchair rugby?

V.C. ALTMANN[a,1], A. HART[b], E. VAN DEN EEDE[a]
[a] *Sint Maartenskliniek, Nijmegen The Netherlands*
[b] *Northern Arizona University, Department of Physical Therapy and Athletic Training, Flagstaff Arizona, USA*

Abstract. Purpose: Clarify eligibility criteria for wheelchair rugby. Methods: There are 467 wheelchair rugby athletes in the international classification database. The data of athletes in the highest sport class (3.5) and athletes who are ineligible (class 4.0 or higher) were reviewed. All remarks about functional skills testing and on court observation were examined to investigate if there are characteristics supporting the decision of eligibility. Results:

Sport class	No. of athletes	Played in game	Description of activities
3.5	19	19	14
4.0	18	6	5

Two sport specific tasks were frequently documented in athletes ruled ineligible and never observed in athletes in the 3.5 sport class. Of a set of ten tasks, only one or two were cited in athletes in the 3.5 class, while three or more were present in athletes ruled ineligible. Conclusion: The classification system for wheelchair rugby is designed for athletes with SCI. As athletes without SCI entered the sport, deficits in the system were noted, most importantly in determining eligibility. If an athlete meets the criteria in the eligibility test and in manual muscle testing, the evaluation continues to functional skills testing and on court observation. Based on review of the database, adequate decisions can be made for all athletes based on several activities.

Keywords. classification, wheelchair rugby, minimum eligibility.

1. Introduction

Wheelchair rugby was developed in 1977 by athletes with tetraplegia due to spinal cord injury (SCI) wanting to play a team sport, and who, due to severe impairment, felt not competitive in wheelchair basketball. Based on the type and severity of impairments causing activity limitation [3], each athlete is given a class, ranging from 0.5 (least ability) to 3.5 (most ability). Athletes with more function than the 3.5 sport class are ineligible for this sport (for example, athletes with paraplegia). There are four players from each team on court at one time; the sum of sport classes of the athletes on each team must equal to or less than 8.0.

Each athlete is classified in a process consisting of manual muscle testing, functional activities testing and on court observation. The classification system is

---

[1] Corresponding author: Viola C Altmann, Sint Maartenskliniek Rehabilitation centre, PO Box 9011, 6500 GM Nijmegen, The Netherlands, v.altmann@maartenskliniek.nl.

described in the International Wheelchair Rugby Federation (IWRF) Classification Manual, 3rd edition, 2008 [1].

To better manage the classification data as well as enable on-going evaluation of the classification system, the classification database was developed.

Like the sport of wheelchair rugby, the classification system was originally developed and designed for people with SCI. Over the years, athletes with other conditions but "tetra equivalent function", such as multiple amputations and neuromuscular disease, started to compete in wheelchair rugby. These athletes are often in the higher sport classes. To improve team outcomes, they are highly sought after and are having a major impact in the game.

Using the current classification system, decisions on eligibility of several athletes without SCI required extensive observation on court. This lengthy process could potentially have a major impact on the outcome of an important tournament as well as on the athlete awaiting a decision. The necessity of having a more clear and efficient way to determine eligibility was obvious [2].

2. Purpose

The purpose of this study is to clarify the criteria on which an athlete is eligible to play wheelchair rugby.

3. Methods

In August 2006, all athletes in the database with an IWRF sport class 3.5 and athletes ruled ineligible were examined. First, we considered the number of athletes within those sport classes, together with diagnosis. Then we looked at the moment of decision making on eligibility and if the athlete had been in the game for observation. The data were examined for written remarks documenting the reason of ineligibility. All remarks upon functional activities testing and on court observation were categorised to determine if there was a sport-specific task or set of sport-specific tasks leading to the decision of ineligibility.

4. Results

There were 19 athletes in the 3.5 sport class and 18 athletes ineligible, out of 467 athletes with an international sport class in the database August 2006.

Table 1. Results

Sport class	No. of athletes with SCI	No. of athletes with other diagnosis	No. of athletes with SCI who played in game	No. of athletes with other diagnosis who played in game	Description of Tasks
3.5	14	5	14	5	14
Ineligible	10	8	0	6	5

The following remarks from functional skills testing and on court observation are documented in at least three of the ineligible athletes.
Chair skills:
- Use of trunk to enhance push and change direction and velocity with use of fingers on both sides.

- Use of trunk to control chair, maintain balance and empower hits in all directions without use of hands.
- Hopping the chair out of blocks.
- Maintain balance in hit protecting the ball at the same time, no use of hands on the chair.

Ball skills:

- Hold ball overhead for 5-10 seconds using both hands, no need for use of one hand to stabilise in chair.
- Passing 15 meters with one or two hands, enhanced by trunk.
- Control ball in all planes with fingers, at least on one side with ability to hold chair with hand on the other side.
- Pass securely and consistently in all directions.
- Reach outside cone of wheelchair in catch, dribble and picking ball from the floor.
- Protecting ball overhead with two hands.

Comparing the remarks on the characteristics of the 3.5 athletes, the following differences were noted:

- In none of the 3.5 athletes is there a description of protecting the ball overhead and controlling the chair at the same time.
- In none of the 3.5 athletes is there a description of ball control and security in all planes with one hand in a challenged situation.

All other characteristics are described, but only a few (one or rarely two) characteristics in the athletes in the 3.5 sport class compared to three or more characteristics documented in athletes ruled ineligible.

5. Conclusion

The current classification system for wheelchair rugby was designed for athletes with SCI. The classification system seems to have deficits in making a clear and efficient decision on eligibility for the increasing numbers of athletes without SCI.

Use of the following criteria is proposed for eligibility decisions. If the athlete is eligible for evaluation as determined by the eligibility test, and after manual muscle testing, is borderline between the 3.5 and 4.0 sport class, the process continues to functional activities testing and on court observation.

1. If the athlete shows one of these two abilities:
    - Perfect ball control in all planes with one hand in challenged situations.
    - Ball protection overhead and at the same time chair control

    and/or.
2. Three or more characteristics in chair and ball skills as mentioned

He or she is ineligible for wheelchair rugby.

References

[1] International wheelchair rugby classification manual 3nd edition October 2008.
     http://www.iwrf.com/classification.htm
[2] IPC Vista conference 2006. Classification: solutions for the future. Conference proceedings.
[3] IPC Classification Code and International Standards 2007.
     http://www.paralympic.org/release/Main_Sections_Menu/Classification/Code/

11.3

Poster Presentations

Rehabilitation: Mobility, Exercise and Sports
L.H.V. van der Woude et al. (Eds.)
IOS Press, 2010
© 2010 The authors and IOS Press. All rights reserved.
doi:10.3233/978-1-60750-080-3-409

30 year sportwheelchair innovation and its implications

K. VAN BREUKELEN
Double Performance, high performance wheelchairs and handbikes, Gouda, The Netherlands

Abstract. Historical overview of technical and ergonomic innovations used in the development of different types of sportswheelchairs throughout the years 1979-2009. In order to get a better understanding which innovations are relevant for performance-enhancement, injury-prevention and improving wheelchair-mobility in general.

Keywords. technical, ergonomic innovations, sportwheelchair, racing chair, handcycle, tennischair, rugby-chair, basketbalchair.

1. Introduction

This article does give an international historical overview from sportwheelchair innovations throughout a 30 year period (1979-2009). When these sport wheelchairs changed during these years (became better), the athlete could perform on a higher level. We do see both technical innovations (frame-changes) and more ergonomical changes (like seatposture-changes). These seatposture-changes do influence on their turn the way these sport wheelchairs were build. Like in the bike- and auto-industry, the sportwheelchair innovations do transfer to the regular wheelchairs, the ones for daily use. For example, the ultimate sportwheelchair of 1993, is now a popular daily use wheelchair.

2. Method

Literature-study and field-research in the wheelchair-industry and in different wheelchairsports: wheelchair racing, wheelchair rugby and handcycling during national and international competition during the period 1979-2009.

3. Innovation highlights

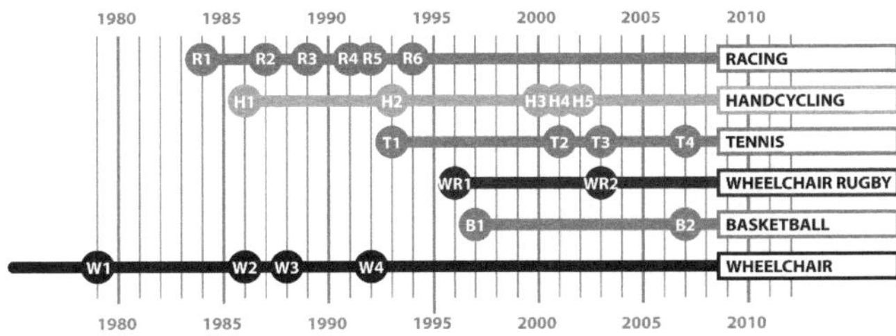

Figure 1. Historical overview sportwheelchair innovation from different wheelchair sports.

The innovation of the sportwheelchair started in 1979 when the Everest and Jennings folding frame was replaced by the first rigid chair with box-frame and axle-plates (W1). Decreasing overall weight, increasing stiffness, and improving seatposition. In 1986 the camberbar was introduced and did often replaced the two axle-plates (W2). Decreasing overall weight and improving stiffness again. Then the ergonomic changes began: the feet were placed vertical (W3) in 1988 and later backwards (W4) in 1992. Both improving seatingposture. From 1993 tennis, rugby and basketball started having their own sport-specific products. Wheelchair racing had already its own sports-specific racing wheelchair: in 1984 (R1) the, stable, bucket seat entered the racing scene and those vehicles had 16 inch frontwheels. The 4-wheel racing chair was replaced over some years by the 3-wheel racing machine starting in 1987 (R2). Making the steering device much easier, preventing toe-inn/toe-out problems and decreasing the overall weight. The wheelbase from the 3-wheel racing-machine was fully enlarged in 1989 (R3), decreasing by that the weight on the 16/18/20 inch frontwheel. Oversized tubing was used for the first time in the year 1991 (R4). Making the frame much stiffer with the result that power is transferred into speed and not into flexibility of the frame. The sit posture changed radically from bucket seat to the aerodynamic kneeling position in 1992 (R5), analogue with the ergonomic changes in the general sport wheelchair. This kneeling position made the powerful butterfly propulsion possible. The last real change in the racing wheelchair was in 1994 when the front fork design changed and the main frame became horizontal (R6), making the frame a little bit more aerodynamic than it already was.

Tennis was the second sport having its own sport specific product. In 1993 the 3-wheel tennis chair was introduced having a longer wheelbase (T1), copied from the racing wheelchair development. Less frontwheel pressure, less rolling resistance. It took until 2001 till the 4-wheel tennis chair get feet on the ground again. But now also with a longer wheelbase (T2), keeping the advantage of the lesser rolling resistance but dropping the disadvantage from the 3-wheel tennischair of losing pressure on the ground from one of the rearwheels when propelling/turning and hanging sidewards in attempting getting the ball. Also here we have seen the ergonomic sit posture changes: the seat changed from the dropped position to the tilted position in 2003 (T3). Improving the seat posture, giving better propulsion- and reaching possibilities and a better orientation to the net. The ATP-(Arm Trunk Power)tennis chair (introduced by Double Performance in 2007) is the ultimate reflection of this ergonomic seat change (T4).

Wheelchair rugby became sport specific when the chairs were made with bumper and wings (1996), making these chairs the heaviest but also toughest among the sport wheelchairs (WR1). Also the axle design changed (2003) in order to resist the impact on the battle-field (WR2).

The basketball world did profit a lot from these former innovations. The basketball sport wheelchair also became a minimal module wheelchair like all other sport wheelchairs: a high performance wheelchair consisting of 2 or 1 module(s) with camberbar, integrated caster pots, longer wheelbase and backwards placed feet inside the mainframe (B1 in 1997). The ergonomic innovation of the ATP-sit posture is also seen in the basketball world from the year 2007 (B2).

Handcycling, compared with the other wheelchair sports the latest developed wheelchair sport, could not start as competition sport untill the sit posture changed from the ordinary wheelchair seat to the lower sit posture with the legs extended forwards (H1) in 1986 ('longseat'). From the recumbent bike industry came, in 1993, the first recumbent handbikes with the long backrest reclined backwarts (H2). These aerodynamic recumbents , also named AP (Arm Power) handbikes, are still very popular specially among athletes with cervical laesions (A division athletes) and athletes with thoracal laesions (B division athletes). In 2000 a new development started, looking back at the sit posture change earlier, 1992, in wheelchair racing. The ATP (Arm Trunk Power) handbikes, also known as kneeling bikes, were developed by Double Performance for the first time and did entered the racing scene (H3). These handcycles are still very popular worldwide among athletes with trunk function (C division athletes). Because these kneel position handcycles did gave the best racing results in that time, also athletes with less function or not able to sit on the knees, tried these ATP handcycles but then sitting with the legs extended forward (H4) in 2001. Later these handbikes disappeared from the racing scene because it became clear that the recumbent bikes were faster because of their excellent aerodynamic characteristics. In 2002 the oval tubing was used for the first time in handcycling (H5), as happened earlier in wheelchair racing. Result of this development is that we have in 2009, two types of competition handcycles: the AP (Arm Power-) bikes (recumbents) and the ATP (Arm Trunk Power-) bikes (knee seat bikes).

All sport wheelchairs changed, first having low pressure tires but later high pressure tires, first tubes, later clinchers. The anti-tip, first used as safety-device, became popular as performance item in most wheelchair sports. Customisation of the chairs to the individual athlete to secure a 'precise' fit became normal and the use of strapping is now seen as a necessity in order to achieve the highest level of performance.

4.　Implications of the innovations

The technical innovations (axle placing forward, introduction/increasing camber, decreasing overall weight, increasing stiffness, increasing wheelbase, introduction high pressure tires, antitip as performance-item) and ergonomic innovations (seatposture- and seatposition-improvement) resulted in performance enhancement through increased sit-stability, acceleration, speed, manoeuvrability and reach in the different wheelchair sports. They resulted also in increased wheelchair mobility and utility through decreasing the rolling resistance, decreasing the needed arm power and increasing the efficiency of the arm power in daily life (-wheelchairs).

Last but not least these innovations do play an important role in injury prevention: reducing shoulder injury's and the stresses on the body.

References

[1]　*Sports on Spokes*, The magazine for wheelchair sports and recreation, Paralyzed veterans of America, 150 issues, 1983-2008

[2]　K. van Breukelen, not published movement-technological research data, Double Performance Gouda, The Netherlands, 1994-2008

[3]　K. van Breukelen, *Rolstoelkunde*, Uitgeverij Lakerveld B.V., Wateringen, The Netherlands, 2008

[4]　Field oriented research brech data gathered in national and international competition of the wheelchair sports racing, rugby and handcycling and in the wheelchair-industry during the period 1979-2009.

Rehabilitation: Mobility, Exercise and Sports
L.H.V. van der Woude et al. (Eds.)
IOS Press, 2010

doi:10.3233/978-1-60750-080-3-412

Does heart rate correlate velocity during wheelchair basketball competition? Some reflections in relation to functional classification

J. PÉREZ [a,1], C. ARAGÓN [a], M. RABADÁN [b], E. NAVARRO [a], J. SAMPEDRO [a]
[a] Faculty of Physical Activity and Sport Sciences - INEF,
Politechnique University of Madrid, Spain
[b] Higher Sports Council. Madrid, Spain

Abstract. Purpose: To study the relationship between individual heart rate and velocity during wheelchair basketball (WB) competition depending players′ functional classification (FC). Methods: Two highly trained players were monitored using a heart rate (HR) monitor during one period of high – level competition match (Eurocup Finals). Physical strain was evaluated from personal percentage of HR (%HRR). At the same time, bidimensional photogrammetry techniques were applied to competition video images and used for kinematic analysis of the players′ movement. 2D coordinates obtained from every player-wheelchair system (one-point mechanical model) respect to a defined inertial reference system were calculated two times per second. Results: For player 1 (class 3 FC, poliomyelitis both legs) mean (± SD) and maximum HRR (%) were 85,5 (±6,1) and 98,4 and for velocity (m/s) were 1,6 (±0,7) and 3,7. For player 2 (class 1 FC, complete spinal injury D5 level) mean and maximum HRR were 75,4 (±16,0) and 95,8 and for velocity were 1,3 (±0,6) and 2,9. Pearson correlation coefficient between HRR and velocity was r=0,21(p<0.05) for player 1 and r=0,06(p=0.48) for player 2. Conclusion: HRR correlates velocity for player 1, but not for player 2. Higher data dispersion in player 2 for this variable seems to be affected by type of disability / functional classification.

Keywords. wheelchair basketball, heart rate, heart rate reserve, velocity, functional classification.

1. Introduction

Wheelchair basketball (WB) has been studied in last decades on the part of Sport Sciences to enhance performance in competition, to specify training and to preserve players′ health, avoiding injury. As team sport, fitness training methodology has to be defined from the evaluation of the physiological demand during competition and related to specific team sport variables; moreover, research in WB as adapted sport, has to take into consideration players′ functional classification [1]. The aim of this

---

[1] Corresponding Author: Javier Pérez Tejero. Faculty of Physical Activity and Sport Sciences – INEF. Politechnique University of Madrid. C/ Martín Fierro n° 7. 28040 Madrid, Spain. Email: j.perez@upm.es

investigation was to study the relationship between individual heart rate (internal load) and velocity (external load) during WB competition regarding players´ functional classification.

2. Methods

Two highly trained players from same team were studied during one period (10 minutes of game) of one high level competition match (Eurocup WB finals, IWBF). For physiological stress assessment, both players were monitored using a heart rate (HR) monitor during competition (data sampling every 5 seconds) and related to personal percentage of HR (%HRR) [2]. For this, maximal personal aerobic parameters were evaluated twelve days before competition with a maximal graded exercise test on a wheelchair ergometry (WERG) using the own sport wheelchair) [3]. For physical stress assessment, bidimensional (2D) photogrammetry techniques from competition images were used for kinematic analysis of the player's movement [4]. To define the geometrical characteristics of the projection, 6 points of reference along the court were obtained, covering the recording/game area. Reference signals were measured directly before the game and, during competition, camera location at the tier had full view of the court and reference system. Sampling frequency determination was 2 images per second. The mechanical model selected was 1 point - 1 system (player + wheelchair). Point's positions were calculated, and, from them, instant velocity, average, maximum individual velocity and individual accumulated distance covered were calculated for both players. Only game/action sequences of competition were studied, so pauses situations were excluded for both analyses. A time criterion was used for data integration: data from both physiological and physical load was averaged every 5 seconds. Velocity was averaged every 10 data and related with every data for individual HR. In total, 13 competition sequences were analyzed, which meant 120 HR data and 1200 velocity data for every player. Mean (X) and standard deviation (SD) for %HRR and velocity are presented for both players. Pearson product correlation coefficient was used to evaluate the degree of association for both variables related player. A "T" test for independent measures was used to evaluate differences between players. SPSS 15.0® software was used for data computing and graphics generation. Confidence level was established at p<0.05.

3. Results

Players´ individual data and laboratory wheelchair ergometry outcomes are presented (tables 1 and 2).

Table 1. Players' individual data

FC IWBF)	Age (years)	Weight (kg)	Height (cm)	Player role	Disability level	Gait	Time since injury (years)	Experience in WB (years)
3	37	48,3	166,2	Playmaker	Polio 2 legs	2 crutches	34	18
1	35	85,5	191	Forward	Paraplegia T5 complete	Wheelchair	14	13

Table 2. Players´data from wheelchair ergometry.

Player	VO$_2$ peak l/min	VO$_2$ peak ml/kg/min	Max HR lat/min	Rest HR lat/min	HR reserve lat/min
1	2,46	51,3	187	60	127
2	2,76	31,9	160	64	96

For player 1 mean (± SD) and maximum %HRR were 85,5 (±6,1) and 98,4 and mean velocity (m/s) was 1,6 (±0,7) and maximum 3,7. For player 2, mean and maximum %HRR were 75,4 (±16,0) and 95,8 and mean velocity was 1,3 (±0,6) and 2,9. Pearson correlation coefficient between %HRR and velocity for player 1 was r=0,21 (p<0.05) and r=0,06 (p=0.48) for player 2. Dispersion graph for both relations is shown in figure 1, where dispersion for player 1 is less extensive than player 2. This fact is corroborated with a significant relationship for both variables in player 1 but not for player 2.

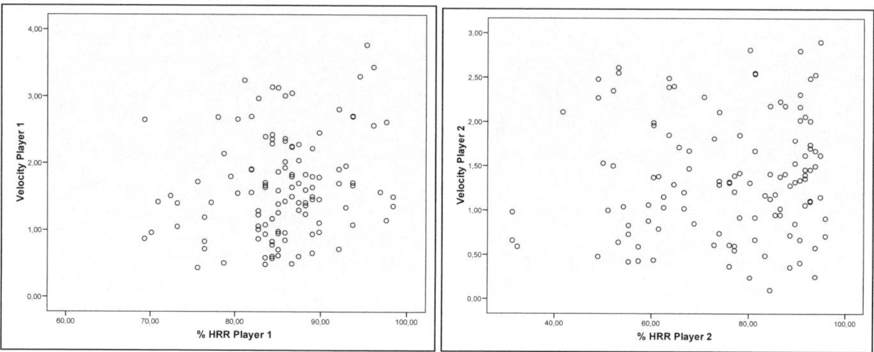

Figure 1. Dispersion graphs for %HRR and velocity for player 1 (left) and player 2 (right).

Moreover, when both players were compared with an independent T test for both variables, there were significant differences between them for %HRR (t (240) = 6,39, p<0,05) and for velocity (t (240) = 2,78, p<0,05). They significantly differ in physiological and physical answer even when they are studied at the same sport context (same team, same temporal cadence and same offensive - defensive patterns). It was demonstrated the different adaptation behaviour of HR in persons with SCI to exercise regarding the pattern of cardiac output [5]. In our opinion, %HRR screening along competition is useful for WB players related physical exigency, but not for players with complete SCI above T6 (class 1 players). More research and sample is needed using this methodology to confirm this answer along the different FC of high level WB players.

References

[1]   J. Pérez, M. Rabadán, J.L. Pacheco, J. Sampedro, Heart rate assessment during wheelchair basketball competition: its relationship with functional classification and specific training design, *Sport for Persons with a disability. Perspectives* (2007), eds. Colin Higgs & Yves Vanladewijck, ICSSPE – IPC, vol. 7, 151 – 174.

[2]   T. Janssen, *Physical strain and physical capacity in men with spinal cord injuries* (1994), Free University of Amsterdam. Published doctoral thesis.

[3]   M. Rabadán, J. Pérez, A. Boraita, M. Hernández, A.E. Díaz, R. Fernández, M.E. Heras, Valoración funcional en baloncesto en silla de ruedas mediante prueba de esfuerzo y protocolo en rampa, *11th European Congress of Sports Medicine*, Oviedo (Spain), November 2001.

[4]   J. Pérez, E. Navarro E., J. Sampedro, Evaluación de los desplazamientos en baloncesto en silla de ruedas mediante técnicas de análisis biomecánico, *Biomecánica aplicada a la actividad física y el deporte* (2007), eds. P. Pérez & S. Llana , Colección Aula Deportiva Técnica, Universidad de Valencia, Spain, 351 – 378.

[5]   M.T.E. Hopman, M. Pistorius I.C.E. Kamerbeek, A. Binkhorst, Cardiac output in paraplegics subjects at high exercise intensities, *International Journal of Applied Physiology* **66** (1993), 531-535.

Rehabilitation: Mobility, Exercise and Sports
L.H.V. van der Woude et al. (Eds.)
IOS Press, 2010

doi:10.3233/978-1-60750-080-3-415

A qualitative examination of wheelchair configuration for optimal sports performance

B.S. MASON[a], L. PORCELLATO[b], L.H.V. VAN DER WOUDE[c],
V.L. GOOSEY-TOLFREY [a]

[a] *School of Sport and Exercise Sciences, Loughborough University, U.K.*
[b] *Faculty of Health and Social Care, Liverpool John Moores University, U.K.*
[c] *Centre for Human Movement Sciences, University Medical Centre Groningen, RUG, Groningen, The Netherlands*

Abstract. The purpose of this investigation was to determine how experienced wheelchair sportsmen perceived areas of wheelchair configuration and subsequent modifications to influence aspects of performance. Nine experienced wheelchair sportsmen from basketball, rugby and tennis were interviewed. Using an Interpretative Phenomenological Analysis, common themes present in the interviews were grouped into three superordinate themes: i) performance indicators, ii) 'principal areas' of wheelchair configuration, c) 'supplementary areas' of wheelchair configuration. Results revealed that participants demonstrated a good understanding as to how making 'general' changes to areas of their wheelchairs configuration influenced their sports performance. Yet, methods for determining their optimal positions were extremely subjective and based predominantly on trial and error. This study therefore identified optimization of wheelchair configuration as a key area for future investigation, with an emphasis on rear wheel camber resulting from participants disparity with regards to its impact upon straight line mobility.

Keywords. interviews, wheelchair tennis, wheelchair rugby, wheelchair basketball, sports equipment, sports performance.

1. Introduction

Research into the ergonomics of manipulating areas of wheelchair configuration has been conducted under daily life propulsion conditions to assist everyday manual wheelchair users. However, very little is known about the consequences of making adjustments to areas of wheelchair configuration upon aspects of sports performance, as only a limited number of studies have been conducted on this area [1, 2].

A qualitative approach can be beneficial when attempting to develop a better understanding of a relatively unknown phenomena due to the more holistic appraisal it can allow [3]. The aim of the current investigation was to establish how experienced wheelchair sportsmen perceived areas of wheelchair configuration to affect aspects of sports performance. It was anticipated that the results of this study could identify areas of wheelchair configuration that are in most need of future research attention, by comparing perceptions between participants and to the results of previous research.

2.　Method

Nine experienced wheelchair sportsmen from basketball [n=3], rugby [n=3] and tennis [n=3] volunteered to participate in the study. To ensure athletes had a profound understanding of the topic area, participants were required to have > 10 years playing experience at an international level. Each participant was interviewed using a semi-structured approach. Interviews were recorded and transcribed into word processing format. An Interpretative Phenomenological Analysis was conducted, whereby emergent themes were clustered into groups with common connections.

3.　Results

Data was grouped into a total of three superordinate themes: a) Performance Indicators; b) Principal Areas of Wheelchair Configuration; c) Supplementary Areas of Wheelchair Configuration.

Performance Indicators

Three key areas were repeatedly identified by participants to be vital for successful mobility performance: a) initial acceleration; b) turning; c) sprinting. However, the area that the majority of participants felt contributed the greatest towards successful performance was stability.

Principal Areas of Wheelchair Configuration

Areas of wheelchair configuration that have received previous research attention were grouped as 'Principal Areas of Wheelchair Configuration' and were comprised of areas relating to the seat and the main wheels..

It became apparent that participants gave greater consideration to match play related factors such as ball handling ahead of mobility related factors when configuring these areas of a sports chair. Participants seemed to be in agreement with regards to how making 'general' modifications to these areas influenced performance. For instance, a good understanding of the advantages and drawbacks of sitting high and low were demonstrated. However, in terms of establishing where optimal settings may lie, it was apparent that players methods were very subjective. Therefore, identifying points when sitting high becomes too high for example, was not particularly clear.

Rear wheel camber was the area of wheelchair configuration that caused the most concern due to the mixed responses provided by participants, even with regards to its 'general' influence upon mobility performance. All participants felt certain that increasing rear wheel camber improved turning and maneuverability. Yet, the effects of camber upon aspects of straight line performance produced varying responses.

Supplementary Areas of Wheelchair Configuration

Areas of configuration which have not been researched extensively in the literature, yet were still thought to have a significant bearing upon performance were grouped under the superordinate theme 'Supplementary Areas of Wheelchair Configuration'. This included areas such as frames, footrest position, strapping, castor wheels and tires.

4. Discussion

It seemed clear from the results of this study that players' understanding of how making general changes to configuration influenced aspects of their performance. However, at the elite level of wheelchair sports, where minor adjustments can potentially affect the injury risk and efficiency of an athlete, it seems essential that a greater understanding of optimal settings are established in relation to the specific anthropometrics and disability level of performers.

The necessity for further research to be conducted into the influence of rear wheel camber, with a particular emphasis on its relationship with straight line performance was also highlighted. The varied responses elicited by participants suggests that this is an area that athletes may require assistance with in order to select a degree of camber that is optimal to each individual. The need for further research into camber is of further importance given the disparity amongst results within the existing literature. Despite considerable differences in methodologies it has been revealed that increasing camber can reduce [4], increase [2] and have no bearing at all [5] upon the rolling resistance during straight line propulsion.

5. Conclusion

The current investigation has identified how complex a process configuring a sports wheelchair can be for athletes. It has been made apparent that the experienced group of wheelchair sportsmen interviewed have a good understanding of the performance consequences of making adjustments to configuration. This is likely to be the result of 'trial and error' having previously been through the process on numerous occasions. However, for those less experienced athletes and in order to optimize players configuration settings it is essential that further objective research is undertaken to help inform athletes and wheelchair manufacturers alike.

References

[1]   Faupin, P. Campillo, T. Weissland, J.P. Micallef, Effect of the wheel camber of a wheelchair on the linear speed and the speed of turning of the wheelchair basketball player, *Cinesiologie* **201** (2002), 4-6.
[2]   Faupin, P. Campillo, T. Weissland, P. Gorce, A.Thevenon, The effects of rear wheel camber on the mechanical parameters produced during the wheelchair sprinting of handibasketball athletes, *Journal of Rehabilitation Research and Development* **41** (2004), 421-28.
[3]   F. Ryan, M. Coughlan, P. Cronin, Step-by-step guide to critiquing research. Part 2: qualitative research, *British Journal of Nursing* **16** (2007), 738-44.
[4]   H.E.J. Veeger, L.H.V. van der Woude, R.H. Rozendal, The effect of rear wheel camber in manual wheelchair propulsion, *Journal of Rehabilitation Research and Development* **26** (1989), 37-46.
[5]   S.M. Buckley, Y.N. Bhambhani, The effects of wheelchair camber on physiological and perceptual responses in younger and older men, *Adapted Physical Activity Quarterly* **15** (1998), 15-24.

Rehabilitation: Mobility, Exercise and Sports
L.H.V. van der Woude et al. (Eds.)
IOS Press, 2010

Subject Index

Rehabilitation: Mobility, Exercise and Sports
L.H.V. van der Woude et al. (Eds.)
IOS Press, 2010

Author Index